Interprofessional Collaboration for Women's Health Issues

Editor

WILLIAM F. RAYBURN

OBSTETRICS AND GYNECOLOGY CLINICS OF NORTH AMERICA

www.obgyn.theclinics.com

Consulting Editor
WILLIAM F. RAYBURN

March 2021 • Volume 48 • Number 1

ELSEVIER

1600 John F. Kennedy Boulevard • Suite 1800 • Philadelphia, Pennsylvania, 19103-2899

http://www.theclinics.com

OBSTETRICS AND GYNECOLOGY CLINICS OF NORTH AMERICA Volume 48, Number 1
March 2021 ISSN 0889-8545, ISBN-13: 978-0-323-79499-2

Editor: Kerry Holland
Developmental Editor: Kristen Helm

Obstetrics and Gynecology Clinics (ISSN 0889-8545) is published quarterly by Elsevier Inc., 360 Park Avenue South, New York, NY 10010-1710. Months of issue are March, June, September, and December. Periodicals postage paid at New York, NY, and additional mailing offices. Subscription price per year is $335.00 (US individuals), $944.00 (US institutions), $100.00 (US students), $404.00 (Canadian individuals), $991.00 (Canadian institutions), $100.00 (Canadian students), $459.00 (international individuals), $991.00 (international institutions), and $225.00 (international students). To receive student/resident rate, orders must be accompanied by name of affiliated institution, date of term, and the signature of program/residency coordinator on institution letterhead. Orders will be billed at individual rate until proof of status is received. Foreign air speed delivery is included in all *Clinics* subscription prices. All prices are subject to change without notice. POSTMASTER: Send address changes to *Obstetrics and Gynecology Clinics*, Elsevier Health Sciences Division, Subscription Customer Service, 3251 Riverport Lane, Maryland Heights, MO 63043. **Customer Service: Telephone: 1-800-654-2452 (U.S. and Canada); 314-447-8871 (outside U.S. and Canada). Fax: 314-447-8029. E-mail: journalscustomerservice-usa@elsevier.com (for print support); journalsonlinesupport-usa@elsevier.com (for online support).**

Reprints. For copies of 100 or more of articles in this publication, please contact the Commercial Reprints Department, Elsevier Inc., 360 Park Avenue South, New York, New York 10010-1710. Tel.: 212-633-3874; Fax: 212-633-3820; E-mail: reprints@elsevier.com.

Obstetrics and Gynecology Clinics of North America is also published in Spanish by McGraw-Hill Interamericana Editores S.A., P.O. Box 5-237, 06500, Mexico; in Portuguese by Reichmann and Affonso Editores, Rio de Janeiro, Brazil; and in Greek by Paschalidis Medical Publications, Athens, Greece.

Obstetrics and Gynecology Clinics of North America is covered in MEDLINE/PubMed (Index Medicus), Excerpta Medica, Current Concepts/Clinical Medicine, Science Citation Index, BIOSIS, CINAHL, and ISI/BIOMED.

Printed in the United States of America.

Contributors

CONSULTING EDITOR

WILLIAM F. RAYBURN, MD, MBA
Adjunct Professor, Department of Obstetrics and Gynecology, College of Graduate Studies, Medical University of South Carolina, Charleston, South Carolina, USA; Associate Dean, Continuing Medical Education and Professional Development, Distinguished Professor and Emeritus Chair, Department of Obstetrics and Gynecology, University of New Mexico School of Medicine, Albuquerque, New Mexico, USA

EDITOR

WILLIAM F. RAYBURN, MD, MBA
Adjunct Professor, Department of Obstetrics and Gynecology, College of Graduate Studies, Medical University of South Carolina, Charleston, South Carolina, USA; Associate Dean, Continuing Medical Education and Professional Development, Distinguished Professor and Emeritus Chair, Department of Obstetrics and Gynecology, University of New Mexico School of Medicine, Albuquerque, New Mexico, USA

AUTHORS

SUZANNE MCMURTRY BAIRD, DNP, RN
Nursing Director, Clinical Concepts in Obstetrics, LLC, Brentwood, Tennessee, USA

RICHARD H. BEIGI, MD, MSc
Professor, Department of Obstetrics, Gynecology, and Reproductive Sciences, University of Pittsburgh School of Medicine, President, University of Pittsburgh Medical Center Magee-Womens Hospital, Pittsburgh, Pennsylvania, USA

NADIA BENADLA, MD
Department of Radiology, Montpellier Cancer Institute, INSERM, U1194, University of Montpellier, Montpellier, France

ALLISON S. BRYANT, MD, MPH
Department of Obstetrics and Gynecology, Associate Professor of Obstetrics, Gynecology and Reproductive Biology, Harvard Medical School, Massachusetts General Hospital, Boston, Massachusetts, USA

ERICA C. CAMARGO, MD, MMSc, PhD
Associate Inpatient Medical Director, Department of Neurology, Massachusetts General Hospital, Instructor, Neurology, Harvard Medical School, Boston, Massachusetts, USA

JAIME L. DALY, MD
Department of Anesthesiology, Assistant Professor of Anesthesiology, University of Colorado School of Medicine, University of Colorado Hospital, Aurora, Colorado, USA

TERESA MARGARIDA CUNHA, MD
Department of Radiology, Instituto Português de Oncologia de Lisboa Francisco Gentil, Lisboa Codex, Portugal

PARDIS HOSSEINZADEH, MD
Section of Reproductive Endocrinology and Infertility, Department of Obstetrics and Gynecology, University of Oklahoma Health and Sciences Center, Oklahoma City, Oklahoma, USA

JALEESA JACKSON, MD
Department of Anesthesia, Critical Care, and Pain Medicine, Clinical Fellow in Anaesthesia, Harvard Medical School, Massachusetts General Hospital, Boston, Massachusetts, USA

DARA G. JAMIESON, MD
Clinical Associate Professor, Department of Neurology, Weill Cornell Medicine, New York, New York, USA

CAROLYN JENKINS, DrPH, MSN, MS, RN, RD, LD
Emeritus Distinguished Professor, College of Nursing and College of Graduate Studies, Medical University of South Carolina, Charleston, South Carolina, USA

MARGARET (BETSY) BABB KENNEDY, PhD, RN, CNE
Associate Dean, Non-Tenure Track Faculty Affairs and Advancement, Professor, Vanderbilt University School of Nursing, Nashville, Tennessee, USA

STEPHANIE MARTIN, DO
Medical Director, Clinical Concepts in Obstetrics, LLC, Scottsdale, Arizona, USA

JENNIFER W. McVIGE, MA, MD
Dent Neurologic Institute, Amherst, New York, USA

REBECCA D. MINEHART, MD, MSHPEd
Department of Anesthesia, Critical Care, and Pain Medicine, Assistant Professor of Anaesthesia, Harvard Medical School, Massachusetts General Hospital, Boston, Massachusetts, USA

MATHIAS NERON, MD
Department of Surgery, Montpellier Cancer Institute, Montpellier, France

STEPHANIE NOUGARET, MD, PhD
Montpellier Cancer Research Institute, Department of Radiology, Montpellier Cancer Institute, INSERM, U1194, University of Montpellier, Montpellier, France

JENNIFER L. PAYNE, MD
Associate Professor of Psychiatry and Behavioral Sciences, Associate Professor of Gynecology and Obstetrics, Director, Johns Hopkins Women's Mood Disorders Center, Johns Hopkins School of Medicine, Baltimore, Maryland, USA

WILLIAM F. RAYBURN, MD, MBA
Adjunct Professor, Department of Obstetrics and Gynecology, College of Graduate Studies, Medical University of South Carolina, Charleston, South Carolina, USA; Associate Dean, Continuing Medical Education and Professional Development, Distinguished Professor and Emeritus Chair, Department of Obstetrics and Gynecology, University of New Mexico School of Medicine, Albuquerque, New Mexico, USA

JESSICA B. ROBBINS MD
University of Wisconsin School of Medicine and Public Health, Madison, Wisconsin, USA

SARAH C. ROGAN, MD, PhD
Assistant Professor, Maternal and Fetal Medicine Division, Department of Obstetrics, Gynecology, and Reproductive Sciences, University of Pittsburgh School of Medicine, Pittsburgh, Pennsylvania, USA

ALISON K. SHEA, MD, PhD, FRCPC
Assistant Professor, Department of Obstetrics and Gynecology, Faculty of Health Sciences, McMaster University, Hamilton, Ontario, Canada

ANGELA D. SHRESTHA, MD
Howard Brown Health Center, Chicago, Illinois, USA

ANEESH B. SINGHAL, MD
Vice Chair, Quality and Safety, Department of Neurology, Director, Comprehensive Stroke Center, Massachusetts General Hospital, Associate Professor of Neurology, Harvard Medical School, Boston, Massachusetts, USA

ROGER P. SMITH, MD
Parkland, Florida, USA

CLAUDIO N. SOARES, MD, PhD, FRCPC, MBA
Professor and Chair, Department of Psychiatry, Queen's University School of Medicine, Providence Care Hospital, Kingston, Ontario, Canada

NADA L. STOTLAND, MD, MPH
Professor of Psychiatry, Rush Medical College, Chicago, Illinois, USA

NAOMI E. STOTLAND, MD
Professor of Obstetrics and Gynecology, University of California, San Francisco, Zuckerberg San Francisco General Hospital, San Francisco, California, USA

ROBERT WILD, MD, MPH, PhD
Section of Reproductive Endocrinology and Infertility, Department of Obstetrics and Gynecology, University of Oklahoma Health and Sciences Center, Oklahoma City, Oklahoma, USA

Contents

> Interprofessional collaboration has the potential to impact our complex, dynamic health care system through team-led or collective core competencies (professionalism, communication, teamwork, interprofessional education) that promote system improvements for quality care and patient safety. Strategies to reduce errors and subsequent adverse outcomes focus on interactive training; simulations and drills; development of protocols, guidelines, and checklists; use of information technology; and relevant interactive educational activities in the workplace. When sustained with a shared vision, good communication, and enthusiasm for the work being done, interprofessional collaboration can lead to measurable improvements in delivery of women's health care.

> Reproductive health care is crucial to women's well-being and that of their families. State and federal laws restricting access to contraception and abortion in the United States are proliferating. Often the given rationales for these laws state or imply that access to contraception and abortion promote promiscuity, and/or that abortion is medically dangerous and causes a variety of adverse obstetric, medical, and psychological sequelae. These rationales lack scientific foundation. This article provides the evidence for the safety of abortion, for both women and girls, and encourages readers to advocate against restrictions.

> Racism in America has deep roots that impact maternal health, particularly through pervasive inequities among Black women as compared with White, although other racial and ethnic groups also suffer. Health care providers caring for pregnant women are optimally positioned to maintain vigilance for these disparities in maternal care, and to intervene with their diverse skillsets and knowledge. By increasing awareness of how structural racism drives inequities in health, these providers can encourage hospitals and practices to develop and implement national bundles for patient safety, and use bias training and teambased training practices aimed at improving care for racially diverse mothers.

Viral infections are common complications of pregnancy. Although some infections have maternal sequelae, many viral infections can be perinatally transmitted to cause congenital or chronic infection in fetuses or infants. Treatments of such infections are geared toward reducing maternal symptoms and complications and toward preventing maternal-to-child transmission of viruses. The authors review updates in the treatment of herpes simplex virus, cytomegalovirus, hepatitis B and C viruses, human immunodeficiency virus, and COVID-19 during pregnancy.

Pregnancy confers a substantially increased risk of stroke, especially during the third trimester and until 6 weeks postpartum. Hypertensive disorders of pregnancy and gestational hypercoagulability are important contributors to obstetric stroke. Preeclampsia and eclampsia confer risk for future cardiovascular disease. Hemorrhagic stroke is the most common type of obstetric stroke. Ischemic stroke can result from cardiomyopathy, paradoxical embolism, posterior reversible encephalopathy, reversible cerebral vasoconstriction syndrome, and dissections. Cerebral venous sinus thrombosis is a frequent complication of pregnancy.

New onset or exacerbation of preexisting neurologic symptoms during pregnancy often necessitates brain or spinal cord imaging. Magnetic resonance techniques are preferred imaging modalities during pregnancy and the postpartum period. Ionizing radiation with computed tomography and intravenous contrast material with magnetic resonance or computed tomography should be avoided during pregnancy. New onset of headaches in the last trimester or in the postpartum period may indicate cerebrovascular disease or a mass lesion, for which brain imaging is necessary. The continuum of cerebrovascular complications of pregnancy and enlarging lesions may produce neurologic symptoms later in pregnancy and after delivery, necessitating imaging.

Active peripartum psychiatric illness is associated with adverse outcomes for exposed pregnancies/children. Likely due to high rates of obesity, pregnant women with psychiatric illness also have higher rates of preeclampsia, cesarean section, and gestational diabetes. Postpartum depression is associated with lower IQ, slower language development, and behavioral problems in exposed children. Discontinuing psychiatric medications for pregnancy increases risk for relapse significantly, and the postpartum time period is high risk for developing psychiatric illness. Obstetricians-gynecologists are front-line providers for psychiatric care of women during peripartum. This article provides a framework and knowledge base for management of psychiatric illness during peripartum.

Hemorrhage remains a leading cause of preventable maternal morbidity and mortality worldwide and in the United States. Postpartum hemorrhage is the number one cause of severe morbidity during hospitalization for birth, despite hospital, state, and national initiatives. In addition, studies show that more than 90% of maternal deaths related to obstetric hemorrhage are preventable. This article reviews relevant physiologic changes of pregnancy that may have an impact on hemorrhage management and describes collaborative approaches for management of hemorrhage in this unique population.

Managing dyslipidemia over a women's life, including a focus on pregnancy, contraception, and atherosclerotic cardiovascular disease risk prevention can decrease the burden of cardiovascular disease.

Benign uterine diseases are very common gynecologic conditions that affect women mostly in reproductive age. Ultrasound examination is the first-line imaging technique, but MRI is more accurate for diagnosis, characterization, and patient management. In this review, we especially highlight the added value of MRI in the diagnosis of benign uterine disease, discuss their imaging characteristics, and describe the therapeutic options and the added value of MRI in the treatment planning.

The World Health Organization estimates that more than 260 million people are affected by depression worldwide, a condition that imposes a significant burden to individuals, their families, and society. Women seem to be disproportionately more affected by depression than men, and it is now clear that some women may experience windows of vulnerability for depression at certain reproductive stages across their life span, including the midlife transition. For some, age, the presence of cardiovascular or metabolic problems, and the emergence of significant, bothersome vasomotor symptoms and sleep problems may result in a compounded, deleterious impact on well-being and overall functioning.

Roger P. Smith and William F. Rayburn

Studies indicate that burnout rates among obstetricians-gynecologists range from 40% to more than 75%, which is in the middle to upper one-third of medical specialties. Symptoms range from feelings of underappreciation and unresolved fatigue, to cynicism, depression, physical symptoms, and illness. Burnout is associated with poor job satisfaction, questioning career choices, and dropping out of practice, impacting workforce concerns and patient access. Awareness of the symptoms and some simple stress and fatigue reduction techniques can decrease the risk of being trapped in the downward spiral of burnout. Successful interventions range from more sleep, to hobbies and vacations, to skilled counseling.

OBSTETRICS AND GYNECOLOGY CLINICS

SERIES OF RELATED INTEREST

Clinics in Perinatology
www.perinatology.theclinics.com

THE CLINICS ARE AVAILABLE ONLINE!
Access your subscription at:
www.theclinics.com

Preface

Interprofessional Collaboration and Its Importance to Women's Health

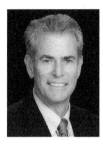

William F. Rayburn, MD, MBA
Editor

It is a pleasure for me to serve as the editor of this special issue of *Obstetrics and Gynecology Clinics of North America* pertaining to "Interprofessional Collaboration to Address Specific Women's Health Issues." The ability to work with professionals from other disciplines and specialties has been identified as a key skill necessary for delivering patient-centered high-quality and safe care. A review of the literature about collaborative practice and teamwork has identified key competencies needed to enable health care professionals to work effectively as part of a team. Probably the most important competency is interprofessional communication.

The intent of this issue was not to follow any one approach but to select and use what we consider to be the best elements to address select women's health issues. This issue represents several reports presented in other specialty *Clinics* issues that were relevant to women's health. As editor, I asked the authors to rewrite their original article with an obstetrician-gynecologist as either a co-author or a reviewer along with myself. References were updated, and key points were intended to reflect the role of the obstetrician-gynecologist as a collaborative team member. The issue is divided into topics that relate to obstetrics, gynecology, and women's health needs in general.

Facilitating team-based collaboration can be challenging and requires skill, experience, and preparation to deal with the various responsibilities and demands involved. Whether involved with small or large groups, facilitators need to focus on team formation and team maintenance, create a nonthreatening environment, and enable all providers to participate and learn equally. However, these aims are more challenging in a multidisciplinary, interprofessional context given the history of social and economic inequalities and any friction that may exist between members of the health and social care professionals.

Obstet Gynecol Clin N Am 48 (2021) xiii–xiv
https://doi.org/10.1016/j.ogc.2020.12.003
0889-8545/21/© 2020 Published by Elsevier Inc.

obgyn.theclinics.com

All authors are engaged in patient care, and many are involved with training medical students and resident physicians. Teaching students how to learn about, from, and with other physicians and health professionals is essential at the onset. Educational offerings at medical schools are focusing more on interprofessional faculty development with the goals of reducing feelings of isolation, developing a more collaborative approach, and providing opportunities to share knowledge, experiences, and innovations.

Articles in this special issue deal with a spectrum of disciplines in response to past failures of interprofessional collaboration that resulted in compromises to patient quality and safety. Through this effort, we attempted to present a more informed understanding of collaborative learning. Systematic reviews have shown that this type of learning has led to positive outcomes in relation to participant's reactions, attitudes, knowledge/skill, behaviors, and practice, as well as patient benefits. Further research can focus on addressing gaps in knowledge relating to the longer-term impacts of interprofessional education on provider behavior, organizational practice (eg, avoiding duplication, avoiding hospitalization, reducing lengths of patient stays, unnecessary patient readmissions), and improvements in women's health.

William F. Rayburn, MD, MBA
Department of Obstetrics and Gynecology
University of New Mexico School of Medicine
MSC 10 5580, 1 University of New Mexico
Albuquerque, NM 87131-0001, USA

E-mail address:
wrayburnmd@gmail.com

Interprofessional Collaboration in Women's Health Care

Collective Competencies, Interactive Learning, and Measurable Improvement

William F. Rayburn, MD, MBA[a],*,
Carolyn Jenkins, DrPH, MSN, MS, RN, RD, LD[b]

KEYWORDS

- Collaboration • Communication • Competencies • Interprofessional learning
- Outcomes improvement • Workplace

KEY POINTS

- In addition to individual clinical competencies in obstetrics and gynecology, learners need to acquire collective competencies to work effectively within health care systems that have embraced team-based models of care.
- Many of the described learning methods focus on improving communication processes between health professionals and being oriented toward the working environment, simulation scenarios, and debriefings about quality of care and patient safety.
- Common interprofessional strategies to enhance outcome improvement deal with development of protocols, guidelines, and checklists; use of information technology; and interactive workplace education.
- To improve measured outcomes-linked performances and continuation of this process, interprofessional collaboration requires leadership, organization support, enthusiasm for the work being done, and a shared vision and understanding of benefits from professional-to-professional learning activities.

INTRODUCTION

Like other fields of care, women's health is becoming increasingly complex because of the rapidly advancing medical technology and knowledge, and the challenge of managing multiple or chronic illnesses. Physicians in general obstetrics and gynecology and in the subspecialties are often asked to address specific needs that demand

[a] Department of Obstetrics and Gynecology, College of Graduate Studies, Medical University of South Carolina, Charleston, SC 29425, USA; [b] College of Nursing and College of Graduate Studies, Medical University of South Carolina, Charleston, SC 29425, USA
* Corresponding author. 1721 Atlantic Avenue, Sullivan's Island, SC 29482.
E-mail address: wrayburnmd@gmail.com

Obstet Gynecol Clin N Am 48 (2021) 1–10
https://doi.org/10.1016/j.ogc.2020.11.010
0889-8545/21/© 2020 Elsevier Inc. All rights reserved.

collaboration and expertise from many disciplines. Additionally, with costs of health care rising, and errors in patient care, although declining but still a concern, the need for improvement in both and quality is a priority.[1] Furthermore, expansion of traditional continuing education is facilitated by an awareness of limitations in disciplinary silos and the need for learning to be designed to effect practice improvement calls for more creative approaches for improving collaboration.[2]

Failures in teamwork and communication account for 70% of sentinel events in obstetrics.[3] Recognizing this, the Joint Commission, American College of Obstetricians and Gynecologists, and Institute of Medicine acknowledge that teamwork and improved communication within the health care team are critical for patient safety.[3–5] As an example, in a labor and delivery setting, the patient and her unborn baby are not cared for solely by her obstetrician, but also by nurses, anesthesia staff, operating room support staff, and other specialists as needed. Formal teamwork training is becoming a part of the orientation of new hospital staff members, with the goal of improving teamwork and communications within the team.[6]

Health care policy makers emphasize that continuing interprofessional collaboration and education play key roles in improving the organization of health care systems and outcomes.[7] Well-documented difficulties with communication within the health care team and professionally isolated approaches to care demonstrate potentially serious compromises in patient safety and the quality of care.[8] In addition to profession-specific clinical competencies, learners need other types of competences to work effectively in developing and improving health care systems that embrace team-based care.[9]

Interprofessional collaboration is when "multiple health workers from different professional backgrounds work together with patients, families, caregivers, and communities to deliver the highest quality of care."[10] As shown in **Fig. 1**, we consider

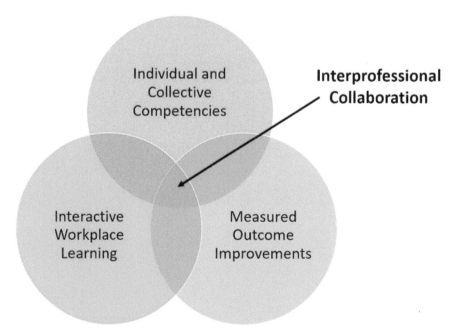

Fig. 1. Essential themes that overlap to embrace interprofessional collaboration.

interprofessional collaboration to entail an overlap of three essential themes: (1) individual and collective competencies, (2) interactive workplace learning, and (3) measured improvements in patient care and health care systems. Overlaps of these themes are intended to enhance skills, knowledge, and behaviors that promote interprofessional communication and teamwork to enhance and measure the patient care they provide. Although each theme is described separately in this article, they must overlap to optimize interprofessional collaboration.

INDIVIDUAL AND COLLECTIVE CORE COMPETENCIES

The Accreditation Council for Graduate Medical Education defined and outlined six core competencies that they identified as cornerstones for all practicing resident physicians.[11] Subsequently, the American Board of Medical Specialties included these six principles into their Maintenance of Certification programs.[12] These standards represent key components in the behavior, attitude, and skill sets required to meet the qualifications for certification and medical practice. The six core competencies involve:

- Practice-based learning and improvement
- Patient care and procedural skills
- Systems-based practice
- Medical knowledge
- Interpersonal and communication skills
- Professionalism

By exhibiting these core competencies, individuals can better understand the importance of their unique skill sets. For this to be interprofessional, there needs to be a cross-collaboration that incorporates collective or team-led competencies in addition to competencies of every provider. It is not sufficient, however, to have individuals on a team who are competent without having the collective competence of the team. For example, during a hurried delivery in response to a nonreassuring fetal heart rate tracing, a competent obstetrician, circulating nurse, anesthesiologist, and pediatrician working independently do not necessarily result in a successful outcome. Instead, the potential for a successful outcome is improved if the interprofessional team has the knowledge, attitudes, skills, and special capabilities in the form of a team with common objectives focused on outcomes for mother and baby.

A goal of interprofessional collaboration is to reach the highest level of performance improvement. To attain this goal, there needs to be collaboration between providers before it can be called "interprofessional." Collective competencies of the team, in addition to individual competencies of every provider, must be present. Interprofessional collaboration requires an exhibition of the following four collective core competencies or pillars:[13]

- A mutual respect of values and ethics
- An understanding of everyone's roles and responsibilities
- Frequent communication among patients, families, communities, and professionals
- Application of relationship-building values to perform and collaborate effectively in different team roles

Success with interprofessional collaboration begins with the selection of a leader in the organization and identification of "champions" with the same collective competencies and dedication to continual evaluation of this process. To ensure progress, a women's health leader is essential to elucidate values and coordinate these collective competencies. Engaging "champions" with different individual competencies is central to generating a sense of shared team skills and interprofessional ownership. Transparent representation of the engaged departments and programs (eg, obstetrics and gynecology, medicine, surgery, nursing, pharmacy, support systems, social services) in planning team-based care ensures that collaborative roles and responsibilities are identified and more likely to be implemented.

It is critical to have an organizational leadership with interest, knowledge, and experience to advance the interprofessional agenda with activities that instill with others a positive attitude to interactive learning and outcomes-linked performances. This "buy-in" leadership is needed from all departments and programs within the organization. Costs of additional time for learning and outcome analyses usually span several different professional or departmental budgets in a health system. Agreement over financial and protected time arrangements is cumbersome but requires investment at the beginning and periodically.

Sustaining interprofessional collaboration is complex. It requires open communication among participants, enthusiasm for the work being done, and a shared vision and understanding of the benefits of introducing or modifying curricula for professional learners. Regular meetings are to be anticipated to gather everyone's perspectives and ensure meaningful levels of discussion and agreement.

INTERACTIVE LEARNING IN THE WORKPLACE

The continuing education of obstetricians-gynecologists and other women's health care providers should not only include learning about the traditional specialty-specific medical knowledge but also interprofessional learning with an exploration of the potential facilitators and barriers. An interprofessional education offering can be defined as an activity undertaken when members of two or more health or social care professionals learn with, from, and about each other with a focus on improving collaboration and the quality of care.[4] Linked to this definition, Reeves and Kitto[14] described the following core educational concepts: (1) promote collaboration, not only between learners but among developers, facilitators, and patients; (2) egalitarian (or equal) learning; (3) learner-led and team oriented; (4) use real-life clinical problems to motivate learners; and (5) shared reflection to provide opportunities for learners to discuss and debrief the successes and challenges in their clinical work.

Interprofessional education is considered one of the approaches in the health system that increases interprofessional collaboration and improves the quality of patient care. Safabakhsh and colleagues[15] sought to design a commonly accepted interprofessional continuing education model. The five themes identified included (1) interprofessional collaboration, (2) needs of community and learners, (3) focus on the patient, (4) use of interactive teaching methods, and (5) feedback.

Essential skills for engagement in interprofessional learning include listening to the views of others, sharing your views, and being willing to negotiate a plan of action. This is like the skill presented in teaching patient-centered cultural competencies through the LEARN model as described originally by Berlin and Fowkes.[16] As shown in **Box 1**, this acronym stands for listen, explain, acknowledge, respect, and negotiate.

Interprofessional strategies to reduce errors and subsequent adverse outcomes have focused on team and individual training using a variety of learning methods: simulations and drills; development of protocols, guidelines, and checklists; use of information technology; facilitated team debriefings; and education.[17] Examples of educational strategies in women's health to reduce errors and subsequent adverse

> **Box 1**
> **Essential learning skills for interprofessional collaboration**
>
> Listen with understanding and respect other's views.
>
> Explain your perspective by providing the data and detail.
>
> Acknowledge and discuss differences and similarities in views.
>
> Recommend solutions.
>
> Negotiate a next step.

outcomes are shown in **Table 1**. These strategies and tools apply to inpatient and office settings. Although most studies describe positive reactions among participants and improvement in knowledge, skills, and behavior, data are limited about their impact on patient outcomes.[17]

A common way to deliver interactive and experiential learning is through simulation training. There are many examples of effective simulation activities in obstetrics and gynecology.[18,19] Simulation training, specifically as it relates to intrapartum conditions (eg, shoulder dystocia, eclampsia, operative vaginal delivery, postpartum hemorrhage, perimortem cesarean delivery) and gynecologic surgery, is among the most promising in medicine for improving clinical outcomes.

Protocols and checklists developed interprofessionally have been shown to reduce patient harm through improved standardization and communication. Recommendations from the American College of Obstetricians and Gynecologists encourage implementation of protocols, guidelines, and standardization of practice into systems of care.[3,18] Protocols and checklists should be recognized as guides to the management of a clinical situation or process of care that would apply to most women. Obstetrician-gynecologists, with input from other members of the interprofessional team, should be engaged in the process of generating and presenting guideline-driven data to foster stakeholder "buy-in" and create consensus to improve adherence.

A worthwhile model of interprofessional learning consists of a practitioner-centered approach that focuses on assessing and improving day-to-day challenges.[17] Workplace learning takes into consideration the context that includes the environment (ie, policy, culture, law) and relationships with the office and hospital staff. This also ensures that the interprofessional learning is outcome-oriented and demonstrates added value for the educational activity.[1] A first step for team-based collaboration is to collectively analyze the overall gaps in the workplace and the challenges and problems in the population or patients that need to be addressed, because local relevance including the challenges and problems of the patient population adds meaning and context for the team.[13]

Shown in **Table 2** are different learning methods and examples of team-based educational activities, as modified and expanded from Barr and colleagues.[17] Certainly, many examples would be incorporated using the different learning methods. Interaction of different health professionals and engagement from patients are critical to optimize practice-based learning and system change. Digital and social media are becoming universal in modern medical practice. The widespread use of social media brings unprecedented connectivity that opens new horizons for physician and other team members with patients and the public.

Interactive, workplace learning has gained much interest in several councils for accredited education. The Accreditation Council for CME, American Nurse Credentialing Center, and Council for Pharmacy Education have a joint accreditation

Table 1
Examples of interprofessional educational strategies to reduce errors and subsequent adverse outcomes in women's health

Educational Strategies	Examples in Women's Health
Simulations and drills	Postpartum hemorrhage; insertion and removal of contraceptive implants; catheter management after pelvic reconstructive surgery; vaginal hysterectomy model
Development of protocols	Diabetes mellitus during pregnancy; induction of labor at 39 wk; midwifery care during home births; gynecologic emergency care
Guidelines	Enhanced recovery after surgery; opioid reduction after delivery or surgery; antibiotic prophylaxis after pelvic surgery; American Society for Colposcopy and Cervical Pathology guidelines for management of precancerous pap test results
Health economics	Medicaid expansion with coverage and access to care for pregnant women; early pregnancy office visits rather than emergency room visits; race and ethnic differences in gynecologic care
Checklists	Minimizing professional liability; standardization of practice to improve outcomes; standardizing cesarean delivery technique
Clinical expert series	Management of select chronic illness during pregnancy; aging women and the office assessment; criteria for selecting contraceptives
Use of information technology	Professional use of digital and social media; televisits; mobile applications
Case-based discussions	Morbidity and mortality conferences; care for transgender and gender diverse individuals; pregnancy termination to reduce maternal mortality
Empowering patients	Home monitoring of blood pressure and glucose; care of surgical wounds; rethinking prenatal care
Peer review	Prolonged hospital admissions; teaching effectiveness; documentation on electronic records
Reducing barriers to care	Over-the-counter access to hormonal contraception; treatment of pregnant women with substance use; pediatric gynecology modules; labor support in incarcerated populations
Chart reviews	Counseling about vaccinations, tobacco and nicotine cessation, obesity, travel precautions; spouse abuse
Promoting wellness	Burnout among women's health practitioners; postpartum depression/post-traumatic stress disorder; boosting female sexual desire

process for team-based, outcome-focused education that focuses on improved clinical care for the patient and improved lifelong learning for the health professionals.[20] These three groups have agreed that continuing interprofessional education must include (1) a decreased focus on didactic learning, (2) an increased focus on workplace learning, (3) demonstration of continuing education's impact on improving outcome-linked performance in the clinical setting, and (4) an emphasis on lifelong learning skills.

Table 2
Learning methods and examples of interprofessional collaboration

Learning Methods	Examples of Interprofessional Collaboration
Action-based	Case-based learning; joint preclinic chart reviews; checkout rounds
Blended	Combining virtual learning with classroom methods
Debates	Controversies surrounding treatment of specific conditions
Electric (e-) learning	Medline searches from different health journals
Exchange-based	Seminar-based panel discussions; surgical debriefing; patient handoffs
Observation-based	Joint visits to patients' homes; visits to other hospitals; assisting on robotic surgery; ultrasonography training
Practice-based	Informal meetings in multidisciplinary clinic setting
Sharing experiences	EdTalk videos engaging leaders in innovative discussions; morbidity and mortality conferences
Simulation-based	Emergent situations; patient counseling; improving communication
Telehealth/telemedicine	Distance peer-to-peer learning; alternative to office visits; mHealth
Reflection/peer review	Anonymous input from patients and peers; huddles debriefings; inpatient rounds with peers; surgery assistance

MEASURING WOMEN'S HEALTH CARE IMPROVEMENT

A goal of interprofessional collaboration is to reach the highest level of performance improvement. Through interprofessional communication and teamwork, individuals can better understand the importance of their unique knowledge and skill set and perhaps provide to patients an improved health care experience. An effective model of improvement can involve not only women's health care delivery but also health system redesign (eg, practice networks, electronic health records, efficiencies, and cost-effectiveness).[21]

To be valued, interprofessional teams require time and encouragement to develop, implement, and sustain programs to evaluate and recommend improvements to delivery of women's health care. This direction requires educating providers to endorse workplace learning activities, such as quality improvement projects and patient safety rounds.[13,22] This generation of practitioners can oversee, advise, and ensure that other health care professionals overcome or minimize any barriers to learning within teams and that all team members display competencies in the workplace.

Interprofessional collaboration can initiate and implement certain measurable strategies that may prove to be effective in reducing error and improving overall quality and satisfaction with care. The ability to implement programs that positively impact clinical outcomes is lacking across many clinical sites and organizations, however. Schot and colleagues[23] identified three distinct ways that health care professionals can contribute to interprofessional collaboration by: (1) bridging professional, social, physical, and task-related gaps; (2) negotiating overlaps in roles and tasks; and (3) creating spaces to be able to do so. Consideration of a program of evaluation warrants a gap and barrier analysis, identification of key stakeholders with assigned tasks, development of consensus on relevant learning methods, creation of dashboards and tracking program performance, administrative and community support, and consideration of logistic assistance from a liability insurer or health system.

Research in women's health care delivery has provided a comprehensive set of insights into interprofessional learning and collaboration. Systematic reviews show that this type of learning can lead to positive outcomes in relation to interprofessional attitudes, knowledge/skills, behaviors, and practice. This growth and its associated publications will develop a better understanding about collaborative practice. There is an important role of understanding social determinants of health and use of social science theories to underpin the development and implementation of such activities. Future interprofessional activities should aim to draw on these theories to strengthen collaborative health care for women.

Much of what has been recommended in the workplace is related to events in the hospital, especially in the labor and delivery unit, surgical suite, and postoperative or postpartum ward. Interprofessional collaboration in the clinic and community seems to be less obvious and perhaps more difficult to examine and measure. Obstetrics and gynecology is moving more toward ambulatory care with more interest in avoiding a nonobstetric hospital admission, emergency department referral, or inpatient surgery.[24] Outpatient consultations seem to be more common between those in general obstetrics and gynecology and the subspecialists. Furthermore, much of women's general health care is provided in the clinics of adult primary care physicians and advanced practitioners, so open communication with obstetrician-gynecologists remains essential.

Moving forward, future investment in continuing collaboration in women's health must be based on interprofessional evidence that is accumulating. Future research can focus on addressing current gaps relating to the longer-term impacts (costs/benefits) on interprofessional behavior, organizational practice (eg, avoiding duplication, avoiding hospitalization, reducing length of patient stays, and unnecessary readmissions), differences in delivering inpatient and outpatient care, and measured improvements to women's health care.

Finally, the fit and function of women's health caregivers have not received enough attention. Historically, the emphasis has been on the actions and outcomes of individual women's health providers, but stressors from health systems affects the well-being of practitioners whose actions help define the effectiveness of the systems themselves.[25] Attention needs to continue on their well-being as performers within the system of care. A gentler, more comprehensive approach is needed to help these practitioners to reconcile stressors pertaining to individual and collective competencies, interactive workplace learning, and improvement in outcomes-led performances.

DISCLOSURE

The authors have no financial disclosures or conflicts of interest to report.

REFERENCES

1. Institute of Medicine. Measuring the impact of interprofessional education (IPE) on collaborative practice and patient outcomes. Washington, DC: National Academies Press; 2015.
2. Reeves S. An overview of continuing interprofessional education. J Contin Educ Health Prof 2009;29:142–6.
3. American College of Obstetricians and Gynecologists Committee on Patient Safety and Quality Improvement. ACOG Committee Opinion No. 447: Patient safety in obstetrics and gynecology. Obstet Gynecol 2009;114:1424.

4. Kohn LT, Corrigan JM, Donaldson MS, editors. Committee on quality of health care in America, Institute of Medicine. To err is human: building a safer health system. Washington, DC: National Academy Press; 1999.

5. Joint Commission on Accreditation of Healthcare Organizations. JCAHO sentinel event alert #30. 2004.

6. Gilligan C, Outram S, Levett-Jones T. Recommendations from recent graduates in medicine, nursing and pharmacy on improving interprofessional education in university programs: a qualitative study. BMC Med Educ 2014;14:52.

7. Institute of Medicine. Interprofessional education for collaboration: learning how to improve health from interprofessional models across the continuum of education to practice. Washington, DC: The National Academies; 2013.

8. The Joint Commission. Sentinel Event Data-Root Causes by Event Type. Available at: http://www.jointcommision.org/sentinel_event_statistics/. Accessed October 21, 2020.

9. Kitto S, Goldman J, Schmitt MH, et al. Examining the intersections between continuing education, interprofessional education and workplace learning. J Interprof Care 2014;28:183–5.

10. World Health Organization. Framework for action on interprofessional education and collaborative practice. Geneva (Switzerland): WHO; 2010.

11. Accreditation Council for Graduate Medical Education. Common Program Requirements. Available at: http://www.acgeme.org/What-We-Do/Accreditation/Common-Program-Requirements. Accessed November 12, 2020.

12. American Board of Medical Specialties. Board Certification Based on Core Competencies. Available at: http://www.abms./org/-/a-trusted-credential/based -on-core-competencies/. Accessed November 12, 2020.

13. Interprofessional Education Collaborative Expert Panel. Core competencies for interprofessional collaborative practice: report of an expert panel. Washington, DC: Interprofessional Education Collaborative; 2011.

14. Reeves S, Kitto S. Collaborating interprofessionally for team-based care. In: Rayburn W, Turco M, Davis D, editors. Continuing professional development in medicine and health care: better education, better patient outcomes. Philadelphia: Wolters Kluwer; 2018. p. 122.

15. Safabakhsh L, Irajpoor A, Yamani N. Designing and developing a continuing interprofessional education model. Adv Med Educ Pract 2018;9:459–62.

16. Berlin EA, Fowkes WC. A teaching framework for cross cultural health care. Application in family practice. West J Med 1983;139:934–8.

17. Barr H, Koppel I, Reeves S, et al. Effective interprofessional education: argument, assumption and evidence. Oxford: Blackwell; 2005.

18. ACOG Committee Opinion Summary. Committee on Patient Safety and Quality Improvement. Clinical guidelines and standardization of practice to improve outcomes. Available at: https://doi.org/10.1097/AOG.0000000000003454. Accessed November 1, 2020.

19. Freeth D, Ayida G, Berridge E, et al. Multidisciplinary obstetric stimulated emergency scenarios (MOSES) promoting patient safety in obstetrics with teamwork-focused interprofessional simulations. J Contin Educ Health Prof 2009;29:98–104.

20. Continuing Education Accreditors in Nursing, Pharmacy, and Medicine Joint Accreditation. Available at: http://www.jointaccrditatio.or/. Accessed September 19, 2020.

21. Davis D, Rayburn W. Integrating continuing professional development with health system redesign: building pillars of support. Acad Med 2016;91:26–9.

22. Davis NL, Davis DA, Rayburn WF. Clinical faculty: taking the lead in teaching quality improvement and patient safety. Am J Obstet Gynecol 2014;211:215–6.
23. Schot E, Tummer L, Noordegraaf M. Working on working together. A systematic review of how healthcare professionals contribute to interprofessional collaboration. J Interprof Care 2020;34:332–42.
24. Rayburn WF, Strunk AL. Profiles about practice settings of American College of Obstetricians and Gynecologists Fellows. Obstet Gynecol 2013;122(6):1295–8.
25. Smith R, Rayburn W. Burnout in obstetrician-gynecologists. Its prevalence, identification, prevention, and reversal. Obstet Gynecol Cl No Am, in press.

Reproductive Rights and Women's Mental Health

Essential Information for the Obstetrician-Gynecologist

Nada L. Stotland, MD, MPH[a], Angela D. Shrestha, MD[b],
Naomi E. Stotland, MD[c],*

KEYWORDS

- Abortion • Abortion effects • Reproductive rights • State laws

KEY POINTS

- Abortion and other reproductive health care are essential to women's well-being and that of their families.
- Restrictions on reproductive health care are increasingly common in the United States and are demonstrably deleterious to women's rights and well-being.
- Restrictions on reproductive health care have no basis in medical science.
- It is incumbent on obstetrician/gynecologists to be aware of existing and proposed restrictions in their states and practice settings, and, as trusted experts, to advise patients, the public, and policy makers of the scientific evidence against such restrictions.

INTRODUCTION

Reproductive rights are fundamental to women's health and overall well-being. Women must have control over their reproductive lives in order to plan and complete their education, make employment decisions and fulfill them, choose life partners, and have children if they desire them, when they think they can provide good care for them. The World Health Organization declares reproductive rights to be essential human rights and has issued many statements and guidelines for their implementation.[1–3] The American College of Obstetricians and Gynecologists (ACOG) has also developed, and strongly advocated for, many reproductive rights.[4–8] Although the right to terminate pregnancy has been hotly contested and challenged, especially in the United States, contraception, sterilization, and perinatal care rights are challenged,

[a] Rush Medical College, Chicago, IL, USA; [b] Howard Brown Health Center 4025 N Sheridan Road, Chicago, IL 60613, USA; [c] University of California, San Francisco, Zuckerberg/San Francisco General Hospital, 1001 Potrero Avenue, San Francisco, CA 94110, USA
* Corresponding author.
E-mail address: naomi.stotland@gmail.com

Obstet Gynecol Clin N Am 48 (2021) 11–29
https://doi.org/10.1016/j.ogc.2020.11.002
0889-8545/21/© 2021 Elsevier Inc. All rights reserved.

and limited, as well. The right to essential education is violated by the failure to provide scientifically accurate sex education, and the dissemination of misinformation, in many school systems. Recent reports indicate that members of gender/sexual and racial minority groups are not accorded the same rights as women in majority populations.[9] It should go without saying that injustices that harm women harm their families and society as a whole.

Reproductive rights include the rights of pregnant women to prenatal care and to choices in childbirth. The differential between black and white women's perinatal care and outcomes is shocking. In the United States, it is illegal to take a single drop of blood from a nonconsenting adult. Considerable attention is paid to the rights of patients to receive information about their medical conditions and to give or withhold consent to proposed interventions. The fetus has not been considered a person under the law. Nevertheless, women have been arrested, tried, and detained because of allegations that their behavior poses risks to their unborn children. They have been accused of murder when a fetus dies. They have been subjected to obstetric interventions that they actively oppose. Minority and underprivileged women constitute most of these cases. Laws limiting access to contraception and abortion or according personhood to the fetus are destructive to women.[10] They are based on the premise that women do not understand straightforward reproductive realities, are unable to make informed decisions, and do not care about the safety of their unborn children. The thousands of proposed and hundreds of enacted laws that mandate specific procedures or require physicians to provide specific misinformation contravene medical ethics and undermine the physician-patient relationship.[11] There are no comparable intrusions into any other area of medicine.

OVERVIEW

This article does not use the term prolife, coined by antiabortion groups, and adopted nearly universally in public discourse. In this context, the term limits the protection of life to the fertilized egg, embryo, and fetus. It does not encompass the abolition of the death penalty in the criminal justice system. It does not propose to protect the life of the child born to an unwilling or unprepared mother, or of any human being once it is born. It makes the life of the pregnant woman secondary or inconsequential. This article is based on reviews of the scientific literature and information about laws, legal cases, and other events. At the same time, it must reflect the authors' deep concern about the disregard for and hostility toward women reflected in attacks on women's reproductive rights. As this article is being written, Roman Catholic hospitals are not permitted to perform abortions even when there is no hope of extrauterine life for the fetus and the pregnant woman's health or life is acutely threatened by the pregnancy.[12] Health care providers may not mention contraception to patients, again, regardless of patient preference, patient religion, or clinical indication.[13] As Governor of the State of Indiana, in 2016, Michael Pence signed into law an act forbidding abortion for genetic defects, making the voluntary donation of fetal tissue a felony, and requiring that all fetal remains, regardless of their origin or stage of gestation, be buried or cremated.[14]

Reproductive rights encompass not only the right not to have a child but also the right to have one, and in circumstances of the woman's choosing. Having a child is not only a personal choice but is also essential in the perpetuation of the society and the species. Most wealthy countries provide an array of support services to families: months or years of parental leave from work; national health insurance to cover obstetric costs and pediatric care; quality early childhood education and care; and even prenatal and postnatal exercise classes and other helpful activities. Some provide cash payments to families with children. Canada offers several of these supports; the United States provides almost none. Most women have little choice of perinatal practitioner or place of delivery. Although there are attempts to make hospital birth (for uncomplicated pregnancies) friendlier, with fewer interventions, some women prefer to deliver at home and/or to be cared for by a midwife rather than an obstetrician. The rates of cesarean delivery in many places are higher than the scientific evidence supports.

In addition, there are the rights of women who are unable to conceive. In some states, health insurance policies are required to cover at least some infertility diagnoses and treatment. The use of reproductive technology is much less regulated in the United States than in Europe. There is little or no protection or follow-up for women who undergo hormone stimulation and egg retrieval in order to donate (for pay) their eggs to others. These women are often young, nulliparous, and in need of funds for their education. The donation of sperm does not require medical intervention. The legal rights of children to full knowledge about the sources of gametes with which they were conceived changes over time. The rights of so-called surrogates, or women who bear a child conceived with the sperm of a man who wishes to raise a child, or an embryo from a couple who wish to have one, are unclear. Surrogacy is not allowed in some countries.

This article addresses the history of reproductive rights and their current status; the assumptions about and attitudes toward women reflected in those rights, or the absence of them; the impact of rights denied on women's well-being; and both the scientific facts and the rampant misinformation about the impact of induced abortion on women's mental health. The article focuses on these issues in the United States, where they are problematic, public, and hotly contested. The United States Supreme Court ruled in 2020 that companies can deny coverage of contraceptives in the health plans offered to their employees if the company owners have a religious objection to them.[15] There is an ongoing history of barriers to the provision of emergency contraception.

The restrictions and requirements relative to reproductive care exacerbate the serious health concomitants of poverty, domestic violence, poor education, and racial discrimination. It is poor women who are most vulnerable to unplanned and untenable pregnancies, and poor women who face the highest barriers to ending those pregnancies. With regard to abortion, there is substantial scientific evidence about its relationship to mental health in particular. With regard to forced intrusions and discriminatory access to care, the authors must rely on our knowledge of the impact of injustice and abuse in general.[16,17]

Obstetrician gynecologists (ob/gyns) are at the interface between women and their reproductive rights. It is ob/gyns who work with patients as they make reproductive decisions and carry them out. Experiences with their ob/gyns leave lasting and powerful effects. The issues involved are often highly emotional, demanding that ob/gyns process their own beliefs and values so as to maintain therapeutic neutrality in clinical care.

HISTORY

The concept of reproductive rights is relatively new. Throughout history, and across societies, women have been expected to marry. Within marriage, women were bound to submit to sexual intercourse, and, thus, to pregnancy. There were penalties for women who became pregnant outside of marriage.

Although effective contraception and safe abortion only became generally available in the mid–twentieth century, historical and anthropologic studies reveal that contraception and abortion were attempted or practiced in a wide variety of times and places. Abortion techniques are described in Egyptian medical papyruses dating from 1700 BC. The Hippocratic Oath is often cited as evidence that abortion was forbidden in ancient Greece. In fact, the oath is evidence that abortion was practiced in ancient Greece; had it not been, there would have been no reason to mention it. Several ancient medical or gynecologic texts describe abortifacient drugs, and ancient tools used for surgical abortions have been discovered.[18,19]

Women's magazines in the nineteenth century routinely carried advertisements for purported abortifacients thinly disguised as menstrual or other remedies.[20] Historical texts seem to imply that herbal and other remedies were effective abortifacients, but no outcome evidence was gathered, and no such effective intervention is now known. As far is known, abortion was fraught with a high risk of physical pain, morbidity, and mortality until the advent of sterile technique, anesthesia, and access to both.

The popular BBC television series Call the Midwife, set in a low-income neighborhood in post–World War II London, included an episode in which the impoverished, married, mother of several young children desperately sought and underwent an illegal abortion apparently induced by a local woman who administered some caustic substance. There was much consternation among the staff at the midwife center over revealing what had happened either to the police or to the physician called in to treat her. The patient's life was barely saved. Nevertheless, through her agonizing pain, the woman only cares about 1 thing: "Has it (the fetus) come away?" The fact is that civil laws, religious prohibitions, pain, and the very real fear of death do not prevent millions of women from attempting abortions. It is estimated that 73.3 million women, worldwide, per year, have abortions, and that more than 30,000 women die from illegal, unsafe abortions.[21] This history, and these statistics, are testimony to the intensity, the desperation, with which women regard control of their procreative functions. Limitations subject women and their families to mental and physical harm.

RELIGION AND ABORTION

Many Americans may mistakenly believe that abortion is forbidden by most or all religions. This belief is not true.[22] A blanket prohibition on abortion is not part of the ancient Judeo-Christian tradition. Traditional Judaism allowed abortion at early stages of pregnancy, at least under some circumstances, including danger to the mother's health. Similar latitude exists in the Islamic tradition. The early Roman Catholic Church regarded abortion as acceptable until the fetus was considered to have a soul, as shown by its movements in utero as perceived by the mother (quickening). Current Church doctrine, although forbidding abortion regardless of the circumstances, also states that there is disagreement among theologians as to when the embryo becomes a person and is thus entitled to the protections due a person. Many nonevangelical Protestant denominations, as well as non-Orthodox Jewish scholars, support latitude in abortion decisions. Although traditional Taoism, Buddhism, and Hinduism explicitly forbid abortion, abortion is widely practiced in India, China, and other countries where these faiths are prominent.[23] In practice, in the United States, women of various religions have abortions in proportion to the occurrence of those religions in society as a whole; that is, women who profess religions opposed to abortion have abortions as often as those who do not profess such religions.

BASIC REPRODUCTIVE KNOWLEDGE

The right to know is central to rights to reproductive health care. Many women cannot draw an accurate representation of their reproductive systems. They do not know when, during their menstrual cycles, they are most fertile. Misinformation about conception and contraception is rife. Some adolescents believe that douching after intercourse with a carbonated beverage can prevent pregnancy, that coitus interruptus prevents pregnancy, and that pregnancy cannot result from first intercourse.[24]

However, much sex education (where there is sex education) in the United States is predicated on the misapprehension that the provision of information about sex encourages sexual activity. The US government funds so-called abstinence-only sex education in schools. This approach is demonstrably counterproductive. To encourage abstinence, the effectiveness of contraceptives is downplayed or denied, and the risks of contraceptives are invented or exaggerated. The students are given no realistic approaches to their own sexuality, and those who do have intercourse are less likely to use contraception. Abstinence-only education does not significantly increase premarital abstinence.[25] Young women are not given the information they need about consent to make their own decisions about sexual activity, or the assertiveness tools to enable them to exercise those rights.

ABORTION IN PRACTICE
Demographics

The Guttmacher Institute, in New York City, gathers and makes available on its Web site (www.guttmacher.org) information about contraception and abortion throughout the world. In the United States, approximately 30% of women have an abortion by age 45 years[26] (**Fig. 1**).

Asked for their reasons, women undergoing abortion report that they have chosen to terminate their pregnancies because of poverty, lack of social support, youth, the need to complete their educations or establish their careers, and/or they are experiencing domestic violence.[27] Lay people, and health care professionals, may assume that pregnancy would be a protection from interpersonal violence; in fact, pregnancy does not diminish, but apparently increases, the incidence of violence against women.[28,29] There are strong links between domestic violence and abortion; abusers may coerce women into intercourse, refuse or forbid the use of contraception, and they inherently make the living situation dangerous for mother and child.[30,31]

ABORTION OUTCOMES

Both published studies and the popular media (and state and national laws and court decisions) fail to recognize that abortion only happens to women who are pregnant, and that, therefore, outcomes of abortion must always be compared with those of ongoing pregnancy, delivery, and motherhood (or relinquishing a child for adoption). In terms of medical morbidity and mortality, uninterrupted pregnancy is 14 times more likely than abortion to cause maternal injury or death.[32] For some decades, adverse mental health outcomes were alleged by antiabortion forces and used as the basis for antiabortion laws. In some states, abortion providers are still required by law to tell women seeking abortion that the procedure will increase their risk of depression, substance abuse, suicide, and failure to bond with future children.

Comprehensive reviews of the published evidence reveal decades of consistently reassuring findings, including reviews by the American Psychological Association and the Royal College of Physicians.[33,34] The American Psychiatric Association, on the grounds of women's mental health, has held a rigorous prochoice position since 1973. There also exists a string of severely methodologically flawed published articles claiming adverse psychiatric sequelae.[35–40] For example, poorly done studies compare the mental well-being of women who have abortions with that of

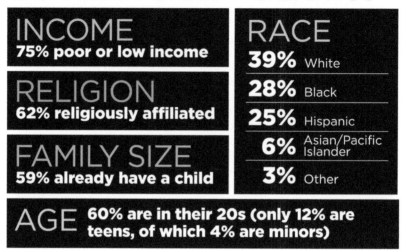

Fig. 1. US abortion patient statistics. (Guttmacher Institute, U.S. Abortion Patients, Infographic, New York: Guttmacher Institute, 2016, https://www.guttmacher.org/infographic/2016/us-abortion-patients.; with permission.)

women who go on to deliver or with women in the general population. They fail to recognize that the circumstances of individuals undergoing abortion are not comparable with either of these supposed control groups. They do not provide baseline data about the mental health of women preceding an abortion.[41,42] They do not take the circumstances that occasioned the abortion decision into account. The reasons women decide to abort are all mental health risk factors: poverty, lack of social supports, domestic violence, rape, incest, overwhelming responsibilities, lack of education, and preexisting mental illness. Methodologically acceptable studies indicate that the strongest predictor of a woman's mental health after an abortion is her mental health before the abortion.[43] Abortion may be associated with alcohol or substance abuse, suicidality, depression, and anxiety, but it does not cause them. Difficulty obtaining an abortion for any reason increases a woman's stress, as does exposure to clinic demonstrators, not to mention criminal attacks on abortion facilities and staff.[44]

The publication of studies claiming negative mental health effects of abortion has led to consternation in the scientific community and the publication of reanalyses revealing gross methodological errors, invalidating the conclusions, and ultimately resulting in the disavowal of 1 such article by the editors of the journal that published it.[45,46] Nevertheless, misinformation and misdirection are rampant.[47,48] For example, a Google search quickly led to a Web site called TeenBreak, which informed hapless pregnant teens, or their adult advisers, that abortion causes depression and suicide. Many of the resources listed at the top of such searches are disguised antiabortion centers. The US government, and some states as well, continue to fund so-called pregnancy crisis centers, which advertise help for pregnant women, but actually exist to deter women from having abortions. They provide misinformation, not only about mental health and other health outcomes but also about the likelihood that the unmarried woman will receive support for the baby from its father. Some centers offer free ultrasonography imaging and deliberately delay conveying the results until it is too late in gestation for an abortion.

Because of the realities discussed earlier, it is difficult to perform methodologically pure studies of abortion outcomes. Pregnant women cannot be randomly assigned to abortion or ongoing pregnancy. In 2020, The Turnaway Study was published. It reports landmark research, comparing women who presented for abortion just days before the legal gestational limit with those who presented just days after that limit and were therefore denied abortion. The subjects were followed for 5 years. There was no evidence that the abortions caused mental illness, and women who were forced to continue their pregnancies were more likely to be poor and otherwise in worse circumstances than those whose pregnancies were terminated.[49]

There is no evidence that women derive any benefit from enforced waiting periods before undergoing abortions or that they are more likely to regret decisions to abort any more than any other life decision. Their feelings about having had an abortion may vary over time. The decision to have an abortion may be easy or difficult. Afterward, women may experience guilt or sadness—feelings, not psychiatric disorders—for a time, but by far the most common reaction is relief.[50]

PSYCHOSOCIAL UNDERPINNINGS AND PUBLIC MANIFESTATIONS OF OPPOSITION TO ABORTION

Strong feelings about mothers in general, and about one's own mother, are core elements of human psychology. For a young child, its mother is the most powerful person on earth. That power can be reassuring or terrifying. Anxiety about one's own wantedness may give rise to objections to abortion. Adoptees may think that, had their biological mothers had access to abortion, they would not exist. Some groups representing people with disabilities oppose abortion because they believe that aborting fetuses with genetic or other defects is evidence that they have no right to exist. For some who oppose it, abortion represents the rejection of women's submissive maternal role, thus threatening both the men who are dominant in society and the women who feel valued only for their reproductive function, and the fulfillment of religious doctrines requiring women to submit to their husbands.

Unplanned pregnancy in a sexual partner can arouse a wide variety of psychological reactions in a man. He may be proud of this evidence of his virility. He may be pleased by the prospect of having a child, and with this partner. If his partner had led him to believe that a pregnancy was not possible, he may feel tricked and trapped. Or he may feel guilty for conceiving the pregnancy and forcing his partner either to abort or give birth. If the pregnancy is unwelcome to him, but his erstwhile sexual partner opts to carry it, he may feel obligated to a lifetime in the relationship and as a father in it. If his partner opts to abort, he may feel helpless to protect, and deprived of, his potential child. In 1 study, men who shared the decision to abort and accompanied their pregnant partners to an abortion clinic thought that this experience was a maturational turning point: the first time that they took responsibility for the consequence of their behavior and made a responsible decision about it.

Attitudes toward women's sexuality color beliefs and attitudes toward contraception and abortion. Although women's ability to force men into sexual intercourse is limited by sexual anatomy and physiology, as well as the differential in physical strength and social power, women have been, and continue to be, held accountable for male sexual aggression. It was Eve who ate the apple, sexually seduced Adam, and occasioned their ouster from the Garden of Eden. Orthodox Judaism, Hinduism, and orthodox Islam enforce gender segregation, limit women's activities, and require women to cover their bodies. Women's sexuality is essentially considered irresistible to men. Rape is blamed on women's dress and behavior. In some cultures, the rape victim may be forced to marry the rapist or murdered by her male relatives because the rape brings dishonor to her family. If it is women's irresponsible lust that is responsible for unplanned and unwanted pregnancies, then her pregnancy, instead of a joy, becomes a just punishment.

What about the psychology of the pregnant woman herself? Of course, women absorb and struggle with the sexual attitudes and mores of their own cultures.[51] Some antiabortion activists, and legislators, assert that women who have abortions have engaged in wanton, lustful sexual intercourse and simply want to rid themselves of the consequences. There is the implication that such women have negative attitudes toward motherhood. In fact, most women respect motherhood and many desire it. Most women who have abortions do so because they respect the responsibilities of motherhood. They think that the decision to continue a pregnancy must take into account the effect on their existing responsibilities, including children they already have, and that they should give birth to a child only when they have maximized the resources—educational, social, financial—they can bring to its care.[52]

Some women oppose abortion in theory but choose to terminate pregnancies they experience as untenable under their current circumstances. At many abortion facilities, demonstrators stand outside with signs depicting babies in utero or dismembered fetuses, shout at incoming patients that they are about to murder their babies, and attempt to approach and dissuade them. Physicians who work at these facilities report that, at least once, one of these demonstrators has asked them for an abortion outside regular working hours. After their abortions, they resume their places as demonstrators. This occurrence is not necessarily an example of hypocrite; it is a psychological function. One part of the psyche opposes abortion on religious grounds and another part of the same psyche finds a particular, personal pregnancy intolerable for some reason. This dual dynamic may help to explain the discordance between the frequency with which women terminate pregnancies and the attitudes they express in person, in opinion polls, and even in voting for political candidates.

Thus, public attitudes toward abortion, as reported in polls, are misleading.[53] It is essential to know precisely how questions were phrased, in what order, and in what context. Most polls offer stark alternatives, sometimes in favor of prohibitions: should abortion be permitted in all circumstances/at all stages of pregnancy or only in cases of rape or incest? Many people's attitudes toward abortion are complex, nuanced, and context dependent. The same individual who endorses a more or less strict prohibition may well, if the question is put another way, agree that no one but the pregnant woman herself, knowing her own resources and circumstances, can determine whether it is a good idea for the pregnancy to continue. Opinion polls that are claimed to show that women oppose abortion are belied by the greater than 30% incidence. Nevertheless, they may influence women contemplating abortion; it may be difficult to take an action that you are told most people oppose.

Expressed attitudes also reflect a superficial resolution of unconscious contradictions. Apparently, more people believe that an embryo or a fetus is a person and that abortion is murder than believe abortion should be illegal in cases of rape or incest. Why should it be acceptable to destroy a fetus/person because it was conceived by rape or incest? This logical lacuna reveals the underlying attitude that being forced to continue a pregnancy is a punishment for a woman's voluntary participation in sexual intercourse; if the participation was not voluntary, the punishment is not indicated, and she need not continue the pregnancy.

ABORTION AND YOUTH

Responses to overly simplistic questions do not allow for consideration of other logical inconsistencies. For example, the reflex answer to the proposition that pregnant adolescents be required to get permission from, or to tell, their parents when they seek an abortion is that adolescents are not mature enough to make this decision, and that therefore their parents have a right, if not an obligation, to be involved in or control the decision. However, consider the adolescent who is pregnant from incest or rape by a family friend or relative, the adolescent in an abusive family, or the adolescent who realistically anticipates severe punishment or exclusion from the family as a result of her pregnancy. Consider most particularly that the adolescent prohibited from having an abortion because she is immature will, in a few months, undergo labor and delivery and assume full legal and social responsibility for a newborn baby. This situation is another example of the failure to recognize that only pregnant women, or girls, have abortions.

The scientific arguments about adolescents' cognitive and emotional capacity to make this decision became confusing because of arguments about the punishment of adolescents who commit crimes. Adolescents do lack adult impulse control (so do many adults) and are therefore vulnerable to the impulse to commit crimes. Studies of brain development support this argument, which has been brought forward by advocates who believe that adolescents who impulsively commit crimes should not be tried and punished as adults.[54] Decisions about pregnancy are not in the impulse category. Adolescents are able to consider pregnancy alternatives. Pregnancy poses far greater obstetric, medical, and psychosocial risks than abortion, especially for adolescents, and there is no evidence that abortion causes mental harm to them.[55–57]

THE RIGHT NOT TO BECOME PREGNANT

The defunding of Planned Parenthood by the national and state governments, which also deprives poor women of basic medical and gynecologic care, is only 1 barrier to contraception access. In the United, States, 10.3 million women have had a partner who tried to make them pregnant against their will or refused to use a condom. More than 2 million women have become pregnant as a result of rape by an intimate partner. Some religiously affiliated health systems and workplaces also have prohibitions against the provision of, or offering insurance coverage of, sterilization and contraception, leaving otherwise insured women at risk for unwanted pregnancy and/or struggling to find the money for these services. Movements to allow over-the-counter oral contraceptives, or allow pharmacists to prescribe them, as supported by ACOG, are a step in a positive direction.[58]

FETAL PERSONHOOD

Another barrier to abortion, and invitation to coercive treatment of pregnant women, is legislation or court decisions designating the fetus, embryo, or even the fertilized egg as a person, with all the rights of a person. This designation of course makes abortion murder. The so-called morning-after pill prevents implantation but is regarded as an abortifacient by those who consider the fertilized egg to be a person. Some states require that a woman undergoing an abortion after a designated gestational stage undergo medically unnecessary, possibly deleterious, general anesthesia, with the scientifically refuted rationale that otherwise the fetus will experience pain. There are laws requiring that the patient be told that the fetus will experience pain.[59]

The starkest evidence of the denial of human rights is the treatment of pregnant women. Women have been subjected to obstetric interventions to which they object on the grounds that the fetus will thereby be protected. Others have been prosecuted and jailed for behaviors allegedly damaging to the fetus. These behaviors include suicide attempts, the use of alcohol or illegal substances, and attempts to self-abort with medication obtained through the Internet. Pregnant women who are brain dead as a result of injury or disease, and who had, when competent, expressed objections to being kept alive if they should succumb, have been kept on artificial life support until the fetus is deemed viable and is delivered surgically. Poor and minority women constitute most of the victims of these interventions.[10,60,61]

It is difficult for obstetric professionals to stand by in cases where a pregnant patient refuses interventions that could protect or save an unborn baby, but they have no right to invade her body or ignore her rights. Again, ACOG has considered the ethics and impacts of these situations and taken carefully reasoned official positions opposing forced interventions and punitive approaches to pregnant women. Aside from considerations of human rights, fear of punishment prevents pregnant women from seeking perinatal care.[62–64]

The concept of fetal personhood poses a major danger to women's rights and women's health. Almost all women who become, and decide to remain, pregnant are highly invested in the welfare of their unborn children. Setting up a legal conflict between woman and fetus disparages that investment and reduces the woman with individual civil rights to an incubator for a potential person.

ANTIABORTION LEGISLATION AND ITS CONSEQUENCES

Canada has chosen not to legislate abortion and not to endow the unborn with the rights of personhood. The controversy over abortion in the United States is unique in magnitude, public attention, motivation, and outcomes. Reference is made earlier to many instances of legislated limitations and prohibitions on abortion. With respect to abortion and other reproductive issues, the United States Supreme Court, in recent decades, has shown itself to be out of touch with both the scientific facts and the realities of women's lives. The Supreme Court's Roe v Wade decision of 1973 is considered to be the fundamental protection for abortion rights in the United States, but the decision has significant limitations. It was decided from privacy rights rather than reproductive rights. It ordered that states could not enact laws that imposed undue burdens on access to abortion before fetal viability, without providing criteria for what is undue. Over the ensuing years, states passed, and the Supreme Court refused to overturn, laws that imposed serious burdens: waiting periods, medically unnecessary interventions, scripted misinformation, outdated and medically deleterious dosage regimens for medical abortions, and rules for facilities and doctors that forced many to close. In 2019, conservative state legislators raced to enact an unprecedented wave of bans on all, most, or some abortions, and, by the end of the year, 25 new abortion bans were signed into law.[65] State laws criminalizing physicians who perform abortions have also been passed.[66] The combined effects of perceived or real popular pressure, danger, and legal limitations have caused many ob/gyns and many health centers to refuse to perform abortions altogether.

In the United States, federal funding of abortion services is prohibited by the Hyde Amendment. In addition to the impact of this prohibition on women on Medicaid, prohibition affects women in the armed services, whose care is federally funded. The Guttmacher Institute reports that, as of September 1, 2020, 12 states restrict coverage of abortion by private insurance plans. Forty-five states allow individual health care providers, and other facility staff, to refuse to participate in abortions, and 42 states allow health institutions to refuse. Eighteen states mandate preabortion counseling including false statements about health effects, breast cancer, or fetal pain. Twenty-six states mandate a waiting period; one-half of these make it necessary to make 2 trips to the facility. Thirty-seven states require that adolescents obtain permission[65,67] (**Fig. 2**).

Both legislation and Supreme Court decisions contain language contravening the evidence of the major medical experts in the country and mandating unprecedented and unparalleled interference with patient care. Although late-term abortions are most safely performed using the extraction technique, the Supreme Court upheld a law calling this "partial-birth abortion" and outlawing it.[66] Antiabortion activists have used this derogatory label for abortions performed earlier in pregnancy as well.

In 2015, a group of antiabortion activists made surreptitious videotapes at Planned Parenthood clinics and falsified the tapes so that they seemed to show clinic personnel selling fetal tissue. Members of the group have been criminally indicted. At the same time, the notions that abortions are being performed so that clinics can

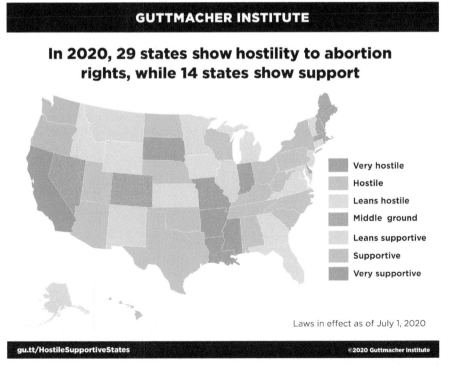

Fig. 2. 2020 US abortion rights statistics. (Guttmacher Institute, State Abortion Policy Landscape: From Hostile to Supportive, Policy Analysis, New York: Guttmacher Institute, 2020, https://www.guttmacher.org/article/2019/08/state-abortion-policy-landscape-hostile-supportive; with permission.)

profit from the sale of fetal tissue has taken hold. A doctor has been murdered by an individual claiming his intent was to protect baby parts. A congressional committee subpoenaed the records of a University of New Mexico research project involving donated fetal tissue, demanding and planning to publish identifying information about every person present or participating—despite the clear evidence that this unnecessary information will subject them to harassment or worse—also in the name of protecting aborted fetuses. The association between Planned Parenthood clinics and abortion in the minds of the public and legislators has resulting in the defunding and closure of many such clinics, depriving women of the contraceptive and general health care that constitute most of the clinics' services.

The United States Food and Drug Administration simplified the medical abortion regimen in 2016.[68] The Governor of Arizona signed a bill mandating the use of the outdated protocol just days before the new guidelines went into effect. This law, like many others, reintroduces the question of the right to privacy into the reproductive rights debate. Some legislation mandates scrutiny and reports of medical records.

With regard to parental involvement in the abortion decisions of their minor children, the Supreme Court has ruled that parental involvement can be mandated by states as long as there is a provision for what is called a judicial bypass. A girl who does not wish, or is afraid, to inform her parents that she plans to have an abortion can go before a judge and assert both the reasons she wants an abortion and evidence of her decisional maturity and/or independence from her parents. This process necessitates that such girls are aware that it exists, can identify and locate the proper court and the days and hours it is in session, absent themselves from their school or jobs or parents' homes, travel to the court, and master the anxiety nearly anyone experiences in anticipation of an appearance in court. Not surprisingly, the decisions of courts in these matters vary widely from state to state.

The Supreme Court has upheld the prerogative of health systems and facilities to refuse to provide reproductive services in the name of religious freedom: theirs, not their patients'.[6,13,69,70] The concept of religious freedom at the founding of the United States was meant to allow everyone to practice, or not to practice, the religion of their individual choice. At present, the concept is used to allow practitioners of one religion to withhold legal services and rights from those of another religion. As of May 2016, 1 in 6 of every acute care hospital bed in the United States is in a Catholic-controlled hospital. In 10 states, more than 30% of hospital beds are in Catholic hospitals, and there are 46 such hospitals that are the sole provider of hospital care in their geographic areas. They require staff to formally agree that they will not even provide information about contraception or abortion. This requirement includes circumstances, which are many, in which contraception or abortion is critical to a patient's care. As mentioned earlier, a Catholic hospital allows a woman to die rather than terminating a pregnancy, even a pregnancy with a fetus with a condition incompatible with extrauterine survival. A patient desiring a tubal ligation at the time of cesarean delivery cannot have one. Catholic hospitals claiming to provide comprehensive care have no legal obligation to inform patients or prospective patients of these restrictions and their implications. Because anyone in a health care system can refuse reproductive services because of their personal beliefs, many pharmacies, both local and parts of national chains, refuse to stock or dispense postcoital contraception.[71]

On June 27, 2016 the Supreme Court announced a decision constituting a major milestone in abortion law. The court struck down a Texas law requiring physicians who perform abortions to have hospital admitting privileges and abortion clinics to meet the building requirements of surgicenters; neither requirement is supported by the scientific literature. The court defined undue burden for the first time as the imposition of restrictions that are not supported by medical or scientific evidence, replacing the appellate court decision that laws may be based on rational suspicion, even if there is contrary evidence. The current composition of state legislatures and the federal judiciary is now such that the antiabortion movement is hoping that the Roe v Wade decision will be overturned. Louisiana recently enacted a law identical to the Texas law, but the Supreme Court refused to uphold it.

Recent data indicate that the passage of antiabortion laws, even when they are quickly or ultimately overturned by the courts, causes sufficient concern and confusion that attendance at Planned Parenthood or other facilities decreases. Abortion is more frequent in countries with laws against it than in countries where it is legal and accessible.

WORLD VIEW

Around the globe, the nations where abortions are safe, legal, and available have the lowest incidences of abortion, and the unsafe abortions in countries where it is illegal are the, or a major, cause of maternal mortality. Millions of children have lost their mothers to illegal procedures their mothers undertook so as to safeguard the resources that those children need. Efforts to make abortion legal and available have been successful in a growing list of countries. Before Uruguay legalized abortion, a group of medical professionals and advocates successfully instituted a program gracefully reconciling a nearly total legal abortion ban with the provision of information and care that saved many lives.[72] Health care professionals refrained from performing or advocating for abortion, but informed pregnant patients about the safe use of abortifacient medication they could obtain outside the health care system, and offered safe follow-up both to patients who terminated and those who maintained their pregnancies.

RESOURCES

The Guttmacher Institute, mentioned earlier, has contraception and abortion data for North America and globally.

The University of Toronto has an International Reproductive and Sexual Health Law Program. In-depth information about laws and studies all over the world is available on their Web site, www.law.utoronto.ca/programs-centres/programs/irshl-reproductive-and-sexual-health-law, and they publish a blog to which readers can subscribe for free.

THE ROLE OF THE OBSTETRICIAN/GYNECOLOGIST

Ob/gyns are not the only clinicians performing abortions, prescribing contraceptives, delivering babies, and providing preventive reproductive health care, but they and their professional organizations are the medical experts about, and advocates for, reproductive rights. Every one of these rights conjures powerful feelings. The first task of the ob/gyn is to come to grips with those feelings. That is not to say or urge that the feelings must be eradicated, because they are valuable human resources; ob/gyns deal with the most emotionally fraught and intimate events in human experience. Looking within is not easy; some feelings are not pretty. When feelings conflict with the reproductive rights discussed in this article, when a clinician cannot conscience providing certain services, that fact must be communicated, without prejudice or judgment, to patients.

When clinical events are painful, mutual support among members of staff is enormously helpful. Sometimes a mental health expert can contribute. For example, a recently delivered mother of 6 who was a Jehovah's Witness developed an internal hemorrhage and soon did not have enough circulating blood to maintain life. Despite being informed of that fact, she steadfastly refused transfusion and maintained that members of her church would sustain her husband and children after she was gone. The entire staff was appalled at the prospect of these children, including the newborn, losing their mother unnecessarily. The psychiatric consultant and hospital lawyer found the patient to be fully informed and competent. The staff had to stand by as she died. After this traumatic experience, they conveyed a conference, with representatives of the Jehovah's Witness church and the psychiatric consultant, to share and work through their feelings of guilt, rage, and sadness. Postscript: the Jehovah's Witnesses were very sensitive to the effect of their beliefs on the obstetric staff; church leaders and the bereaved father brought the baby and all its siblings back to the hospital months later to show that, indeed, all were lovingly cared for.

Group sharing is also helpful as members of the specialty, like all clinicians—and all people—begin to grapple with the realities of discrimination against people of color, immigrants, and members of the LGBTQ (lesbian, gay, bisexual, transsexual, queer) community. Dreadful disparities in outcome cannot be blamed on external circumstances. LGBTQ patients die of untreated diseases because their experiences with health care professionals have frightened them away. Mothers of color die in disproportionate numbers. The clinical scenarios that lead to these deaths have to be painfully dissected and the problems remedied. Staff members of color and LGBTQ status also have experienced unacceptable interactions with patients, their families, and other staff. In most cases, the offending individual has not been aware of the injury that was caused. These events cannot be reduced or eliminated until they are aired and faced.

The most important clinical application is listening while attempting to recognize assumptions and stereotypes and withholding judgment. Ob/gyns need to know the current laws and regulations in their own states and communities, and, when relevant, communicate them to patients. Patients need to know their rights; when they do, they are more forthcoming about their own histories, signs, symptoms, and clinical preferences.

Ob/gyns—the experts—are also the ideal sources of information for the public and for the government. ACOG statements are superb resources; the research and the contemplation have been performed. Use them for teaching, clinical care, and for op-ed pieces in newspapers, media interviews, and testimony before policy and law-making bodies.

CLINICAL CARE POINTS

- If, in the course of contraception or abortion care, a patient expresses concern about religious restrictions, she can be offered the references cited in this article. She can also be told that women belonging to every faith use contraception and have abortions as often as members of the public as a whole.
- Of course, clinicians inform patients about the risks of any anticipated procedure. However, patients should understand that any risks of abortion must be compared with those of continuing the pregnancy.
- Help young patients who have not told their parents about their pregnancies think through their decisions. Ultimately, they can and should make their own assessments and decisions, but some can use help informing and involving parents who will be supportive and helpful.
- It is stressful when pregnant women refuse interventions clinicians deem necessary for the benefit of the fetus. Nevertheless, those patients have the same right to refuse as non-pregnant patients. The best approach, after the nature of and

reason for the proposed intervention has been explained, is not to threaten or pressure the patient, is to ask her why she is refusing and listen respectfully and empathically to her response.

- Needless to say, clinicians working in institutions or organizations that restrict aspects of reproductive healthcare, even the provision of information about those restrictions, must acknowledge that patients are thus deprived of their rights — and their health.
- The American College of Obstetricians and Gynecologists, representing the profession within the United States, has been at the forefront of efforts to protect the reproductive rights and health of women. It falls to individual clinicians to educate about, advocate for, and I mplement those rights in their own institutions and communities.

REFERENCES

1. Inchley J, Currie D, Young T, et al. Growing up unequal: gender and socioeconomic differences in young people's health and well-being. Health behaviour in school-aged children (HBSC) study: International report from the 2013/2014 survey. Denmark: World Health Organization; 2016.
2. Erdman JN, DePiñeres T, Kismödi E. Updated WHO guidance on safe abortion: Health and human rights. Int J Gynecol Obstet 2013;120(2):200–3. Available at: https://www.clinicalkey.es/playcontent/1-s2.0-S0020729212005735.
3. World Health Organization. Reproductive, maternal, newborn and child health and human rights: a toolbox for examining laws, regulations and policies. Switzerland: Department of Reproductive Health and Research, World health Organization; 2014.
4. Over-the-counter access to hormonal contraception: ACOG committee opinion, number 788. Obstet Gynecol 2019;134(4):e96–105.
5. ACOG Committee on Ethics. ACOG committee opinion no. 439: informed consent. Obstet Gynecol 2009;114(2 Pt 1):401–8.
6. American College of Obstetricians and Gynecologists. ACOG committee opinion no. 385 November 2007: the limits of conscientious refusal in reproductive medicine. Obstet Gynecol 2007;110(5):1203–8. Available at: http://ovidsp.ovid.com.proxy.cc.uic.edu/ovidweb.cgi?T=JS&NEWS=n&CSC=Y&PAGE=fulltext&D=ovft&AN=00006250-200711000-00050.
7. American College of Obstetricians and Gynecologists' Committee on Ethics. Committee opinion no. 664: refusal of medically recommended treatment during pregnancy. Obstet Gynecol 2016;127(6):175.
8. Committee on Health Care for Underserved Women. ACOG committee opinion no. 613: increasing access to abortion. Obstet Gynecol 2014;124(5):1060–5.
9. Davis D. Reproductive injustice: racism, pregnancy, and premature birth. Social Forces 2020. https://doi.org/10.1093/sf/soaa067.
10. Paltrow LM, Flavin J. Arrests of and forced interventions on pregnant women in the united states, 1973–2005: Implications for women's legal status and public health. J Health Polit Policy Law 2013;38(2):299–343. Available at: https://search.datacite.org/works/10.1215/03616878-1966324.
11. Weinberger SE, Lawrence HC, Henley DE, et al. Legislative interference with the Patient–Physician relationship. N Engl J Med 2012;367(16):1557–9. Available at: https://doi.org.proxy.cc.uic.edu/10.1056/NEJMsb1209858.
12. Merton AH. Enemies of choice: The right-to-life movement and its threat to abortion. Boston: Beacon Press; 1982.

13. Cohen IG, Lynch HF, Curfman GD. When religious freedom clashes with access to care. N Engl J Med 2014;371(7):596–9. Available at: https://doi.org.proxy.cc.uic.edu/10.1056/NEJMp1407965.

14. State of indiana. HB 1337, 2016. Available at: https://legiscan.com/IN/bill/HB1337/2016.

15. Rovner J. High court allows employers to opt out of ACA's mandate on birth control coverage. LNP; 2020. Available at: https://search-proquest-com.proxy.cc.uic.edu/docview/2421426877.

16. Chakraborty A, McKenzie K. Does racial discrimination cause mental illness? Br J Psychiatry 2002;180(6):475–7. Available at: https://dx-doi-org.proxy.cc.uic.edu/10.1192/bjp.180.6.475.

17. Major B, Dovidio JF, Link BG. The oxford handbook of stigma, discrimination, and health. New York: Oxford University Press; 2018. Available at: http://bvbr.bib-bvb.de:8991/F?func=service&doc_library=BVB01&local_base=BVB01&doc_number=030121848&sequence=000001&line_number=0001&func_code=DB_RECORDS&service_type=MEDIA.

18. Mead M. A study of abortion in primitive societies. A typological, distributional, and dynamic analysis of the prevention of birth in 400 preindustrial societies. George Devereux. Q Rev Biol 1977;52(4):457.

19. Riddle JM. Contraception and abortion from the ancient world to the renaissance. Cambridge (MA): Harvard Univ. Press; 1992.

20. Brodie JF. Contraception and abortion in nineteenth-century America. Ithaca (NY): Cornell Univ. Press; 1994. 1. publ. ed.

21. Bearak J, Popinchalk A, Ganatra B, et al. Unintended pregnancy and abortion by income, region, and the legal status of abortion: estimates from a comprehensive model for 1990–2019. Lancet Glob Health 2020;8(9):e1152–61. Available at: https://doi.org.proxy.cc.uic.edu/10.1016/S2214-109X(20)30315-6.

22. Pew forum: religious groups' official positions on abortion. 2008. Available at: https://www.pewforum.org/2013/01/16/religious-groups-official-positions-on-abortion/.

23. Damian CI. Abortion from the perspective of eastern religions: Hinduism and buddhism. Rev Rom Bioet 2010;8(1):125–36. Available at: https://search-proquest-com.proxy.cc.uic.edu/docview/1286680900.

24. Lundsberg LS, Pal L, Gariepy AM, et al. Knowledge, attitudes, and practices regarding conception and fertility: a population-based survey among reproductive-age united states women. Fertil Steril 2014;101(3):767–74.e2. Available at: https://search.datacite.org/works/10.1016/j.fertnstert.2013.12.006.

25. Ott MA, Santelli JS. Abstinence and abstinence-only education. Curr Opin Obstet Gynecol 2007;19(5):446–52. Available at: https://search.datacite.org/works/10.1097/gco.0b013e3282efdc0b.

26. Jerman J, Jones RK, Onda T. Characteristics of U.S. abortion patients in 2014 and changes since 2008. Guttmacher Institute; 2016.

27. Finer LB, Frohwirth LF, Dauphinee LA, et al. Reasons U.S. women have abortions: quantitative and qualitative perspectives. Perspect Sex Reprod Health 2005;37(3):110–8. Available at: https://search.datacite.org/works/10.1363/3711005.

28. Finnbogadóttir H, Dykes A. Increasing prevalence and incidence of domestic violence during the pregnancy and one and a half year postpartum, as well as risk factors: -A longitudinal cohort study in southern sweden. BMC Pregnancy Childbirth 2016;16(1):327. Available at: https://search.datacite.org/works/10.1186/s12884-016-1122-6.

29. Silverman JG, Decker MR, Reed E, et al. Intimate partner violence victimization prior to and during pregnancy among women residing in 26 U.S. states: associations with maternal and neonatal health. Am J Obstet Gynecol 2006;195(1):140–8. Available at: https://search.datacite.org/works/10.1016/j.ajog.2005.12.052.

30. Glander S, Moore M, Michielutte R, et al. The prevalence of domestic violence among women seeking abortion. Obstet Gynecol 1998;91(6):1002–6. Available at: https://doi.org.proxy.cc.uic.edu/10.1016/S0029-7844(98)00089-1.

31. Felipe Russo N, Denious JE. Violence in the lives of women having abortions. Prof Psychol Res Pract 2001;32(2):142–50. Available at: https://search-proquest-com.proxy.cc.uic.edu/docview/614352757.

32. Raymond EG, Grimes DA. The comparative safety of legal induced abortion and childbirth in the united states. Obstet Gynecol 2012;119(2, Part 1):215–9. Available at: https://search.datacite.org/works/10.1097/aog.0b013e31823fe923.

33. Royal College of Psychiatrists. Induced abortion and mental health: a systematic review of the mental health impact of induced abortion. Royal College of Physicians; 2011.

34. Major B, Appelbaum M, Beckman L, et al. Abortion and mental health. Am Psychol 2009;64(9):863–90. Available at: https://search.datacite.org/works/10.1037/a0017497.

35. Foster DG, Steinberg JR, Roberts SCM, et al. A comparison of depression and anxiety symptom trajectories between women who had an abortion and women denied one. Psychol Med 2015;45(10):2073–82. Available at: https://dx-doi-org.proxy.cc.uic.edu/10.1017/S0033291714003213.

36. Major B, Cozzarelli C, Cooper ML, et al. Psychological responses of women after first-trimester abortion. Arch Gen Psychiatry 2000;57(8):777–84. Available at: https://doi.org.proxy.cc.uic.edu/10.1001/archpsyc.57.8.777.

37. Biggs MA, Neuhaus JM, Foster DG. Mental health diagnoses 3 years after receiving or being denied an abortion in the united states. Am J Public Health 2015;105(12):2557–63. Available at: https://search.datacite.org/works/10.2105/ajph.2015.302803.

38. Munk-Olsen T, Laursen TM, Pedersen CB, et al. Induced first-trimester abortion and risk of mental disorder. N Engl J Med 2011;364(4):332–9. Available at: https://doi.org.proxy.cc.uic.edu/10.1056/NEJMoa0905882.

39. Adler NE, David HP, Major BN, et al. Psychological responses after abortion. Science 1990;248(4951):41–4. Available at: http://www.sciencemag.org.proxy.cc.uic.edu/cgi/content/abstract/248/4951/41.

40. Dagg PK. The psychological sequelae of therapeutic abortion–denied and completed. Am J Psychiatry 1991;148(5):578–85. Available at: https://doi.org.proxy.cc.uic.edu/10.1176/ajp.148.5.578.

41. Cougle JR, Reardon DC, Coleman PK. Depression associated with abortion and childbirth: a long-term analysis of the NLSY cohort. Med Sci Monit 2003;9(4):CR105. Available at: https://www-ncbi-nlm-nih-gov.proxy.cc.uic.edu/pubmed/12709667.

42. Coleman PK, Coyle CT, Shuping M, et al. Induced abortion and anxiety, mood, and substance abuse disorders: Isolating the effects of abortion in the national comorbidity survey. J Psychiatr Res 2009;43(8):770–6. Available at: https://search.datacite.org/works/10.1016/j.jpsychires.2008.10.009.

43. Major B, Cozzarelli C, Sciacchitano AM, et al. Perceived social support, self-efficacy, and adjustment to abortion. J Pers Soc Psychol 1990;59(3):452–63. Available at: https://www-ncbi-nlm-nih-gov.proxy.cc.uic.edu/pubmed/2231279.

44. Cozzarelli C, Major B. The effects of anti-abortion demonstrators and pro-choice escorts on women's psychological responses to abortion. J Soc Clin Psychol 1994;13(4):404–27. Available at: https://search-proquest-com.proxy.cc.uic.edu/docview/848840344.

45. Steinberg JR, Finer LB. Coleman, coyle, shuping, and rue make false statements and draw erroneous conclusions in analyses of abortion and mental health using the national comorbidity survey. J Psychiatr Res 2012;46(3):407–8. Available at: https://search.datacite.org/works/10.1016/j.jpsychires.2012.01.019.

46. Kessler RC, Schatzberg AF. Commentary on abortion studies of steinberg and finer (social science & medicine 2011; 72:72–82) and coleman (journal of psychiatric research 2009;43:770–6 & journal of psychiatric research 2011;45:1133–4). J Psychiatr Res 2012;46(3):410–1. Available at: https://search.datacite.org/works/10.1016/j.jpsychires.2012.01.021.

47. Rowlands S. Misinformation on abortion. Eur J Contracep Reprod Health Care 2011;16(4):233–40. Available at: https://search.datacite.org/works/10.3109/13625187.2011.570883.

48. Stotland NL. The myth of the abortion trauma syndrome. JAMA 1992;268(15):2078–9. Available at: https://doi.org.proxy.cc.uic.edu/10.1001/jama.1992.03490150130038.

49. Foster DG. The turnaway study. New York: Scribner; 2020. Available at: https://ebookcentral-proquest-com.proxy.cc.uic.edu/lib/[SITE_ID]/detail.action?docID=6199332.

50. Stotland NL. Abortion: facts and feelings. Washington, DC: American Psychiatric Press; 1998.

51. Major B, Gramzow RH. Abortion as stigma: cognitive and emotional implications of concealment. J Pers Soc Psychol 1999;77(4):735–45.

52. Moore AM, Singh S, Bankole A. Do women and men consider abortion as an alternative to contraception in the united states? an exploratory study. Glob Public Health 2011;6(sup1):S25–37. Available at: http://www.tandfonline.com.proxy.cc.uic.edu/doi/abs/10.1080/17441692.2011.568948.

53. Pew Research Center. Public opinion on abortion: views on abortion, 1995-2019. Washington, DC: Pew Research Center; 2019. Available at: https://www.pewforum.org/fact-sheet/public-opinion-on-abortion/.

54. Steinberg L, Cauffman E, Woolard J, et al. Are adolescents less mature than adults? Am Psychol 2009;64(7):583–94. Available at: https://search.datacite.org/works/10.1037/a0014763.

55. Pope LM, Adler NE, Tschann JM. Postabortion psychological adjustment: are minors at increased risk? J Adolesc Health 2001;29(1):2–11. Available at: https://doi.org.proxy.cc.uic.edu/10.1016/S1054-139X(01)00212-9.

56. Leppälahti S, Heikinheimo O, Kalliala I, et al. Is underage abortion associated with adverse outcomes in early adulthood? A longitudinal birth cohort study up to 25 years of age. Hum Reprod 2016;31(9):2142–9. Available at: https://www-ncbi-nlm-nih-gov.proxy.cc.uic.edu/pubmed/27402909.

57. Henshaw SK, Kost K. Parental involvement in minors' abortion decisions. Fam Plann Perspect 1992;24(5):196–213. Available at: https://search.datacite.org/works/10.2307/2135870.

58. Yang YT, Kozhimannil KB, Snowden JM. Pharmacist-prescribed birth control in oregon and other states. JAMA 2016;315(15):1567–8. Available at: https://doi.org.proxy.cc.uic.edu/10.1001/jama.2016.2327.

59. Lee SJ, Ralston HJP, Drey EA, et al. Fetal pain: a systematic multidisciplinary review of the evidence. JAMA 2005;294(8):947–54. Available at: https://doi.org.proxy.cc.uic.edu/10.1001/jama.294.8.947.

60. Pollitt K. Pro: reclaiming abortion rights. Picador; 2015. Available at: http://www.vlebooks.com/vleweb/product/openreader?id=none&isbn=9781250055842&uid=none.

61. KATHA POLLITT. Abortion and punishment. New York Times (Online) Web site. 2016. Available at: https://search-proquest-com.proxy.cc.uic.edu/docview/1777651084. Accessed September 14, 2020.

62. American College of Obstetricians and Gynecologists' Committee on Ethics. Committee opinion no. 664: refusal of medically recommended treatment during pregnancy. Obstet Gynecol 2016;127(6):e175–82. Available at: http://ovidsp.ovid.com.proxy.cc.uic.edu/ovidweb.cgi?T=JS&NEWS=n&CSC=Y&PAGE=fulltext&D=ovft&AN=00006250-201606000-00045.

63. American Psychiatric Association. Position statement on legislative intrusion and reproductive choice, official action. American Psychiatric Association; 2013.

64. Tuerkheimer D. How not to protect pregnant women. The New York Times 2015;A19.

65. The Guttmacher Institute. An overview of abortion laws. The Guttmacher Institute; 2020.

66. ACOG. Statement regarding abortion procedure bans. American College of Obstetricians and Gynecologists; 2015.

67. LINDA GREENHOUSE. The abortion map today. The New York Times 2016. Available at: https://global.factiva.com/en/du/article.asp?accessionno=NYTF000020160414ec4e0003a.

68. Greene MF, Drazen JM. A new label for mifepristone. N Engl J Med 2016;374(23):2281–2. Available at: https://doi.org.proxy.cc.uic.edu/10.1056/NEJMe1604462.

69. Sonfield A. Learning from experience: where religious liberty meets reproductive rights. Guttmacher Policy Review 2016;19(1):1.

70. ACOG. Open letter to Texas legislators: get out of our exam rooms. States News Service; 2013.

71. Kaye J, Amiri B, Melling L, et al. Health care denied: patients and physicians speak out about catholic hospitals and the threat to women's health and lives. American Civil Liberties Union; 2016.

72. Patrick A. From uruguay, a model for making abortion safer. New York Times (Online) Web site. Available at: https://search-proquest-com.proxy.cc.uic.edu/docview/1799811021. 2016. Accessed September 14, 2020.

Racial/Ethnic Inequities in Pregnancy-Related Morbidity and Mortality

Rebecca D. Minehart, MD, MSHPEd[a],*, Allison S. Bryant, MD, MPH[b],
Jaleesa Jackson, MD[a], Jaime L. Daly, MD[c]

KEYWORDS

- Maternal mortality • Severe maternal morbidity • Racial disparities • Obstetrics
- Obstetric anesthesia

KEY POINTS

- Black women die at a staggering rate of 3 to 4 times greater as compared with their White counterparts, regardless of socioeconomic factors.
- Systemic and institutionalized racism is the predominant cause of Black women's inequities in accessing care and dramatic underrepresentation in research.
- Hospital factors and provider bias play a large role in Black women suffering more morbidity and mortality.
- Women's health care providers are uniquely positioned to help erase some of these inequities by focusing on these vulnerabilities.

INTRODUCTION

There is no denying that racial inequities in health care continue to afflict citizens of the United States; the rates at which the severe acute respiratory syndrome novel coronavirus 2 infection disproportionately affects minority communities[1,2] serve as evidence of this disturbing fact. For pregnant women in America, these inequities existed before this pandemic, with maternal morbidity and mortality rates that have continued to increase over the past 2 decades.[3–5] As recently as May 2019, the Centers for Disease Control and Prevention (CDC) issued a Morbidity and Mortality Weekly Report that included data demonstrating that pregnant or postpartum women of color die at a

[a] Department of Anesthesia, Critical Care, and Pain Medicine, Harvard Medical School, Massachusetts General Hospital, 55 Fruit Street, GRJ 440, Boston, MA 02114, USA; [b] Department of Obstetrics and Gynecology, Harvard Medical School, Massachusetts General Hospital, 55 Fruit Street, Founders 4, Boston, MA 02114, USA; [c] Department of Anesthesiology, University of Colorado School of Medicine, University of Colorado Hospital, 12605 East 16th Avenue, Aurora, CO 80045, USA
* Corresponding author.
E-mail address: rminehart@mgh.harvard.edu
Twitter: @RDMinehart (R.D.M.); @asbryantmantha (A.S.B.); @jjacksonMD (J.J.)

Obstet Gynecol Clin N Am 48 (2021) 31–51
https://doi.org/10.1016/j.ogc.2020.11.005
0889-8545/20/© 2020 Elsevier Inc. All rights reserved.

staggering rate of 3 to 4 times greater as compared with their White counterparts, regardless of socioeconomic factors,[6] although these inequities were not new. This report and others like it renewed demands for answers as to why these women were dying at such disparate rates, as National Public Radio,[7] the Harvard Business Review,[8] the Associated Press[9] and others, including community voices, called for the medical profession's accountability. Reports from health care professional societies like the American College of Obstetricians and Gynecologists' (ACOG) Committee Opinion on racial and ethnic disparities in maternal care[10] and a toolkit for postpartum care[11,12] attempt to raise awareness of inequities and suggest possible solutions, but clearly there remains an enormous need for understanding why these inequities exist, particularly between White and Black mothers, where the disparities are the greatest.[6]

Health care providers caring for pregnant women have an imperative to improve maternal care. A deeper understanding of why these racial inequities exist and an acknowledgment of the historic and current contributions may inspire real change throughout our complex system of health care. Actively restructuring how health care is provided is the surest way to dismantle systemic racism, from individual provider (eg, addressing unconscious provider bias, granting agency to Black women and other women of color as experts about their bodies, and partnering with health care providers for relationship-centered care[13]), to health care fields themselves (eg, regaining patient trust in the medical professions, making health care jobs more accessible and more representative of our diverse population). This review focuses on what inequities exist and what are the potential drivers of these inequities, with a brief overview of potential solutions.

INEQUITIES IN MATERNAL HEALTH OUTCOMES VERSUS INEQUITIES IN PROVISION OF MATERNAL CARE

The definition of a health disparity is a health difference seen in groups, whereas inequity is a disparity specifically arising from unfairness and discrimination in social, economic, environmental, or health care resources.[14] Before considering reasons why Black mothers are becoming sicker and dying at higher rates than White mothers, we first consider inequities in 2 categories: outcomes and the provision of care.

Inequities in Outcomes

Inequities in maternal health outcomes can be highlighted through outlining the obstetric conditions leading to severe maternal morbidity (SMM) and mortality for which there are disparities. SMM, which has no formally accepted definition,[15] has alternately been described as "a life-threatening diagnosis or the need to undergo a life-saving procedure during a delivery hospitalization"[16,17] and as "unintended outcomes of the process of labor and delivery that result in significant short-term or long-term consequences to a woman's health."[18] The ACOG and others[18] have proposed conditions and criteria for SMM, which may serve as an initiation point for building consensus among professional organizations (**Table 1**). Although the categorization and inclusion of these morbidities may need adjustment, this list fills an undeniable need for better classifying and understanding the extent of SMM through careful research.

Holdt Somer and colleagues[15] attempted to identify gaps in the existing literature on disparities in SMM. Although their list of SMM definitions were not entirely congruent with the ACOG definitions, these authors demonstrated a significant increase in SMM for multiple racial groups, predominantly Black women as compared with their White

Table 1
Example list of diagnoses and complications constituting severe maternal morbidity

SMM	Not Severe Morbidity (Insufficient Evidence if This Is the Only Criterion)
Hemorrhage	
Obstetric hemorrhage with ≥4 units of the blood cells transfused	
Obstetric hemorrhage with 2 units of red blood cells and 2 units of fresh frozen plasma transfused (without other procedures or complications) if not judged to be overexuberant transfusion	Obstetric hemorrhage with 2 units of red blood cells and 2 units of fresh frozen plasma transfused and judged to be "overexuberant"
Obstetric hemorrhage with <4 units of blood products transfused and evidence of pulmonary congestion that requires >1 dose of furosemide	Obstetric hemorrhage with <4 units of blood products transfused and evidence of pulmonary edema requiring only 1 dose of furosemide
Obstetric hemorrhage with return to operating room for any major procedure (excludes dilation)	
Any emergency/unplanned peripartum hysterectomy, regardless of number of units transfused (includes all placenta accreta spectrum conditions)	Planned peripartum hysterectomy for cancer/neoplasia
Obstetric hemorrhage with uterine artery embolization, regardless of number of units transfused	
Obstetric hemorrhage with uterine balloon or uterine compression suture placed and 2–3 units of blood products transfused	Obstetric hemorrhage with uterine balloon or uterine compression suture placed and ≤1 unit of blood products transfused
Obstetric hemorrhage admitted to ICU for invasive monitoring or treatment (either medication or procedure, not just observed overnight)	Any obstetric hemorrhage who went to the ICU for observation only without further treatment
Hypertension/neurologic	
Eclamptic seizure(s) or epileptic seizures that were "status"	
Continuous intravenous infusion of an antihypertensive medication	
Nonresponsiveness or loss of vision, permanent or temporary (but not momentary), documented in physician's progress notes	
Stroke, coma, intracranial hemorrhage	
Preeclampsia with difficult-to-control severe hypertension (>160 mm Hg systolic blood pressure or >110 mm Hg diastolic blood pressure) that requires multiple intravenous doses, persistent ≥48 h after delivery, or both	Chronic hypertension that drifts up to severe range and needs postoperative medication dose alteration; preeclampsia blood pressure control with oral medications ≥48 h after delivery

(continued on next page)

Table 1 *(continued)*	
SMM	**Not Severe Morbidity (Insufficient Evidence if This Is the Only Criterion)**
Liver or subcapsular hematoma or severe liver injury admitted to the ICU (bilirubin >6 or liver enzymes >600)	Abnormal liver function requiring extra prolonged postpartum length of stay but not in the ICU
Multiple coagulation abnormalities or severe hemolysis, elevated liver enzymes, and low platelet count (HELLP) syndrome	Severe thrombocytopenia (<50,000) alone that does not require a transfusion or ICU admission
Renal	
Diagnosis of acute tubular necrosis or treatment with renal dialysis	Oliguria treated with intravenous fluids(no ICU admission)
Oliguria treated with multiple doses of furosemide	Oliguria treated with 1 dose of furosemide (no ICU admission)
Creatinine ≥2.0 in a woman without preexisting renal disease OR a doubling of the baseline creatinine in a woman with preexisting renal disease	
Sepsis	
Infection with hypotension with multiple liters of intravenous fluid or pressors used (septic shock)	Fever >38.5 °C with elevated lactate alone without hypotension
Infection with pulmonary complications such as pulmonary edema or acute respiratory distress syndrome	Fever >38.5 °C with presumed choriometritis/endometritis with elevated pulse but no other cardiovascular signs and normal lactate
	Positive blood culture without other evidence of significant systemic illness
Pulmonary	
Diagnosis of acute respiratory distress syndrome, pulmonary edema, or postoperative pneumonia	Administration of oxygen without a pulmonary diagnosis
Use of a ventilator (with either intubation or noninvasive technique)	
Deep vein thrombosis or pulmonary embolism	
Cardiac	
Preexisting cardiac disease (congenital or acquired)with ICU admission for treatment	Preexisting cardiac disease (congenital or acquired) with ICU admission for observation only
Peripartum cardiomyopathy	Preexisting cardiac disease (congenital or acquired) without ICU ad mission for observation only
Arrhythmia requiring >1 dose of intravenous m education but not ICU admission	Arrhythmia requiring 1 dose of intravenous medication but no ICU admission

(continued on next page)

Table 1 **(continued)**	
SMM	**Not Severe Morbidity (Insufficient Evidence if This Is the Only Criterion)**
ICU/invasive monitoring	
Any ICU admission that includes treatment or diagnostic or therapeutic procedure	ICU admission for observation of hypertension that does NOT require intravenous medications
Central line or pulmonary catheter used to monitor a complication	ICU admission for observation after general anesthesia
Surgical, Bladder, and Bowel Complications	
Bowel or bladder injury during surgery beyond minor serosal tear	
Small-bowel obstruction, with or without surgery during pregnancy/ postpartum period	
Prolonged ileus for ≥4 d	Postoperative ileus that resolved without surgery in ≤3 d
Anesthesia complications	
Total spinal anesthesia	
Aspiration pneumonia	Failed spinal anesthesia that requires general anesthesia
Epidural hematoma	Spinal headache treated with a blood patch

Abbreviations: HELLP, hemolysis, elevated liver enzymes, and low platelet count; ICU, intensive care unit.

Adapted from American College of Obstetricians and Gynecologists and Society for Maternal-Fetal Medicine, Kilpatrick SK, Ecker JL, et al. Severe maternal morbidity: screening and review. Obstetric Care Consensus No. 5. Obstet Gynecol 2016;128:e54-60; with permission.

counterparts. **Table 2** lists the disparities as well as gaps in the authors' literature search on a variety of morbid conditions. Specific conditions, such as inherited thrombophilias and sickle cell diseases, have a clear genetic basis, although their severity and treatment reflect other influences. The overwhelming majority of other conditions and their outcomes may be attributed to myriad factors involving the interplay between race and health, notably the impact of systemic and structural racism, which we explore elsewhere in this article.

Inequities in the Provision of Care

Outside of outright SMM and mortality, the provision of maternal care is also rife with inequities and contributes to disparities in outcomes. Black and Asian women are more likely to have higher cesarean delivery rates overall as compared with White women, and more likely for subjective indications.[19] A recent article reviewing racial disparities using the Robson Ten-Group Classification System revealed that Black women had the highest rates of cesarean delivery of any group, and specifically the highest rates in Robson Groups 1 to 4, typically thought of as low risk and most favorable for a vaginal delivery. The authors further postulated that this could be due to the "lack of appropriate care"[20] and needs further scrutiny.

Access to doula support for pregnant and postpartum Black women has historically also been limited,[21] despite the known benefits, such as lower rates of cesarean

Table 2
Examples of racial/ethnic disparities in health outcomes classified by SMM indicator

SMM Indicator	Disparities Identified in Current Literature Search
Acute MI	Increased cardiovascular risk factors among Black women; some literature finds increased MI risk among non-Hispanic White and Black women
ARF	Increased among Black and American Indian/Alaska native; additionally, black and Hispanic women with lupus erythematosus at increased risk of ARF
Acute respiratory distress syndrome	Increased among Black and American Indian/Alaska native women
Amniotic fluid embolism	Conflicting reports in the literature; some suggest an increase among Black woman
Aneurysm	No literature exists
Blood transfusion	Increased among Black women
Cardiac arrest or ventricular fibrillation	Increased among Black women
Cardio monitoring	Increased among Black, Hispanic, Asian/Pacific Islander, and American Indian/Alaska native women
Conversion of cardiac rhythm	Increased among Black women
Disseminated intravascular coagulation	Increased among Black, Hispanic, Asian/Pacific Islander, and American Indian/Alaska native women
Eclampsia	Increased among Black and Hispanic women
Heart failure during procedure or surgery	Increased among Black, Hispanic, and Asian/Pacific Islander women
Hysterectomy	Increased among Black, Hispanic, and Asian/Pacific Islander women
Internal injuries of thorax, abdomen, and pelvis	Increased among Black women
Intracranial injuries	No literature exists
Operations on heart and pericardium	Increased among Black women
Puerperal cerebrovascular disorders	Subarachnoid hemorrhage increased among Black and Hispanic women, intracerebral hemorrhage and stroke increased among Black women
Pulmonary edema	Increased among Black and Asian/Pacific Islander women
Sepsis	Increased among Black and Hispanic women
Severe anesthesia complications	Increased among Black women; use of general anesthesia may also be increased among Black women

(continued on next page)

Table 2 **(continued)**	
SMM Indicator	**Disparities Identified in Current Literature Search**
Shock	Increased among Black, Asian/Pacific Islander, and American Indian/Alaska native women
Sickle cell anemia with crisis	Increased among Black women
Temporary tracheostomy	Increased among Black women
Thrombotic embolism	Increased among Black women; thrombotic risk factors differ non-Hispanic White and Black women
Ventilation	Increased among Black, Hispanic, Asian/Pacific Islander, and American Indian/Alaska native women
Additional indicators of morbidity	
Cardiomyopathy	Increased among Black women
Preeclampsia/HELLP	Increased among Black and American Indian/Alaska native women
Hemorrhage	Increased among Hispanic and Asian/Pacific Islander women; conflicting data regarding Black women

Abbreviations: ARF, acute renal failure; HELLP, hemolysis, elevated liver enzymes, and low platelet count; MI, myocardial infarction

Adapted from Holdt Somer SJ, Sinkey RG, et al. Epidemiology of racial/ethnic disparities in severe maternal morbidity and mortality. Semin Perinatol 2017;41:258-65; with permission.

delivery, lower rates of forceps or vacuum deliveries, improved birth experiences, and decreased maternal stress.[22] Doula services are not usually covered under traditional, currently available health insurance plans,[21] which likely contributes considerably to inequities in access.

Black and Hispanic women also receive epidural analgesia for labor at lower rates than White women.[23–25] The reasons for this are multifactorial,[24] and are postulated to be:

- Minority patients are less likely to have the same access to care as nonminority patients
- The possibility of provider bias in favor of nonminority patients exists
- Minority patients may be more likely to mistrust the medical system, which may limit adherence to recommendations
- Nonminority patients may demand more care than minority patients[26]

Lower use of labor epidural analgesia may be a precipitating factor for Black women being more likely to receive general anesthesia for cesarean delivery.[25] Recent links have demonstrated higher rates of morbidity in women who were deemed to be candidates to receive neuraxial anesthesia for cesarean delivery, yet received general anesthesia instead.[27] In their study, Guglielminotti and colleagues[27] found that racial or ethnic minority women were more likely to receive a potentially avoidable general anesthetic than White mothers, highlighting another area for improving care discrepancies through understanding and addressing problems present. For a subgroup of racially diverse women who did not prefer epidural analgesia for their labor and delivery, 60% of Black women reported that they felt pressure from their providers to accept an epidural, as compared with 40% of White women.[28] Even when Black and Hispanic women received epidural analgesia, they were much more likely to report analgesic failure than White women.[28]

Postpartum pain evaluation and management continues to be problematic for Black women. In 2 recent studies, Black women had higher pain scores as compared with White women, they were assessed less frequently for pain as compared with White women, and they received fewer opioids than White women,[29,30] including receiving a prescription for opioids at discharge.[29] These factors have significant consequences, because undertreated pain after childbirth can impair women's recovery and infant bonding.[31] As such, all providers should be cognizant of these disparities in pain assessment and treatment.

All providers would benefit from accurate information regarding racial inequities in care outcomes as well as how we provide care. For example, fewer than one-half of maternal–fetal medicine specialists identified inequities accurately in 6 of 7 survey questions, and fewer than one-third agreed (strongly or somewhat) that their personal biases may affect how they cared for patients.[32] Much of the care given on labor, delivery, and postpartum units is delivered by nurses, for whom an accurate knowledge of SMM and potential racial inequities in care is also highly relevant. A recent survey assessed postpartum nurses' reported knowledge and practices and found that only 54% of nurses knew of increasing maternal mortality and 93% misattributed hemorrhage as the leading cause of death, rather than cardiovascular disease.[33] Overall, the gaps in knowledge from the multidisciplinary group caring for pregnant women must be acknowledged and addressed systematically.

In 2018, committee members representing the ACOG, the Association of Women's Health, Obstetric and Neonatal Nurses, the Society for Maternal-Fetal Medicine, the American College of Nurse-Midwives, the Society for Obstetric Anesthesia and Perinatology, the American Academy of Family Physicians, the Association of Maternal & Child Health Programs, and the University of Michigan School of Public Health authored a patient safety bundle addressing racial and ethnic disparities from multiple angles,[34] which we describe elsewhere in this article. This collaboration between the leading women's health organizations represented a pivotal moment of solidarity against such inequities (see **Table 2**).

THE LINKS BETWEEN RACE AND HEALTH

Race is a hotly debated topic, with many scholars advocating that it is "an unscientific, societally constructed taxonomy that is based on an ideology that views some human populations as inherently superior to others on the basis of external physical characteristics or geographic origin,"[35] but that nevertheless critically impacts myriad outcomes, including health, longevity, and social status attainment.[35,36] In 2016, the National Health Interview Survey conducted by the CDC revealed that White males and females had consistently higher reports of health than Black males and females.[37] To better visualize the relationship between race and health, Williams and colleagues[35] developed a framework (**Fig. 1**, **Table 3**) that is still useful to consider today. We focus on a subset of these factors, primarily racism, biological factors, and risk factors and resources, as they relate to maternal health and well-being. As will explain further elsewhere in this article, there is a considerable overlap and intertwining influence between these categories.

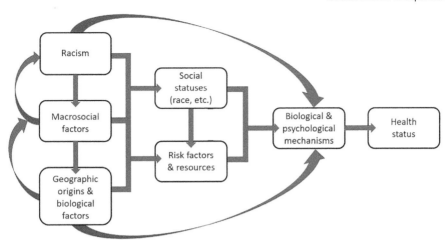

Fig. 1. A framework for understanding the relationship between race and health. (*Adapted from* Williams DR, Lavizzo-Mourey R, Warren RC. The concept of race and health status in America. Public Health Rep 1994;109(1):26-41; with permission.)

Table 3
Types of factors involved in the relationship between race and health

Factor	Definitions	Examples
Racism	Racial ideology (categorization or ranking), prejudice, or discrimination (individual or institutional)	A Black mother is not prescribed adequate opioid pain relief because her provider believes black women do not experience as much pain.
Macrosocial factors	Historical conditions, economic structures, political order, legal codes, and social cultural institutions	Black people are generally under-represented in medical research given their historical mistreatment and abuse, and therefore are more distrustful of medical researchers.
Biological factors	Morphologic, physiologic, biochemical, or genetic factors	Chronic stress manifested physically results in higher rates of chronic hypertension, diabetes, and other cardiovascular comorbidities in Black mothers than in White mothers.
Social status	Race or ethnicity, socioeconomic status, sex, social roles, geographic location, or age	Black mothers are more likely to live in impoverished environments as compared to White mothers, and are more likely to be uninsured.
Risk factors and resources	Health behaviors, stress, medical care, social ties, or psychological, cultural, or religious factors	Black mothers are more likely to deliver in hospitals with much higher rates of SMM and mortality.

Adapted from Williams DR, Lavizzo-Mourey R, Warren RC. The concept of race and health status in America. Public Health Rep 1994;109(1):26-41; with permission.

Racism

Although there are many historically relevant racial and ethnic narratives that are likely responsible for other disparities, each of which deserves equally thorough coverage, we focus our discussion on Black women given the current enormous gap in maternal care. As late as 1972, the United States was still involved in the Tuskegee Syphilis study, where Black men were withheld known effective treatment for syphilis.[38] This egregious display of governmentally backed, morally and ethically corrupt, prolonged and formalized racism is one of many that cultivated a deep distrust in many Black Americans of the health care system. This distrust persists today and may be partially responsible for lower rates of participation in medical research by Black patients, who reported much higher rates of distrust in the medical research process.[39,40] Clearly, this factor leaves a knowledge vulnerability at the intersection of racial disparities in SMM with Black women's potential unwillingness to participate in prospective research studies,[18,39,40] especially given that an overwhelming number of obstetric and women's health providers (eg, obstetricians, anesthesiologists, nurse midwives, certified registered nurse anesthetists, physician assistants, and nurses) are White.[41–45]

Disparities in maternal care in the United States must include a conversation of the historical treatment of Black women, specifically African Americans. For these women, certain historical medical practices which shaped their interactions with health care have been collapsed by Prather and colleagues[46] into 4 distinct periods: during legalized slavery (AD 1619–1865), Black Codes/Jim Crow laws (AD 1865–1965), during the Civil Rights movement (AD 1955–1975), and the post-Civil Rights era (AD 1975-present) and included institutional abuse, rape, and experimentation for perfecting surgical techniques, often without anesthesia (**Table 4** for details). The horrors that these women endured resulting from systematic and continued racism and disenfranchisement cannot be forgotten nor discounted, because they impact the current and future public health initiatives aimed at decreasing these disparities.[4] An unsettling and enlightening recent *New York Times Magazine* edition, *The 1619 Project*, contained a collection of essays describing the previously untold sufferings of many Black men and women in America that augmented many people's understanding of the torture they endured, not just during slavery, but for the 4 centuries since then.[47] In addition, many tools developed and used in obstetrics have ignominious roots. The Sims retractor, for example, was named for J. Marion Sims, known as the "father of modern gynecology," whose work was based on experimenting on Black enslaved women during the mid-1800s.[48] Other women in racial and ethnic minority groups may have complicated relationships with health care as a profession, especially when women are undocumented immigrants.

As early as 2003, the Institute of Medicine highlighted racism, prejudice, and provider bias as drivers of health disparities in their sentinel report, *Unequal Treatment: Confronting Racial and Ethnic Disparities in Health Care*, which described that the effects of socioeconomic differences could not explain the imbalance in care for conditions even with well-established, straightforward guidelines, such as cardiovascular catheterization, cancer diagnostic tests, and antiretroviral therapy for human immunodeficiency virus, to name a few.[49] Even the hint of racism and prejudice can interfere with the provision of care; this dynamic may be overcome by pairing Black physicians with Black patients, who are more likely to undergo recommended preventative tests, with a potential cardiovascular mortality benefit estimated at nearly 20%.[50] Recent work has shown this situation to be true also for newborns, where mortality rates were halved when Black newborns were cared for by Black physicians, although in

Table 4
Historical and contemporary sexual- and reproductive-related health and health care experiences of Black women

Period	Timespan	No. of Years	Personal Experiences of AA Women that Contribute to Disparities in Sexual and Reproductive Health	Health Care Experiences of AA Women that Contribute to Disparities
Slavery	1619–1865	246	Public, nude physical auction examinations to determine reproductive ability; raped for sexual pleasure and economic purpose; purposely aborting pregnancies where rape occurred; Jezebel stereotype emerged of Black women being hypersexual; generational poverty	Nonconsensual gynecologic and reproductive surgeries performed at times repeatedly on female slaves without anesthesia, including cesarean sections and ovariotomy to perfect medical procedures
Black Codes/ Jim Crow	1865–1965	100	Rape; lynching (genitalia/ reproductive mutilation); uncertain/unequal civil rights; stereotypes and negative media portrayals continued; generational poverty	Nonconsensual medical experiments continued; poor or no health care for impoverished Blacks; compulsory sterilization; Jim Crow laws enforced lack of access to quality health care services and opportunities; effects of Tuskegee Untreated Syphilis Study on women (eg, some wives of untreated subjects acquired syphilis and their children suffered consequences of congenital syphilis)
Civil Rights	1955–1975	20	Lynching, uncertain/ unequal civil rights and violence against women to show superiority and control; stereotypes and negative hypersexual medial portrayals continued; generational poverty	Nonconsensual medical experiments continued; compulsory sterilization for recipients of federal funding; effects of Tuskegee Untreated Syphilis Study on women; unequal health care services as a result of both overt and subtle racism
Post-Civil Rights	1975–2018	43	Black exploitation movies, media's hypersexual images continued; generational poverty	Unequal health care continued; targeted sterilizations, hysterectomies, abortions, and birth control

Adapted from Prather C, Fuller TR, Jeffries WL, et al. Racism, African American women, and their sexual and reproductive health: a review of historical and contemporary evidence and implications for health equity. Health Equity 2018;2(1):249-59; with permission.

the same study population, a survival benefit was not extended to decrease their Black mothers' mortality.[51]

Overt racism may not be the sole reason behind widespread provider-driven disparities; much research into biases has shared that provider bias may be explicit (obvious, expressed openly) or implicit (hidden, subconscious). Although racism itself may be classified as an explicit bias, implicit biases act in a more insidious manner, often existing "at the margins of awareness," directing behavior even while one is not fully conscious of the negative bias.[52] Implicit biases are ubiquitous and are accentuated anywhere complex decisions are made and the need for cognitive shortcuts or heuristics is high, such as in the criminal justice system and law enforcement,[53] because biases are a primary pathway for the brain to pattern recognize, without the process of slower, analytical thinking.[54] It is well-known that explicit biases can be spread easily through verbal messages.[55] However, what is striking is how pervasive these implicit biases can be, as seen through a social learning theory lens, which posits that nonverbal cues are influential in defining attitudes toward others. Thus, implicit biases can be created and perpetuated in everyday social interactions where people's nonverbal behaviors (body language, facial expressions) are shared.[55] Researchers have attempted to determine how much implicit bias shapes medical practice, but a recent systematic review revealed serious methodologic limitations in the published medical literature, much of which was lacking a strong theoretic basis.[52] A potential source of robust theory may come from the social psychology and organizational behavior literature on racial diversity, which has spent decades determining what processes are at play between individuals of different races and creating standardized tools to study those processes and interactions.[56–60]

Although provider bias training is advocated,[52] it has not shown to change outcomes in bias when given in small "doses" related to raising awareness of bias,[61] underscoring a true need for culture change and widespread adoption with likely more regular and critical application. Only intensive behavior change techniques have been shown to be effective in altering implicit racial biases, which involve considerable time, financial, and personnel resources,[56,62] all of which must be granted for systems to undergo real change. By dedicating resources to improving our theoretic approaches, applying behavior change principles in the "doses" needed, and exploring new frontiers (eg, automated technology using risk stratification), we will begin to mitigate and modify implicit biases.

Biological Factors

The deceptive allure of a simple explanation for racial differences in health outcomes, especially related to genetic factors, seems to be hypnotic, despite multitudinous evidence to the contrary.[35,36,50] As mentioned elsewhere in this article, except for heritable diseases such as certain thrombophilias and hemoglobinopathies, much of the biological changes are in fact thought to be due to chronic exposure to stress through experiences of prejudice and discrepancies in social standing, which manifests in tangible ways to produce "weathering," also known as the "physical consequence of social inequality."[63] Weathering is rarely found among White mothers, and overwhelmingly is seen in Black women in poor neighborhoods; this process was manifested by low birthweight neonates, preterm birth, and small-for-gestational age births, and mitigated when Black mothers were situated in the upper one-half of neighborhoods for income and had also never resided in low-income neighborhoods.[64]

Inequities and stress harm DNA. A possible biological explanation for this weathering is due to leukocyte chromosomal telomere shortening from enhanced telomerase activity, leading to accelerated aging; telomeres are otherwise known as protective "caps" at the end of chromosomes that consist of repeated nucleotides.[65] A link has been established between telomere shortening and both the duration and amount of stress experienced by mothers caring for an ill child,[66] and with shorter telomere length for Black women (but not men) living in poor and racially segregated neighborhoods.[67] More recently, the magnitude of distrust and anger expressed was associated with decreased telomere length in Black women involved in the Jackson Heart Study.[68] Additionally, telomere length is heritable to some degree, as demonstrated by Black mothers having shorter telomeres than Whites, and Black male neonates having shorter telomeres than White male neonates.[69] It is unclear whether telomere length itself is the appropriate measure; Needham and colleagues[70] demonstrated attenuation in racial and ethnic differences for telomere length when baseline telomere length was taken into consideration for 1169 participants in the Multi-Ethnic Study of Atherosclerosis (MESA), and the majority of telomere shortening was eventually seen in older people and in men when adjusting for baseline length. Clearly, there is an urgent need to understand the links between psychological and physical stress and resulting mechanisms that lead to disease manifestation and worse health for Black mothers.

Risk Factors and Resources

This final category we explore is broad and includes both patient-related factors as well as system-wide influences; the factors influencing hospital care are presented in **Fig. 2**.[71] This area is also ripe for dramatic improvement to prevent SMM and mortality, as enormous between-hospital differences in care exist, even within the same

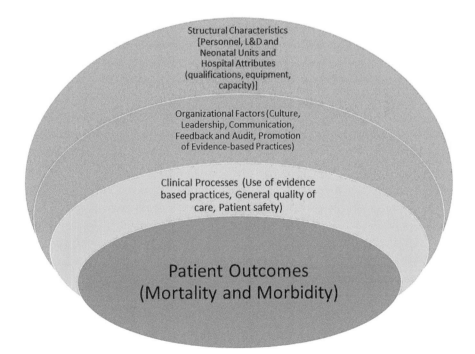

Fig. 2. Hospital quality and SMM: structural factors. L&D, labor and delivery. (*Adapted from* Howell EA, Zeitlin J. Improving hospital quality to reduce disparities in severe maternal morbidity and mortality. Semin Perinatol 2017;41(5):266-72; with permission.)

large metropolitan city (such as New York City), and these racial differences may account for nearly 48% of the racial inequity seen there.[71,72]

Black women may deliver in hospitals that primarily serve a Black population, and these hospitals have been shown to have higher rates of SMM when compared with hospitals primarily serving Whites.[73] This difference may stem from a variety of factors, including organizational issues such as leadership influences, a culture of safety, active teamwork practices, and the use of bundles to improve maternal care.[71] Safety practices such as bundle implementation are critical for maternal safety, because they have been shown to empower all health care providers to initiate critical steps to mitigate delays in treatment[34,74] and improve safety culture.[34,75,76] Improving continuous labor support access (including access to doulas) has been trialed, showing early promise, and should be advocated for Black women's use.[22]

Recent work has also highlighted the need for cultural humility among providers, with a focus of self-reflection on the provider–patient relationship and its sources of power imbalance.[77] Additionally, structural competency is highlighted, which acknowledges the systems and cultural structures that produce health inequities and calls for learning and advocacy to repair longstanding damage from these systems.[78] Widespread adoption of curricula addressing culture seems to be one of the fundamental prerequisites for change.

WHAT ELSE IS BEING DONE NATIONALLY TO COMBAT RACIAL INEQUITIES IN OBSTETRICS?

Multiple national efforts have been made to improve racial inequities in peripartum care. Traditionally, mothers have been stratified and transported to care centers based on concerns for neonatal well-being. Fetal deaths (>20 weeks estimated gestational age) continue to be unacceptably high for Black mothers. Black women's fetuses die at a rate of 10.8 per 1000 as of 2016, which is the highest of all racial and ethnic groups, and more than double that of White mothers (at 5 per 1000).[79] The CDC created the National Network of Perinatal Quality Collaboratives in 2016 to address critical perinatal health issues, for which the National Institute for Children's Health Quality was awarded oversight in 2017.[80]

Although this perinatal focus remains essential, the historical focus on fetal health and status has likely inadvertently made providers systematically neglectful of mothers, especially Black mothers. The 2015 ACOG/Society for Maternal-Fetal Medicine Levels of Maternal Care initiative aimed to risk stratify women based on comorbidities and consolidate services for women who may need escalated care using additional resources[81] (and this was reaffirmed with revisions in 2019[82]). Subsequently in 2018, the Society for Obstetric Anesthesia and Perinatology developed and implemented a designation for "Centers of Excellence"[83] for hospitals and health systems who practice evidence-based obstetric anesthesia care within a culture of safety. That same year, the Preventing Maternal Deaths Act of 2018 was passed, which improved funding and supported the CDC in working with state and tribal mortality review committees to better understand pregnancy-related deaths.[84]

The multiprofessional provider group representing all major women's health organizations created the 2018 Maternal Safety Consensus Bundle mentioned earlier,[34] which provided a concept map to reducing peripartum racial and ethnic disparities by considering the 5 following themes:

- An inability to assess disparities because they are not reliably measured
- A lack of recognition of disparities at both the personal and systems level

- Specific knowledge of the magnitude of racial and ethnic disparities that exist within a health care system
- Communication barriers
- Differences in the structure of care[34]

Within the bundle, multiple evidence-based strategies were provided for each theme, such as improving accurate and respectful data collection on identity to link to outcomes, address implicit biases through a combination of cognitive and behavioral therapies, applying coaching and education to raise awareness throughout a hospital system, uncovering local or systems-based biases through the routine use of quality assurance tools, encouraging shared decision making with patients, and addressing fragmentation of care by improving preconception health, among other suggestions.[34] Taken as a whole, this national, significant focus on inequities is the largest effort to date in facing the deep roots of systemic racism.

WHAT CAN TEAM MEMBERS DO TO IMPROVE MATERNAL CARE AND OUTCOMES FOR BLACK MOTHERS?

Obstetric care is inherently team based, and all providers have the potential to improve care. Women's health providers comprise a diverse group of professionals with a common goal to improve the health and well-being of women. For pregnant women, obstetric services have a long history of leading team training efforts aimed at developing a shared understanding of teamwork and communication, including understanding how different providers communicate under stressful conditions[85] and proactively designing interventions to facilitate best teamwork practices, including speaking up.[86,87] Teamwork training in hospitals has been largely associated with better patient outcomes,[75,88] and large malpractice insurers, such as the Risk Management Foundation of the Harvard Teaching Institutions (also known as Controlled Risk Insurance Company, or CRICO) have incentivized a malpractice insurance premium reduction for anesthesiologists, obstetricians, and certified nurse midwives who undergo yearly team-based simulation training and drills in obstetric emergencies.[89,90] These same educational and quality improvement tools can be used to address bias in the workplace as a critical priority; a roadmap for Readiness, Recognition, Response, and Reporting & Systems Learning has been provided by the Maternal Safety Consensus Bundle.[34] Quality assurance processes should be tailored to seek out and address inequities in delivery of care, as well as in outcomes. Systems-wide provider bias training should be incorporated into the cultures of all clinical and community areas where pregnant women are being cared for, in addition to raising awareness of structural competency.[91,92] By educating providers and holding each other accountable for improving care for racially and ethnically diverse women, we may begin to shift the narrative in racial inequities at large.

SUMMARY

Racism in America has deep and tangled roots that impact maternal health, particularly through pervasive inequities among Black women as compared with White, although inequities exist for other racial and ethnic groups. Health care providers caring for pregnant women are optimally positioned to maintain vigilance for these disparities in maternal care, and to intervene with their unique, comprehensive, and complementary skills. As leaders in patient safety, women's health care providers should drive hospitals and practices to implement national bundles for safer obstetric care and use team-based training practices aimed at improving all settings where we care for racially diverse mothers.

CLINICS CARE POINTS

- Evaluate local practices for evidence of racial inequities in obstetric care delivery and outcomes through quality assurance practices.
- Institute provider anti-bias training on a programmatic level with regular intervals of training, rather than a single session.
- Improve diversity in provider groups caring for women to strengthen care delivered and combat inequities.
- Seek opportunities to capture and incorporate obstetric patients' feedback related to inclusivity of practice.

DISCLOSURE

The authors have nothing to disclose.

REFERENCES

1. Moore JT, Ricaldi JN, Rose CE, et al. Disparities in incidence of COVID-19 among underrepresented racial/ethnic groups in counties identified as hotspots during June 5–18, 2020 — 22 States, February–June 2020. MMWR Morb Mortal Wkly Rep 2020;69:1122–6.
2. Goldfarb IT, Clapp MA, Soffer MD, et al. Prevalence and severity of coronavirus disease 2019 (COVID-19) illness in symptomatic pregnant and postpartum women stratified by Hispanic ethnicity. Obstet Gynecol 2020;136(2):300–2.
3. Kassebaum N. Global, regional, and national levels of maternal mortality, 1990-2015: a systematic analysis for the Global Burden of Disease Study 2015. Lancet 2016;388(10053):1775–812.
4. MacDorman MF, Declercq E, Cabral H, et al. Recent increases in the U.S. maternal mortality rate: disentangling trends from measurement issues. Obstet Gynecol 2016;128(3):447–55.
5. Maternal Mortality Estimation Inter-Agency Group (MMEIG). Maternal mortality in 2000-2017: United States of America. Available at: https://www.who.int/gho/maternal_health/countries/usa.pdf?ua=1. Accessed September 8, 2020.
6. Petersen EE, Davis NL, Goodman D, et al. Vital signs: pregnancy-related deaths, United States, 2011–2015, and strategies for prevention, 13 states, 2013–2017. MMWR Morb Mortal Wkly Rep 2019;68:423–9. Available at: https://doi.org/10.15585/mmwr.mm6818e1. Accessed September 8, 2020.
7. Neighmond P. Why racial gaps in maternal mortality persist. National Public Radio 2019. Available at: https://www.npr.org/sections/health-shots/2019/05/10/722143121/why-racial-gaps-in-maternal-mortality-persist. Accessed September 8, 2020.
8. Delbanco S, Lehan M, Montalvo T, et al. The rising U.S. maternal mortality rate demands action from employers. Harv Bus Rev 2019. Available at: https://hbr.org/2019/06/the-rising-u-s-maternal-mortality-rate-demands-action-from-employers. Accessed September 8, 2020.
9. Stobbe M, Marchione M. US pregnancy deaths are up, especially among minorities. New York: Associated Press; 2019. Available at: https://www.apnews.com/4907da5c58c84a708a548c4ea18fc5c7. Accessed September 8, 2020.

10. Racial and ethnic disparities in obstetrics and gynecology. Committee Opinion No. 649. American College of Obstetricians and Gynecologists. Obstet Gynecol 2015;126:e130–4.

11. ACOG Postpartum Toolkit. Racial disparities in maternal mortality in the United States: the postpartum period is a missed opportunity for action 2018. Available at: acog.org/about/our-commitment-to-changing-the-culture-of-medicine-and-eliminating-racial-disparities-in-womens-health-outcomes/our-commitment-to-changing-the-culture-of-medicine-resources. Accessed September 8, 2020.

12. Black Mamas Matter Alliance. 2020. Available at: http://blackmamasmatter.org/. Accessed September 8, 2020.

13. Hardeman RR, Karbeah J, Kozhimannil KB. Applying a critical race lens to relationship-centered care in pregnancy and childbirth: an antidote to structural racism. Birth 2020;47(1):3–7.

14. Braveman P. What are health disparities and health equity? We need to be clear. Public Health Rep 2014;129:5–8.

15. Holdt Somer SJ, Sinkey RG, Bryant AS. Epidemiology of racial/ethnic disparities in severe maternal morbidity and mortality. Semin Perinatol 2017;41:258–65.

16. Admon LK, Winkelman TNA, Zivin K, et al. Racial and ethnic disparities in the incidence of severe maternal morbidity in the United States, 2012-2015. Obstet Gynecol 2018;132:1158–66.

17. Callaghan WM, Creanga AA, Kuklina EV. Severe maternal morbidity among delivery and postpartum hospitalizations in the United States. Obstet Gynecol 2012; 120:1029–36.

18. American College of Obstetricians and Gynecologists and Society for Maternal-Fetal Medicine, Kilpatrick SK, Ecker JL, Callaghan WM. Severe maternal morbidity: screening and review. Obstetric Care Consensus No. 5. Obstet Gynecol 2016;128:e54–60.

19. Edmonds JK, Yehezkel R, Liao X, et al. Racial and ethnic differences in primary, unscheduled cesarean deliveries among low-risk primiparous women at an academic medical center: a retrospective cohort study. BMC Pregnancy Childbirth 2013;13:168.

20. Valdes EG. Examining cesarean delivery rates by race: a population-based analysis using the Robson ten-group classification system. J Racial Ethn Health Disparities 2020. https://doi.org/10.1007/s40615-020-00842-3.

21. Kozhimannil KB, Attanasio LB, Jou J, et al. Potential benefits of increased access to doula support during childbirth. Am J Manag Care 2014;20(8):e340–52.

22. Thomas MP, Ammann G, Brazier E, et al. Doula services within a healthy start program: increasing access for an underserved population. Matern Child Health J 2017;21(Suppl 1):59–64.

23. Glance LG, Wissler R, Glantz C, et al. Racial differences in the use of epidural analgesia for labor. Anesthesiology 2007;106:19–25.

24. Toledo P, Caballero JA. Racial and ethnic disparities in obstetrics and obstetric anesthesia in the United States. Curr Anesthesiol Rep 2013;3:292–9.

25. Lange EMS, Rao S, Toledo P. Racial and ethnic disparities in obstetric anesthesia. Semin Perinatol 2017;41:293–8.

26. Clark-Hitt R, Malat J, Burgess D, et al. Doctors' and nurses' explanations for racial disparities in medical treatment. J Health Care Poor Underserved 2010;21(1):386–400.

27. Guglielminotti J, Landau R, Li G. Adverse events and factors associated with potentially avoidable use of general anesthesia in cesarean deliveries. Anesthesiology 2019;130(6):912–22.

28. Morris T, Schulman M. Race inequality in epidural use and regional anesthesia failure in labor and birth: an examination of women's experience. Sex Reprod Healthc 2014;5(4):188–94.

29. Badreldin N, Grobman WA, Yee LM. Racial disparities in postpartum pain management. Obstet Gynecol 2019;134(6):1147–53.

30. Johnson JD, Asiodu IV, McKenzie CP, et al. Racial and ethnic inequities in postpartum pain evaluation and management. Obstet Gynecol 2019;134(6):1155–62.

31. Postpartum pain management. ACOG Committee Opinion No. 742. American College of Obstetricians and Gynecologists. Obstet Gynecol 2018;132. https://doi.org/10.1097/AOG.0000000000002683.

32. Moroz L, Riley LE, D'Alton M, et al. SMFM special report: putting the "M" back in MFM: addressing education about disparities in maternal outcomes and care. Am J Obstet Gynecol 2018;218(2):B2–8.

33. Suplee PD, Bingham D, Kleppel L. Nurses' knowledge and teaching of possible postpartum complications. MCN Am J Matern Child Nurs 2017;42(6):338–44.

34. Howell EA, Brown H, Brumley J, et al. Reduction of peripartum racial and ethnic disparities: a conceptual framework and maternal safety consensus bundle. Obstet Gynecol 2018;131(5):770–82 [published correction appears in Obstet Gynecol. 2019 Jun;133(6):1288].

35. Williams DR, Lavizzo-Mourey R, Warren RC. The concept of race and health status in America. Public Health Rep 1994;109(1):26–41.

36. Dressler WW, Oths KS, Gravlee CC. Race and ethnicity in public health research: models to explain health disparities. Annu Rev Anthropol 2005;34:231–52.

37. U.S. Department of Health and Human Services, Centers for Disease Control and Prevention, National Center for Health Statistics. Summary Health Statistics. National Health Interview Survey, 2016. Table A-11a, pages 1-9. Available at: https://ftp.cdc.gov/pub/Health_Statistics/NCHS/NHIS/SHS/2016_SHS_Table_A-11.pdf. Accessed September 8, 2020.

38. Kennedy BR, Mathis CC, Woods AK. African Americans and their distrust of the health care system: healthcare for diverse populations. J Cult Divers 2007;14(2):56–60.

39. Corbie-Smith G, Thomas SB, George DMM St. Distrust, race, and research. Arch Intern Med 2002;162(21):2458–63.

40. Shavers VL, Lynch CF, Burmeister LF. Racial differences in factors that influence the willingness to participate in medical research studies. Ann Epidemiol 2002;12:248–56.

41. Association of American Medical Colleges. 2018 Physician Specialty Data Report. 1.3. Active Physicians by Sex and Specialty, 2017. Available at: https://www.aamc.org/data/workforce/reports/492560/1-3-chart.html. Accessed September 8, 2020.

42. Medscape lifestyle report 2017: race and ethnicity, bias and burnout. Available at: https://www.medscape.com/sites/public/lifestyle/2017. Accessed September 8, 2020.

43. Data USA: registered nurses. Available at: https://datausa.io/profile/soc/registered-nurses#demographics. Accessed September 8, 2020.

44. Data USA: nurse practitioners & nurse midwives. Available at: https://datausa.io/profile/soc/2911XX/#demographics. Accessed September 8, 2020.

45. National Commission on Certification of Physician Assistants. 2018 Statistical Profile of Certified Physician Assistants by Specialty Annual Report. Available at: http://prodcmsstoragesa.blob.core.windows.net/uploads/files/2018StatisticalProfileof CertifiedPAsbySpecialty1.pdf. Accessed September 8, 2020.

46. Prather C, Fuller TR, Jeffries WL, et al. Racism, African American women, and their sexual and reproductive health: a review of historical and contemporary evidence and implications for health equity. Health Equity 2018;2(1):249–59.

47. The 1619 Project. The New York Times Magazine 2019. Available at: https://www.nytimes.com/interactive/2019/08/14/magazine/1619-america-slavery.html. Accessed September 8, 2020.

48. Wall LL. The controversial Dr. J. Marion Sims (1813-1883). Int Urogynecol J 2020; 31(7):1299–303.

49. Institute of Medicine. Unequal treatment: Confronting racial and ethnic disparities in health care (with CD). Washington, DC: The National Academies Press; 2003. https://doi.org/10.17226/12875. Accessed September 8, 2020.

50. Alsan M, Garrick O, Graziani GC. Does diversity matter for health? Experimental evidence from Oakland. Working Paper 24787, NBER Working Paper Series, Revised May 2019. Available at: https://www.nber.org/papers/w24787. Accessed September 8, 2020.

51. Greenwood BN, Hardeman RR, Huang L, et al. Physician-patient racial concordance and disparities in birthing mortality for newborns. Proc Natl Acad Sci U S A 2020;117(35):21194–200.

52. Hall WJ, Chapman MV, Lee KM, et al. Implicit racial/ethnic bias among health care professionals and its influence on health care outcomes: a systematic review. Am J Public Health 2015;105(12):e60–76.

53. Pereda B, Montoya M. Addressing implicit bias to improve cross-cultural care. Clin Obstet Gynecol 2018;61(1):2–9.

54. Stiegler MP, Tung A. Cognitive processes in anesthesiology decision making. Anesthesiology 2014;120(1):204–17.

55. Skinner AL, Perry S. Are attitudes contagious? exposure to biased nonverbal signals can create novel social attitudes. Pers Soc Psychol Bull 2020;46(4):514–24.

56. Hagiwara N, Elston Lafata J, Mezuk B, et al. Detecting implicit racial bias in provider communication behaviors to reduce disparities in healthcare: challenges, solutions, and future direction for provider communication training. Patient Educ Couns 2019;102:1738–43.

57. Boon H, Steward M. Patient-physician communication assessment instruments: 986 to 1996 in review. Patient Educ Couns 1998;35:161–76.

58. Schirmer JM, Mauksch L, Lang F, et al. Assessing communication competence: a review of current tools. Fam Med 2005;37:184–92.

59. Foldy EG, Rivard P, Buckley TR. Power, safety, and learning in racially diverse groups. Acad Manage Learn Educ 2009;8(1):25–41.

60. Avery DR, Richeson JA, Hebl MR, et al. It does not have to be uncomfortable: the role of behavioral scripts in black-white interracial interactions. J Appl Psychol 2009;94:1382–93.

61. Devine PG, Forscher PS, Austin AJ, et al. Long-term reduction in implicit race bias: a prejudice habit-breaking intervention. J Exp Soc Psychol 2012;48: 1267–78.

62. Gawronski B, Bodenhausen GV. Associative and propositional processes in evaluation: an integrative review of implicit and explicit attitude change. Psychol Bull 2006;132:692–731.

63. Geronimus AT. Black/white differences in the relationship of maternal age to birthweight: a population-based test of the weathering hypothesis. Soc Sci Med 1996; 42(4):589–97.

64. Love C, David RJ, Rankin KM, et al. Exploring weathering: effects of lifelong economic environment and maternal age on low birth weight, small for gestational

age, and preterm birth in African-American and White women. Am J Epidemiol 2010;172(2):127–34.

65. Aubert G, Landsorp PM. Telomeres and aging. Physiol Rev 2008;88(2):557–79.

66. Epel ES, Blackburn EH, Lin J, et al. Accelerated telomere shortening in response to life stress. Proc Nat Acad Sci 2004;101(49):17312–5.

67. Gebreab SY, Riestra P, Gaye A, et al. Perceived neighborhood problems are associated with shorter telomere length in African American women. Psychneur-oendocrinology 2016;69:90–7.

68. Jordan CD, Glover LM, Gao Y, et al. Association of psychosocial factors with leukocyte telomere length among African Americans in the Jackson Heart Study. Stress Health 2019;35(2):138–45.

69. Weber KA, Heaphy CM, Joshu CE, et al. Racial differences in maternal and umbilical cord blood leukocyte telomere length and their correlations. Cancer Causes Control 2018;29(8):759–67.

70. Needham BL, Wang X, Carroll JE, et al. Sociodemographic correlates of change in leukocyte telomere length during mid- to late-life: the Multi-Ethnic Study of Atherosclerosis. Psychoneuroendocrinology 2019;102:182–8.

71. Howell EA, Zeitlin J. Improving hospital quality to reduce disparities in severe maternal morbidity and mortality. Semin Perinatol 2017;41(5):266–72.

72. New York City Department of Health and Mental Hygiene. Bureau of Maternal and Child Health. Pregnancy-Associated Mortality New York City, 2006–2010. New York: 2015.

73. Howell EA, Egorova N, Balbierz A, et al. Black-white differences in severe maternal morbidity and site of care. Am J Obstet Gynecol 2016;214(1):122,e1-7.

74. U.S. Department. of Health and Human Services Agency for Healthcare Research and Quality. Patient safety primer: maternal safety. 2019. Available at: https://psnet. ahrq.gov/primers/primer/50/Maternal-Safety. Accessed September 8, 2020.

75. Manser T. Teamwork and patient safety in dynamic domains of healthcare: a review of the literature. Acta Anaesthesiol Scand 2009;53:143–51.

76. Edmondson AC. Psychological safety and learning behavior in work teams. Administrative Sci Q 1999;44:350–83.

77. Murray-García J, Tervalon M. The concept of cultural humility. Health Aff (Millwood) 2014;33(7):1303.

78. Davis S, O'Brien AM. Let's talk about racism: strategies for building structural competency in nursing. Acad Med 2020. https://doi.org/10.1097/ACM. 0000000000003688.

79. Healthy People 2020, Fetal deaths (per 1,000 live births plus fetal deaths, 20+ weeks gestation) by race/ethnicity (of mother). Available at: HealthyPeople.gov https://www.healthypeople.gov/2020/data/Chart/4823?category=3&by=Race/Ethnicity%20(of%20mother)&fips=-1. Accessed September 8, 2020.

80. Centers for Disease Control and Prevention. National Network of Perinatal Quality Collaboratives. Available at: https://www.cdc.gov/reproductivehealth/maternalinfanthealth/nnpqc.htm. Accessed September 9, 2020.

81. American College of Obstetricians and Gynecologists and Society for Maternal-Fetal Medicine, Menard MK, Kilpatrick S, et al. Levels of maternal care. Am J Obstet Gynecol 2015;212(3):259–71.

82. American Association of Birth Centers; Association of Women's Health, Obstetric and Neonatal Nurses; American College of Obstetricians and Gynecologists; Society for Maternal-Fetal Medicine, Kilpatrick SJ, Menard MK, Zahn MC, et al. Obstetric care consensus #9: levels of maternal care: (replaces obstetric care

consensus number 2, February 2015). Am J Obstet Gynecol 2019;221(6): B19–30.

83. Society for Obstetric Anesthesia and Perinatology. Centers of Excellence. Available at: https://soap.org/grants/center-of-excellence/. Accessed September 8, 2020.

84. 115th Congress of the United States. H.R. 1318. Public Law No. 115-344. Preventing Maternal Deaths Act of 2018. Available at: https://www.congress.gov/bill/115th-congress/house-bill/1318. Accessed September 8, 2020.

85. Minehart RD, Pian-Smith MC, Walzer TB, et al. Speaking across the drapes: communication strategies of anesthesiologists and obstetricians during a simulated maternal crisis. Simul Healthc 2012;7(3):166–70.

86. Pian-Smith MC, Simon R, Minehart RD, et al. Teaching residents the two-challenge rule: a simulation-based approach to improve education and patient safety. Simul Healthc 2009;4(2):84–91.

87. Raemer DB, Kolbe M, Minehart RD, et al. Improving anesthesiologists' ability to speak up in the operating room: a randomized controlled experiment of a simulation-based intervention and a qualitative analysis of hurdles and enablers. Acad Med 2016;91(4):530–9.

88. Hughes AM, Gregory ME, Joseph DL, et al. Saving lives: a meta-analysis of team training in healthcare. J Appl Psychol 2016;101(9):1266–304.

89. Gardner R, Walzer TB, Simon R, et al. Obstetric simulation as a risk control strategy: course design and evaluation. Simul Healthc 2008;3(2):119–27.

90. CRICO. CRICO OB Patient Safety Program. 2018. Available at: https://www.rmf.harvard.edu/Clinician-Resources/Article/2012/OB-Risk-Reduction-Program. Accessed September 9, 2020.

91. Bateman BT, Carvalho B. Addressing Racial and Ethnic Disparities in Pain Management in the Midst of the Opioid Crisis. Obstet Gynecol 2019;134(6):1144–6.

92. Davis S, O'Brien AM. Let's talk about racism: strategies for building structural competency in nursing. Acad Med 2020. https://doi.org/10.1097/ACM.0000000000003688.

Management of Viral Complications of Pregnancy
Pharmacotherapy to Reduce Vertical Transmission

Sarah C. Rogan, MD, PhD[a], Richard H. Beigi, MD, MSc[b],*

KEYWORDS

- Viral infections • Pregnancy • Herpes simplex virus • Cytomegalovirus
- Viral hepatitis • Human immunodeficiency virus • COVID-19
- Maternal-to-child transmission

KEY POINTS

- Viral infections are common complications of pregnancy. Although some infections have maternal sequelae, many viral infections can be perinatally transmitted to fetuses or infants.
- Safe and effective treatments are available to treat many viral infections during pregnancy.
- Antiviral therapy is indicated to reduce maternal-to-child transmission of diseases, such as herpes simplex virus, chronic hepatitis B virus, and human immunodeficiency virus.
- Research is ongoing to further clarify the role of treatments for cytomegalovirus, chronic hepatitis C virus, and COVID-19 during pregnancy.

INTRODUCTION

Viral infections are common complications of pregnancy, with a wide range of obstetric, fetal, and neonatal sequelae. Many viruses can be vertically transmitted to the fetus or neonate. In some cases, this transmission can cause a congenital syndrome or severe neonatal illness, as is the case for viruses, such as cytomegalovirus (CMV) and herpes simplex virus (HSV). For other viruses, including hepatitis B (HBV), hepatitis C (HCV), and human immunodeficiency virus (HIV), vertical transmission causes chronic disease in offspring. From a public health standpoint, this maternal-to-child

[a] Maternal and Fetal Medicine Division, Department of Obstetrics, Gynecology, and Reproductive Sciences, University of Pittsburgh School of Medicine, 300 Halket Street, Pittsburgh, PA 15213, USA; [b] Department of Obstetrics, Gynecology, and Reproductive Sciences, University of Pittsburgh School of Medicine, University of Pittsburgh Medical Center Magee-Womens Hospital, 300 Halket Street, Pittsburgh, PA 15213, USA
* Corresponding author.
E-mail address: beigrh@upmc.edu

Obstet Gynecol Clin N Am 48 (2021) 53–74
https://doi.org/10.1016/j.ogc.2020.12.001   **obgyn.theclinics.com**
0889-8545/21/© 2020 Elsevier Inc. All rights reserved.

transmission (MTCT) of chronic illnesses creates a viral reservoir, as these children are at risk for further transmission of the virus across their lifespan.

Treatment of viral infections in pregnancy involves management of maternal symptoms, optimization of obstetric outcomes, and reduction or prevention of vertical transmission. Women often engage in health care more frequently and reliably during pregnancy; thus, for women with chronic illnesses, such as HIV or chronic hepatitis, pregnancy is an ideal time to ensure appropriate treatment and to optimize their health. In this review, the authors address the treatment of several viral infections, including HSV, CMV, HCV, HBV, and HIV. Finally, they discuss emerging data on severe acute respiratory syndrome coronavirus 2 (SARS-CoV-2), the virus that causes COVID-19 disease.

HERPES SIMPLEX VIRUS

HSV infection is common among reproductive-aged adults and is caused by either of 2 strains, HSV-1 or HSV-2. These viruses infect the oropharyngeal and genital tracts and then remain latent in sensory neural ganglia; both strains can cause genital HSV. In the United States, the prevalence of HSV-1 and HSV-2 among reproductive-aged adults is 47.8% and 11.9%, respectively.[1]

During pregnancy, maternal primary HSV has the most significant clinical consequences. Approximately 2% of seronegative pregnant women acquire primary HSV during pregnancy, and although up to 60% of these infections are asymptomatic, primary HSV disease can be severe.[2] In addition to the typical painful or pruritic genital vesicular lesions and ulcerations, patients may present with dysuria and systemic symptoms, including fever, malaise, headache, and lymphadenopathy. Women may also present with their first episode of genital herpes but serologic evidence of prior infection with a different HSV strain. This nonprimary disease is typically less severe than primary disease.

Nucleoside Analogues for Treatment and Suppression of Herpes Simplex Virus

The mainstays of HSV treatment are nucleoside analogues, including acyclovir, its prodrug valacyclovir, and less commonly, famciclovir. Compared with acyclovir, valacyclovir has the benefit of better oral bioavailability and a longer half-life and thus enables less frequent and more convenient oral dosing, but it is more expensive than acyclovir. There are no concerns regarding teratogenicity of these medications or other adverse reactions that would limit their use in pregnancy. Data on first-trimester exposure from a large, population-based retrospective cohort study in Denmark[3] and from the International Acyclovir in Pregnancy Registry[4] demonstrate no association between nucleoside analogue use and birth defects.

Treatment of maternal disease includes acetaminophen, topical anesthetics, sitz baths, and hygienic measures to relieve symptoms. Maternal outbreaks are often self-limited, but antiviral therapy can shorten the duration and severity of symptoms and can limit the duration of viral shedding. Oral treatment regimens typically include acyclovir or valacyclovir. Standard treatment regimens endorsed by the Centers for Disease Control and Prevention (CDC)[5] and the American College of Obstetricians and Gynecologists (ACOG)[6] for maternal symptomatic infection are listed in **Table 1**. For severe primary infections, intravenous acyclovir can also be used.

Although vertical transmission of HSV can occur in utero, fetal infection via transplacental or transcervical passage of the virus is rare. Neonatal infection acquired peripartum is the more significant concern, as it can result in disseminated, lethal disease. Neonatal infection is more common in cases of primary maternal infection

Table 1
Oral treatment regimens for herpes simplex virus infection during pregnancy

Clinical Indication	Acyclovir	Valacyclovir	Treatment Duration
Primary first-episode genital HSV	200 mg 5 times daily *or* 400 mg 3 times daily	1000 mg twice daily	7–10 d
Primary non–first-episode or recurrent genital HSV	400 mg 3 times daily *or* 800 mg twice daily	500 mg twice daily *or* 1000 mg daily	5 d
HSV suppression	400 mg 3 times daily	500 mg twice daily	From 36 wk' gestation until delivery

Data from Refs.[5,6]

during pregnancy, particularly if genital HSV is acquired shortly before labor, as such infections are associated with higher rates of viral shedding in the lower genital tract.[2,7] Notably, patients without active clinical outbreaks can still experience asymptomatic viral shedding.

In addition to its use to improve maternal severity of disease, antiviral therapy is also used with a goal of minimizing the risk of peripartum MTCT of HSV. Acyclovir and valacyclovir are routinely administered prophylactically in the late third trimester until the onset of labor to decrease complications from HSV at time of delivery in women with a history of genital HSV (see **Table 1** for suppressive therapy regimens). The goals of this prophylaxis are to decrease the risk of active HSV disease at the time of delivery and to reduce asymptomatic viral shedding. A metaanalysis of randomized clinical trials concluded that prophylactic acyclovir beginning at 36 weeks' gestation reduced clinical HSV recurrence at delivery by 75%, reduced cesarean deliveries for recurrent genital HSV by 70%, and reduced the risk of HSV viral shedding and total HSV detection at delivery by 91% and 89%, respectively.[8] Results are similar for valacyclovir.[9] Notably, prophylaxis does not eliminate HSV viral shedding or lesions at time of delivery[10] nor does it absolutely prevent neonatal transmission of disease.[11]

CYTOMEGALOVIRUS

CMV is a common infection among reproductive-aged women and is the most common cause of congenital infectious morbidity.[12] This virus, like HSV-1 and HSV-2, is a member of the Herpesviridae family of viruses. Primary CMV infection in immunocompetent adults is generally asymptomatic but can present as a flulike illness. Like HSV, CMV can remain latent, primarily in monocytes, following primary infection and can reactivate to cause an asymptomatic secondary infection and viral shedding; reinfection with a new CMV strain can also occur. Although CMV infection has limited maternal sequelae, in utero vertical transmission of CMV results in fetal infection. The sequelae of congenital CMV vary depending on the gestational age at fetal infection but have the potential to be devastating.

The seroprevalence of CMV among reproductive-aged women is high with rates of 50% to 85% in developed countries, including the United States. Women in minority groups with lower socioeconomic status tend to have higher rates of seroprevalence.[13,14] Approximately 1% to 7% of seronegative at-risk pregnant women will develop a primary infection during pregnancy.[15] The overall birth prevalence of infants with congenital CMV is estimated at 0.6% to 1.08%; between 8% and 12% of these infections are symptomatic at birth.[16–18] Vertical transmission is significantly more likely in cases of primary CMV than recurrent or reactivated disease (32 vs 1.4%[18]); however, because of the high prevalence of CMV seropositivity and the overall low incidence of primary CMV during pregnancy, approximately 75% of cases of congenital CMV are due to nonprimary disease in the mother.[19] Fortunately, congenital CMV is generally less severe when due to recurrent or reactivated disease, and most neonates are asymptomatic at birth in such cases. When primary infection does occur during pregnancy, the risk of congenital infection depends on the gestational age of the fetus at the time of maternal infection and fetal transmission. Transmission rates range from 36% to 40% in the first and second trimesters to 65% in the third trimester[20]; earlier infections generally have more sequelae than infections acquired during the third trimester.[20,21] Largely, severe congenital CMV is secondary to first trimester transmission.[12]

Congenital CMV has a variety of ultrasonographic manifestations, including placentomegaly, hepatosplenomegaly, echogenic bowel, ascites, intracranial calcifications, ventriculomegaly, microcephaly, growth restriction, and stillbirth.[12,22,23] Infants with CMV are at risk for hyperbilirubinemia and jaundice, thrombocytopenia and petechial rashes, hepatitis, hearing loss, and death.[24] Up to 30% of severely affected infants will die of complications of CMV infection, and 80% of survivors will have major morbidity.[24] More commonly, infants are asymptomatic at birth, but they are still at risk for sensorineural hearing loss and other complications later in childhood.[12,24,25] Sensorineural hearing loss is the most common sequelae to develop in asymptomatic infants, and congenital CMV accounts for 15% to 20% of cases of sensorineural hearing loss.[26]

Treatment of Cytomegalovirus and Prevention of Vertical Transmission

Given the potentially devastating consequences of vertical transmission of CMV and the significant public health burden of its sequelae, prevention of vertical transmission and treatment of fetal infection are the focus of much research. The 2 primary therapeutic avenues under investigation are passive immunization with hyperimmune globulin (HIG) and administration of antiviral drugs. The current state of the research into potential therapies is reviewed here.

Early studies on passive immunization with CMV HIG were promising, but more recent data suggest a potential lack of efficacy. It is hypothesized that HIG reduces maternal and placental viral loads to prevent fetal infection, and in cases whereby infection has already occurred, it likely reduces placental and fetal inflammation to improve outcomes.[27] Observational studies of HIG infusions to pregnant women with primary CMV infection in early pregnancy have found reductions in vertical transmission. Nigro and colleagues[27] reported a decrease in vertical transmission of CMV from 40% to 16% following monthly infusions of HIG, and Kagan and colleagues[28] reported a decrease in vertical transmission from 32.5% in historical controls to 7.5% in their study population following biweekly infusions of a higher dose of HIG than was used in the former study. Other observational studies have demonstrated a reduction in neonatal and childhood symptoms following HIG administration to women with confirmed fetal infection.[27,29,30] These observational studies were met with enthusiasm and generated a scientific imperative for more robust efficacy data.

In contrast and importantly, 2 randomized controlled trials (RCTs) have failed to demonstrate a benefit of HIG infusion and have raised concerns about adverse obstetric outcomes associated with this therapy. The phase 2 CHIP trial, a double-blinded RCT of HIG or placebo infusion to women with primary CMV infection, found a nonsignificant decrease from 44% to 30% in vertical infection rates, and women who received HIG had a trend toward a higher rate of obstetric complications, including preterm birth, intrauterine growth restriction, and preeclampsia.[31] More recently, a multicenter phase 3 RCT in the United States (#NCT01376778) was halted early for futility after an interim analysis of 399 cases demonstrated equivalent transmission rates in the HIG and placebo groups.[32] Although preterm birth rates were similar in the 2 groups, a secondary analysis demonstrated an increased risk of a composite outcome of disorders associated with placental dysfunction in the treatment arm.[33] Thus, both RCTs investigating monthly HIG infusions to women with primary CMV in early pregnancy have failed to show a reduction in fetal transmission and have identified a trend of adverse obstetric outcomes associated with this treatment. There remain questions about the optimal timing of HIG administration in relation to timing of infection, dosage of HIG, and frequency of HIG treatments to maximize efficacy,[12] but the current state of the research would indicate that other therapeutic avenues should be pursued.

To that end, antiviral drugs are possible therapeutic agents for the prevention of vertical transmission of CMV and the treatment of fetal infection to minimize fetal and postnatal morbidity. Given the aforementioned safety of valacyclovir in pregnancy, research into antiviral therapy for congenital CMV has focused on this drug. In a pilot study, patients with confirmed fetal infection were treated with valacyclovir 8 g daily and then underwent amniocentesis and fetal blood sampling. Therapeutic concentrations of drug were detected in amniotic fluid and in fetal blood with reductions in fetal viral load.[34] Subsequently, in an open-label phase 2 trial, patients with ultrasound findings of congenital CMV were treated with 8 g daily of valacyclovir from the time of diagnosis until delivery. Women treated with valacyclovir were nearly twice as likely to deliver an asymptomatic neonate compared with historical controls. The treatment regimen required women to take 16 pills per day, but adherence was high, and the dosage was well tolerated.[35] A phase 2-3 RCT conducted in Israel investigated the use of valacyclovir (8 g daily) to reduce vertical transmission in women with periconception or first-trimester seroconversion. This trial found a 71% reduction in vertical transmission with the rate decreasing from 30% in the control group to 11% in the valacyclovir-treated group without any adverse effects.[36] This trial was small, with data reported on only 90 women, but the large effect size without adverse obstetric events suggests promise for this treatment.

As a whole, the current published data on prevention and treatment of congenital CMV are inconclusive. No treatment has definitively been shown to be both safe and efficacious. At present, consensus guidelines from ACOG,[37] the Society for Maternal Fetal Medicine,[38] and the International Congenital Cytomegalovirus Recommendations Group[39] recommend that administration of HIG and antiviral agents for prevention and treatment of congenital CMV be restricted to research trial protocols. Notably, vaccine development is another promising avenue of prevention for CMV under consideration.

VIRAL HEPATITIS

Viral hepatitis, including infections with HBV and HCV, is a global public health concern. Worldwide in 2015, there were 257 million and 71 million people living with HBV and HCV, respectively.[40] The World Health Organization has called for the elimination of viral hepatitis as a public health threat by 2030.[40] Children with vertically acquired viral hepatitis become chronic carriers at a high rate and represent an important source of further societal viral transmission. In addition, they can develop complications, such as cirrhosis, liver failure, and hepatocellular carcinoma, later in life at great cost to the public health system. Treatment of pregnant women with HBV and HCV to prevent MTCT and its sequelae is a promising global health strategy to limit the viral reservoir and to prevent these sequelae of chronic disease.

Treatment of Hepatitis B Virus

Although widespread administration of the HBV vaccine to infants and children has significantly reduced the incidence of HBV,[41] most new cases still occur in children who acquire the virus via MTCT or through contact with other infected children.[40] Screening for HBV infection by testing for hepatitis B surface antigen is a routine component of prenatal care, and it is standard of care in the United States to administer both the HBV vaccine and the HBV immunoglobulin within 12 hours of birth to children born to HBV-positive mothers.[42–44] This strategy is highly effective yet does not eliminate MTCT. Studies have demonstrated that the risk of failure of this passive-active immunization strategy is directly related to the presence of maternal e antigen (hepatitis B e antigen [HBeAg]) and to maternal viral load, with a viral load greater than 6 $\log_{10}$ copies/mL being the most important determinant of MTCT.[45–51] Targeting women with high viral loads for antiviral treatment could further reduce MTCT of HBV.

The antiviral drugs tenofovir, lamivudine, and telbivudine are well studied in pregnancy and have reassuring safety profiles. There is no evidence of teratogenicity or adverse obstetric or neonatal outcomes associated with their use.[52,53] Available data indicate that antiviral treatment is an effective prevention strategy for MTCT of HBV. A metaanalysis of 26 studies enrolling 3622 pregnant women found an improvement in maternal viral suppression at delivery and a corresponding 70% reduction in MTCT of HBV for women treated with lamivudine, telbivudine, or tenofovir disoproxil fumarate (TDF).[52] Because of concerns regarding resistance to lamivudine and telbivudine, TDF is the preferred antiviral drug for use in pregnancy, and women who conceive on another medication should consider transitioning to TDF during pregnancy if they continue therapy.[54] For TDF in particular, an RCT allocated mothers who were both HBeAg-positive and had an HBV DNA level greater than 200,000 IU/mL to TDF or usual care from 30 to 32 weeks of gestation until 4 weeks' postpartum. At delivery, maternal viral suppression less than 200,000 IU/mL increased from 2% among controls to 69% among TDF-treated women, and at 28 weeks' postpartum, MTCT decreased from 18% in infants of control to 5% in infants of TDF-treated women. There were no teratogenic effects, but mothers in the TDF group had elevations in their creatinine kinase and alanine aminotransferase levels after discontinuation of TDF.[55] Another RCT conducted in Thailand failed to demonstrate a significant decrease in MTCT following maternal TDF treatment, but the transmission rate in their control group was only 2%[56]; thus, there are methodological and generalizability concerns about the data from this trial.[57,58]

Given the effectiveness of the use of antivirals to decrease MTCT, the excellent safety data, and analyses that suggest such an approach is cost-effective,[59,60] TDF is now recommended as first-line treatment to decrease MTCT for pregnant women with an HBV viral load greater than 6 $\log_{10}$ copies/mL or 200,000 IU/mL.[42,54,61,62]

Treatment of Hepatitis C Virus

The incidence of HCV infection is on the increase in the United States, with cases of acute HCV increasing by 71% between 2014 and 2018. This increase is highest among reproductive-aged adults, largely because of the opioid crisis and intravenous drug use.[41] Thus, an increasing number of pregnant women are entering pregnancy with HCV infection. The CDC and the US Preventive Service Task Force recently issued new guidelines recommending routine screening for HCV infection in early pregnancy.[63,64] Identifying HCV infection in pregnant women allows for those women to be referred for appropriate surveillance and treatment and helps to identify infants who are at risk of MTCT so that they can receive the appropriate evaluation and follow-up.

Although observational studies have demonstrated an association between HCV infection and adverse obstetric[65–69] and neonatal[65] outcomes, pregnancy has not been shown to affect disease progression.[70] Women with chronic HCV infection tolerate pregnancy well. The risk of MTCT of HCV is approximately 5% and is essentially restricted to women with viremia; women who are coinfected with HIV have a higher rate of transmission.[70–75] Currently, there are no approved treatments to mitigate this risk.[76,77]

Historical treatment of HCV in nonpregnant adults included pegylated interferon-α and ribavirin. This regimen required a long duration of therapy (24–48 weeks), had low efficacy, and was poorly tolerated.[78,79] Moreover, both these medications are contraindicated in pregnancy. In 2011, direct-acting antiviral drugs (DAAs) were introduced and have revolutionized the treatment of HCV in the general population. These antiviral agents target specific enzymes and proteins required for the viral lifecycle, and this specificity for viral proteins limits their toxicity. These agents require only 8 to 12 weeks of therapy to induce a sustained virologic response rate (SVR), or a sustained undetectable viral load for 6 months after completion of treatment.[77,78] In other words, DAAs can cure HCV infection.

At this time, DAAs are not improved for use during pregnancy because of a lack of safety and efficacy data. Animal studies have not demonstrated fetal risk,[76] and a small retrospective study of women inadvertently exposed to DAAs during pregnancy did not reveal any evidence of teratogenicity or adverse neonatal effects.[80] A recently published phase 1 clinical trial provides early evidence in support of the use of DAAs during pregnancy. In this study of 8 pregnant women who completed a 12-week course of ledipasvir-sofosbuvir during the second and third trimesters, pharmacokinetic data were promising; the medications were well tolerated without significant adverse effects, and perhaps most notably, 100% of participants had an SVR at 12 weeks after completion of therapy, indicating disease cure.[81] This study suggests that HCV treatment during pregnancy is safe, feasible, and effective. Larger trials are clearly warranted to better investigate this therapeutic option.

From a global health perspective, pregnancy is an intriguing window of opportunity for treatment of HCV.[82] First, treatment theoretically could reduce obstetric and neonatal complications associated with HCV in pregnancy. Second, treatment of pregnant women might reduce MTCT, which subsequently could limit the viral reservoir, prevent complications of chronic HCV infection in offspring of affected women, and reduce health care costs across the lifespan of these children. Third, pregnancy represents a unique time to engage HCV-positive women in health care. Only 7.4% of people with HCV actually receive treatment,[40] despite national and international recommendations to assess everyone with chronic HCV infection for treatment. Young women are more likely to commit to health care during pregnancy, and with the short duration of therapy required to treat HCV with DAAs, full treatment and cure could be achieved during pregnancy. Ongoing and future investigations will better delineate the role of DAA therapies in pregnancy.

HUMAN IMMUNODEFICIENCY VIRUS

The management of HIV infection in pregnancy represents one of the great public health achievements of the last 25 years. In the United States, there were approximately

245,000 women living with HIV at the end of 2018,[83] and an estimated 5000 HIV-positive women give birth annually.[84] However, there were only 65 cases of perinatal HIV transmission in the United States in 2018, and between 2014 and 2018, the rate of perinatal transmission of HIV decreased from 1.5 to 0.9 per 100,000 live births.[85] Similarly low perinatal transmission rates have been observed in other developed countries.[86] This reduction in perinatal transmission is directly related to the widespread use of combination antiretroviral therapy (ART) in pregnancy. A complete review of ART and the management of HIV in pregnancy is beyond the scope of this article, but the authors highlight several key features of ART in pregnancy.

Principles of Antiretroviral Therapy

ART prevents MTCT of HIV through a combination of several mechanisms: reduction in maternal viremia, fetal preexposure prophylaxis via transplacental passage of antiretroviral drugs, and neonatal postexposure prophylaxis. To enable this 3-pronged approach, ART should be administered antenatally and intrapartum to all pregnant women and to infants postnatally, regardless of maternal viremia or CD4 count.

Ideally, women should be on ART with a suppressed viral load before conception. The perinatal HIV transmission risk correlates with the duration of ART and with maternal HIV RNA level.[87–89] Women on ART before conception have a 0.2% to 0.7% risk of transmission[90,91] and that risk increases with every trimester delay in initiation of ART.[90] Importantly, women who present late in gestation do derive benefit from short-course therapy.[92] Moreover, women should be on combination therapy with multiple drugs, as this approach yields the lowest rates of MTCT, compared with single- or dual-agent therapy.[88,91–93] In 1 study, the odds ratio of MTCT was 0.27 (95% confidence interval, 0.08–0.94) in women on ART compared with women treated with zidovudine alone.[88]

Suppressed maternal viremia does not ensure protection of the fetus from infection. Indeed, in the French Perinatal Cohort, 20% of infected children were born to mothers with plasma viral loads less than 500 copies/mL.[94] Genital viral shedding is an independent risk factor for MTCT[95] and can persist despite initiation of ART and despite undetectable maternal viral loads.[96–98] In some studies, HIV was detected in the genital tract of nearly 40% of women with undetectable plasma viral loads.[99,100] Preexposure prophylaxis of the fetus via placental transport of antiviral drugs is thought to be protective against exposure to these genital secretions intrapartum and thereby to reduce HIV transmission. The nucleoside/nucleotide reverse transcriptase inhibitors (NRTIs) abacavir, lamivudine, and emtricitabine have high placental transfer and achieve approximately equal or higher concentrations in cord blood compared with maternal plasma, whereas tenofovir and zidovudine reach levels in cord blood of at least 80% of maternal plasma levels.[101] Thus, all pregnant women should take at least one of this group of NRTIs with high transplacental passage to provide fetal preexposure prophylaxis.[102] Moreover, women should continue their oral ART intrapartum. Among women with unsuppressed viral loads (HIV RNA >1000 copies/mL), retrospective data suggest that intrapartum or precesarean intravenous zidovudine reduces perinatal HIV transmission.[103]

Specific regimens of ART for pregnancy need to meet several other specific criteria.[102] First, they should have demonstrated efficacy in clinical trials. Second, they should have an acceptable safety profile for women, fetuses, and newborns. Third, there should be pregnancy-specific pharmacologic data to guide their use, particularly regarding pharmacokinetic changes in pregnancy and transplacental passage. Viral genotype and resistance patterns; prior antiretroviral drug exposure;

patient compliance; and the convenience, interactions, and side-effect profiles of each regimen are other considerations. Generally, women entering pregnancy on ART with suppression of viremia should continue their current regimen in pregnancy. For drug-naïve women, recommended treatment regimens to initiate in pregnancy consist of a dual NRTI backbone and either a boosted protease inhibitor or an integrase inhibitor. First-line and alternative drugs in each class of medications are listed in **Table 2**. Detailed guidelines for prescribing and managing ART in pregnancy are available from the Department of Health and Human Services.[102] When caring for HIV-infected pregnant women, obstetricians should work collaboratively with infectious disease providers who have extensive clinical experience with selection and use of ARTs.

Teratogenicity and Adverse Obstetric Outcomes Associated with Antiretrovirals

Overall, data support the safety of ART in pregnancy, and the benefits in maternal health and the reduction of perinatal transmission outweigh current safety concerns. There are specific teratogenicity concerns for some of the first-line agents, but data are inconsistent. In addition, some adverse pregnancy outcomes, such as preterm birth or delivering a low-birth-weight (LBW) or small-for-gestational-age (SGA) infant, might be more common among women on ART.

In 2018, preliminary data from a prospective study in Botswana suggested a possible increase in the risk of neural tube defects (NTD) among infants exposed to dolutegravir in utero. In total, 5 neural tube defects were identified among 1683 deliveries (0.30%) to women with periconceptional dolutegravir use, which was higher than the rate of NTDs among infants born to women on other drug regimens (0.10%) or to women without HIV (0.08%).[104] Importantly, food in Botswana is not fortified with folate. Data from countries with routine folate fortification of food do not support a similar association.[53,105,106] At this time, dolutegravir remains a preferred agent for use during pregnancy, but decisions regarding the choice of ART should be a result of shared decision making between a woman and her provider.[102] Other specific

Table 2
Preferred and *alternative* first-line agents for initiation of antiretroviral therapy for human immunodeficiency virusin drug-naïve pregnant women

Drug Class	Drug
Nucleoside reverse transcriptase inhibitor backbones	Abacavir + lamivudine TDF + emtricitabine TDF + lamivudine Zidovudine + lamivudine
Nonnucleoside reverse transcriptase inhibitors	Efavirenz
Integrase strand transfer inhibitors	Raltegravir Dolutegravir
Protease inhibitors	Atazanavir/ritonavir Darunavir/ritonavir Lopinavir/ritonavir

The drug regimen should include a dual NRTI backbone and either an integrase strand transfer inhibitor or a ritonavir-boosted protease inhibitor.

Data from Panel on Treatment of Pregnant Women with HIV Infection and Prevention of Perinatal Transmission. Recommendations for the Use of Antiretroviral Drugs in Pregnant Women with HIV Infection and Interventions to Reduce Perinatal HIV Transmission in the United States. Available at: https://clinicalinfo.hiv.gov/sites/default/files/inline-files/PerinatalGL.pdf. Accessed October 21, 2020.

teratogenicity concerns include a report of a 2.6-fold increased risk of microcephaly among children with in utero efavirenz exposure,[107] an association between raltegravir and all birth defects,[106] an association between atazanavir and musculoskeletal and skin defects,[108] and an association between zidovudine and congenital heart disease.[109,110] This association with zidovudine and cardiac malformations has not been confirmed in other analyses.[111] At present, atazanavir and raltegravir remain preferred medications, and efavirenz and zidovudine are alternative medications for initiation in pregnancy; women who enter pregnancy on these medications should usually continue them.[102]

An important source of data on the safety of antiretroviral medications is the Antiretroviral Pregnancy Registry (APR). The APR is a prospective study of pregnancies exposed to ART and now contains outcome data on more than 21,000 pregnancies between 1989 and 2020. The rate of birth defects among women exposed to ART in the first trimester is 2.8%, which is not significantly different from the rate among women initially exposed later in gestation or from US population-based comparator rates. The APR contains sufficient power to exclude a 1.5- to 2.0-fold increase in the rate of birth defects with first-trimester exposure to many individual ART agents recommended for use in pregnancy.[53] The APR Advisory Committee Consensus states, "In reviewing all reported defects from the prospective registry, informed by clinical studies and retrospective reports of antiretroviral exposure, the Registry finds no apparent increases in frequency of birth defects with first trimester exposures compared to exposures starting later in pregnancy and no pattern to suggest a common cause. While the Registry population exposed and monitored to date is not sufficient to detect an increase in the risk of relatively rare defects, these findings should provide some assurance when counseling patients. However, potential limitations of registries such as this should be recognized. The Registry is ongoing. Because of the data from an observational study in Botswana, the Registry continues to closely monitor cases of neural tube defects with periconception exposures to dolutegravir and other integrase inhibitors. Given the use of new therapies about which data are still insufficient, health care providers are strongly encouraged to report eligible patients to the Registry at SM_APR@APResgistry.com via the data forms available at http://www.APRegistry.com."

Some evidence suggests that ART might be associated with adverse obstetric outcomes, but the data are contradictory and vary by specific drug regimen. For example, although some studies have shown that multiagent ART is associated with increased odds of preterm birth compared with dual- or single-agent therapy[93,112] and that preconception and first-trimester ART exposure slightly increases the risk of preterm birth compared with later initiation,[113] other studies have shown ART might be protective against preterm birth.[114] Longitudinal data from a large American cohort spanning 1989 to 2004 demonstrate that as ART administration to HIV-positive pregnant women increased from 2% to 84%, preterm birth declined from 35% to 22%.[115] Some studies have particularly implicated protease inhibitors in preterm birth.[113,116,117] The effect size varies among studies, ranging from a 1.2- to 3.4-fold increased risk of preterm delivery associated with ART use.[102] Data are similarly conflicting for infant birth weight, with some studies finding an association between ART and LBW/SGA[118–120] and other studies failing to identify such an association.[121–124] Importantly, untreated HIV predisposes women to adverse perinatal outcomes, including preterm birth, LBW/SGA infants, and stillbirth[125]; thus, such adverse outcomes should not be considered an indication to withhold therapy but may prompt enhanced antenatal fetal surveillance. Future research should be geared toward determining which ART regimens have the best risk-benefit profile in pregnancy.

Antiretroviral Therapy in Breastfeeding Women

HIV is transmissible through breastmilk at rates as high 24%.[126] Therefore, in the United States and other high-income countries where safe and nutritious alternatives to maternal breast milk are available (eg, formula, donor breastmilk), avoidance of breastfeeding is the standard of care. In some low-resource settings, particularly where malnutrition and diarrhea are common, alternative feeding strategies are often not safe or feasible, because of either the cost and availability of formula or the lack of clean water with which to constitute the formula. In these settings, infant mortality is lower among breastfed infants,[127] and the risk of HIV transmission through breastmilk is often outweighed by the potential benefits of breastfeeding. The transmission risk for breastfed infants depends on maternal viral load, CD4 cell count, and on the viral load of breast milk[128] and may be as low as 1% to 3%.[129,130] The World Health Organization recommends that health authorities decide on a national or subnational level whether to primarily support breastfeeding and use of ART to reduce transmission through breastmilk or whether to primarily support avoidance of breastfeeding and alternative infant feeding strategies.[131]

SEVERE ACUTE RESPIRATORY SYNDROME CORONAVIRUS 2: AN EMERGING INFECTION

In late 2019 and early 2020, COVID-19 disease, caused by the SARS-CoV-2 virus, emerged as a global pandemic. By October 2020, there were more than 34 million cases and 1 million deaths reported worldwide.[132] Pregnant women are at increased risk of complications from a variety of respiratory infections because of physiologic and immunologic changes of pregnancy. During the 2009 H1N1 influenza pandemic, pregnant women had an increased risk of mortality from the virus.[133,134] Thus, the maternal and fetal/neonatal implications of COVID-19 are of significant interest. Data are still limited on COVID-19 infections in pregnancy, but emerging evidence indicates some reasons for modest concern.

First, pregnant women with COVID-19 appear to be more likely to be hospitalized than nonpregnant women.[135–137] In the United States, data from a cohort of 91,412 reproductive-aged women with COVID-19 found a hospitalization rate of 31.5% among pregnant women and 5.8% among nonpregnant women.[137] Importantly, it is unclear to what extent that increase in hospitalizations is secondary to consequences of COVID-19 illness rather than basic obstetric indications and to what extent there is a bias toward admitting pregnant women for observation. Risk factors for hospitalization during pregnancy include minority race or ethnicity, obesity, and medical morbidities.[135,136,138] Data on intensive care unit (ICU) admission rates and mechanical ventilation rates also suggest that pregnant women are at increased risk for severe disease. In a study of 598 hospitalized pregnant women with COVID-19 in the United States, 16.2% of patients required ICU admission, and 8.5% of patients required mechanical ventilation.[135] After controlling for age, race/ethnicity, and comorbidities, pregnant women with COVID-19 have a 1.5-fold increased risk of ICU admission and a 1.7-fold increased risk of mechanical ventilation compared with nonpregnant women with COVID-19.[137] There are no current data to suggest that pregnant women with COVID-19 have an increased risk of death; maternal outcomes might depend on local medical resources.[139] Maternal COVID-19 has been associated with adverse obstetric outcomes in several studies. Increased rates of preterm birth, cesarean delivery, neonatal ICU admission, and intrauterine fetal demise have been reported.[135,136,140–142] The severity of disease is associated with the magnitude of risk increase for these adverse outcomes.[141] Ongoing data collection and analysis will better delineate the presence and/or extent of pregnancy-specific risks from COVID-19.

A key question regarding the SARS-CoV-2 virus in pregnancy is the potential for MTCT. Both SARS-CoV-2 DNA and anti–SARS-CoV-2 immunoglobulin M antibodies have been detected in umbilical cord blood, and the viral genome has also been detected in term placentas.[143–145] These findings suggest that in utero vertical transmission can occur, but this mechanism is thought to be very rare. The literature is limited to case reports and small case series. It is unknown whether the risk of in utero transmission depends on the severity or timing of maternal infection. Moreover, it is unclear what effect, if any, in utero vertical transmission has on the fetus or neonate. Viral DNA has also been reported in vaginal secretions,[143,146] which raises the possibility of intrapartum transmission of the virus. However, most MTCT of the SARS-CoV-2 virus likely occurs postnatally through exposure to respiratory droplets. This risk seems to be low. In the United Kingdom, 5% of liveborn infants of women with COVID-19 tested positive for the SARS-CoV-2 virus, and half of these infections were detected in the first 12 hours of life.[138] In a cohort of 101 neonates born to women infected with the SARS-CoV-2 virus in New York City, only 2% of neonates tested positive for the virus, and none of those infants had clinical evidence of disease despite rooming-in and breastfeeding.[147] This rate is similar to that reported in a metaanalysis of data from 936 neonates that reported a pooled proportion of 3.2% for vertical transmission.[145] Importantly, most neonates who test positive for the SARS-CoV-2 virus are asymptomatic.[148] These data suggest that infected mothers and infants do not need to be separated, and breastfeeding is likely safe.

At this time, management of severe COVID-19 disease in pregnancy should be similar to management of nonpregnant adults. Maternal stabilization should be the focus of interventions, as fetal well-being depends on maternal status. Dexamethasone reduces mortality in nonpregnant patients requiring respiratory support and likewise should be used in pregnancy when indicated.[149] Preliminary data on compassionate use of remdesivir in 86 pregnant and postpartum women indicate that the medication is well tolerated with high recovery rates.[150] Currently, although investigations into treatments for COVID-19 are in the early stages, and the best therapy for pregnant women is still unknown, obstetric care during this pandemic should focus on preventative measures, such as social distancing, mask-wearing, and hand hygiene. Pregnant women should be counseled about their modestly increased risk of severe illness to reinforce the importance of preventative measures. These same measures should be recommended postpartum to reduce MTCT of the SARS-CoV-2 virus. As the pandemic evolves, better-quality prospective data and RCTs will provide additional insight into therapeutic options for pregnant women.

VACCINATION IN PREGNANCY

A discussion of viral infections in pregnancy would not be complete without attention to the importance of currently recommended vaccines as well as developing immunizations that offer both proof (for approved vaccines) and the promise (for vaccines under development) for prevention of disease in both mothers and their infants. A listing of pregnancy-specific, current vaccine recommendations is included in **Table 3**.

All pregnant women (lacking contraindication) should receive an inactivated influenza vaccine as well as the current tetanus, diphtheria, and pertussis vaccine (Tdap) during each pregnancy.[151,152] Given the proven benefits of influenza and Tdap vaccines for both maternal and neonatal disease prevention, this practice should

Table 3
Recommended, acceptable, and contraindicated vaccines during pregnancy

Universally Recommended	Acceptable if Indicated	Contraindicated
Inactivated influenza	Hepatitis A	Live-attenuated (intranasal) influenza
Tetanus toxoid, diphtheria toxoid, and acellular pertussis (Tdap)	Hepatitis B Inactivated poliovirus	Measles-mumps-rubella (MMR) Live-inactivated (oral) poliovirus
	Meningococcal	Varicella
	Pneumococcal	Smallpox
	Rabies	
	Yellow fever	

Data from Refs.[151,152]

be endorsed by all obstetrics care providers. As the race for a vaccine against SARS-CoV-2 evolves, pregnant women should be included in trials for vaccines that demonstrate promising early safety data. As described, early studies indicate that women are at risk for severe complications of this disease, and maternal vaccination will likely improve maternal outcomes and protect neonates through transplacental antibody transfer.

Importantly, given the time-recognized concept of maternal immunization primarily for neonatal benefit via transplacental transfer of protective maternal antibody, there has been a resurgence of interest in recent years in development of various vaccines that have such promise. Some examples of such vaccines include, but are not limited to respiratory syncytial virus, group B streptococcus (a bacterium), potentially CMV, and Zika virus. The optimal window for use of the latter two is still under deliberation; nevertheless, this renewed interest and active investigation during pregnancy are likely to generate important new advances in this rapidly changing field.

SUMMARY

Practice guidelines have been reviewed as well as recent advances in the treatment of important viral infections impacting pregnancy. For the infections described herein, maternal treatment during pregnancy has as the primary goal prevention of perinatal transmission and its sequelae, in addition to offering improved maternal health. The management of viral infections in pregnancy is a constantly evolving field. Despite the challenges of conducting research during pregnancy, further study is needed to fill in current knowledge gaps and improve medical care for pregnant women and their unborn children.

CLINICS CARE POINTS

- Viral infections in pregnancy should be treated with the standard medications available.
- In many cases treatment improves the health of both the mother and the unborn baby.
- More research of medications in pregnancy will help Obstetrical providers improve the evidence base for therapies.

DISCLOSURE

The authors have nothing to disclose.

REFERENCES

1. McQuillan G, Kruszon-Moran D, Flagg EW, et al. Prevalence of herpes simplex virus type 1 and type 2 in persons aged 14–49: United States, 2015–2016. NCHS data brief, no 304. Hyattsville (MD): National Center for Health Statistics; 2018.
2. Brown ZA, Selke S, Zeh J, et al. The acquisition of herpes simplex virus during pregnancy. N Engl J Med 1997;337(8):509–16.
3. Pasternak B, Hviid A. Use of acyclovir, valacyclovir, and famciclovir in the first trimester of pregnancy and the risk of birth defects. JAMA 2010;304(8):859.
4. Stone KM, Reiff-Eldridge R, White AD, et al. Pregnancy outcomes following systemic prenatal acyclovir exposure: conclusions from the International Acyclovir Pregnancy Registry, 1984-1999. Birth Defects Res A Clin Mol Teratol 2004;70(4): 201–7.
5. Workowski KA, Bolan GA, Centers for Disease Control and Prevention. Sexually transmitted diseases treatment guidelines, 2015. MMWR Recomm Rep 2015; 64(RR-03):1–137.
6. ACOG Committee on Practice Bulletins. ACOG practice bulletin. Clinical management guidelines for obstetrician-gynecologists. No. 82 June 2007. Management of herpes in pregnancy. Obstet Gyecol 2007;109(6):1489–98.
7. Brown ZA, Benedetti J, Ashley R, et al. Neonatal herpes simplex virus infection in relation to asymptomatic maternal infection at the time of labor. N Engl J Med 1991;324(18):1247–52.
8. Sheffield JS, Hollier LM, Hill JB, et al. Acyclovir prophylaxis to prevent herpes simplex virus recurrence at delivery: a systematic review. Obstet Gynecol 2003;102(6):1396–403.
9. Hollier LM, Wendel GD. Third trimester antiviral prophylaxis for preventing maternal genital herpes simplex virus (HSV) recurrences and neonatal infection. Cochrane Database Syst Rev 2008;(1):CD004946.
10. Watts DH, Brown ZA, Money D, et al. A double-blind, randomized, placebo-controlled trial of acyclovir in late pregnancy for the reduction of herpes simplex virus shedding and cesarean delivery. Am J Obstet Gynecol 2003;188(3): 836–43.
11. Pinninti SG, Angara R, Feja KN, et al. Neonatal herpes disease following maternal antenatal antiviral suppressive therapy: a multicenter case series. J Pediatr 2012;161(1):134–8.e3.
12. Leruez-Ville M, Foulon I, Pass R, et al. Cytomegalovirus infection during pregnancy: state of the science. Am J Obstet Gynecol 2020;223(3):330–49.
13. Cannon MJ, Schmid DS, Hyde TB. Review of cytomegalovirus seroprevalence and demographic characteristics associated with infection. Rev Med Virol 2010;20(4):202–13.
14. Bate SL, Dollard SC, Cannon MJ. Cytomegalovirus seroprevalence in the United States: the national health and nutrition examination surveys, 1988-2004. Clin Infect Dis 2010;50(11):1439–47.
15. Hyde TB, Schmid DS, Cannon MJ. Cytomegalovirus seroconversion rates and risk factors: implications for congenital CMV. Rev Med Virol 2010;20(5):311–26.

16. Dollard SC, Grosse SD, Ross DS. New estimates of the prevalence of neurological and sensory sequelae and mortality associated with congenital cytomegalovirus infection. Rev Med Virol 2007;17(5):355–63.

17. Mussi-Pinhata MM, Yamamoto AY, Moura Brito RM, et al. Birth prevalence and natural history of congenital cytomegalovirus infection in a highly seroimmune population. Clin Infect Dis 2009;49(4):522–8.

18. Kenneson A, Cannon MJ. Review and meta-analysis of the epidemiology of congenital cytomegalovirus (CMV) infection. Rev Med Virol 2007;17(4):253–76.

19. Wang C, Zhang X, Bialek S, et al. Attribution of congenital cytomegalovirus infection to primary versus non-primary maternal infection. Clin Infect Dis 2011;52(2):e11–3.

20. Picone O, Vauloup-Fellous C, Cordier AG, et al. A series of 238 cytomegalovirus primary infections during pregnancy: description and outcome. Prenat Diagn 2013;33(8):751–8.

21. Enders G, Daiminger A, Bäder U, et al. Intrauterine transmission and clinical outcome of 248 pregnancies with primary cytomegalovirus infection in relation to gestational age. J Clin Virol 2011;52(3):244–6.

22. Guerra B, Simonazzi G, Puccetti C, et al. Ultrasound prediction of symptomatic congenital cytomegalovirus infection. Am J Obstet Gynecol 2008;198(4): 380.e1-7.

23. Picone O, Teissier N, Cordier AG, et al. Detailed in utero ultrasound description of 30 cases of congenital cytomegalovirus infection. Prenat Diagn 2014;34(6): 518–24.

24. Stagno S, Whitley RJ. Herpesvirus infections of pregnancy. N Engl J Med 1985; 313(20):1270–4.

25. Fowler KB, Stagno S, Pass RF, et al. The outcome of congenital cytomegalovirus infection in relation to maternal antibody status. N Engl J Med 1992;326(10): 663–7.

26. Grosse SD, Ross DS, Dollard SC. Congenital cytomegalovirus (CMV) infection as a cause of permanent bilateral hearing loss: a quantitative assessment. J Clin Virol 2008;41(2):57–62.

27. Nigro G, Adler SP, La Torre R, et al. Passive immunization during pregnancy for congenital cytomegalovirus infection. N Engl J Med 2005;353(13):1350–62.

28. Kagan KO, Enders M, Schampera MS, et al. Prevention of maternal-fetal transmission of CMV by hyperimmunoglobulin (HIG) administered after a primary maternal CMV infection in early gestation. Ultrasound Obstet Gynecol 2019; 53(3):383–9.

29. Visentin S, Manara R, Milanese L, et al. Early primary cytomegalovirus infection in pregnancy: maternal hyperimmunoglobulin therapy improves outcomes among infants at 1 year of age. Clin Infect Dis 2012;55(4):497–503.

30. Nigro G, Adler SP, Parruti G, et al. Immunoglobulin therapy of fetal cytomegalovirus infection occurring in the first half of pregnancy–a case-control study of the outcome in children. J Infect Dis 2012;205(2):215–27.

31. Revello MG, Lazzarotto T, Guerra B, et al. A randomized trial of hyperimmune globulin to prevent congenital cytomegalovirus. N Engl J Med 2014;370(14): 1316–26.

32. Hughes BL. Randomized trial to prevent congenital cytomegalovirus. Am J Obstet Gynecol 2019;221(6):670–1.

33. Saade G. The effect of treatment of maternal CMV infection on the development of placental syndrome. Am J Obstet Gynecol 2020;222(1):S2–3.

34. Jacquemard F, Yamamoto M, Costa J-M, et al. Maternal administration of vala-ciclovir in symptomatic intrauterine cytomegalovirus infection. BJOG 2007; 114(9):1113–21.
35. Leruez-Ville M, Ghout I, Bussières L, et al. In utero treatment of congenital cyto-megalovirus infection with valacyclovir in a multicenter, open-label, phase II study. Am J Obstet Gynecol 2016;215(4):462.e1-e10.
36. Shahar-Nissan K, Pardo J, Peled O, et al. Valaciclovir to prevent vertical trans-mission of cytomegalovirus after maternal primary infection during pregnancy: a randomised, double-blind, placebo-controlled trial. Lancet 2020;396(10253): 779–85.
37. American College of Obstetricians and Gynecologists. ACOG Practice Bulletin No. 151: cytomegalovirus, parvovirus B12, varicella zoster, and toxoplasmosis in pregnancy. Obstet Gynecol 2015;125(6):1510–25.
38. Hughes BL, Gyamfi-Bannerman C, Gyamfi-Bannerman C. Diagnosis and ante-natal management of congenital cytomegalovirus infection. Am J Obstet Gyne-col 2016;214(6):B5–11.
39. Rawlinson WD, Boppana SB, Fowler KB, et al. Congenital cytomegalovirus infection in pregnancy and the neonate: consensus recommendations for pre-vention, diagnosis, and therapy. Lancet Infect Dis 2017;17(6):e177–88.
40. World Health Organization. Global hepatitis report 2017. Geneva (Switzerland): World Health Organization; 2017. Available at: http://www.who.int/hepatitis/publications/global-hepatitis-report2017/en/. Accessed October 19, 2020.
41. Centers for Disease Control and Prevention. Viral hepatitis surveillance – United States, 2018. 2020. Available at: https://www.cdc.gov/hepatitis/statistics/SurveillanceRpts.htm. Accessed October 19, 2020.
42. Dionne-Odom J, Tita ATN, Silverman NS. #38: hepatitis B in pregnancy screening, treatment, and prevention of vertical transmission. Am J Obstet Gy-necol 2016;214(1):6–14.
43. American College of Obstetricians and Gynecologists. ACOG Practice Bulletin no. 86: viral hepatitis in pregnancy. Obstet Gynecol 2007;110(4):941–56.
44. Mast EE, Margolis HS, Fiore AE, et al. A comprehensive immunization strategy to eliminate transmission of hepatitis B virus infection in the United States: rec-ommendations of the Advisory Committee on Immunization Practices (ACIP). Part 1: immunization of infants, children, and adolescents. MMWR Recomm Rep 2005;54(RR-16):1–31.
45. Burk RD, Hwang LY, Ho GY, et al. Outcome of perinatal hepatitis B virus expo-sure is dependent on maternal virus load. J Infect Dis 1994;170(6):1418–23.
46. del Canho R, Grosheide PM, Mazel JA, et al. Ten-year neonatal hepatitis B vaccination program, The Netherlands, 1982-1992: protective efficacy and long-term immunogenicity. Vaccine 1997;15(15):1624–30.
47. Wiseman E, Fraser MA, Holden S, et al. Perinatal transmission of hepatitis B vi-rus: an Australian experience. Med J Aust 2009;190(9):489–92.
48. Lin X, Guo Y, Zhou A, et al. Immunoprophylaxis failure against vertical transmis-sion of hepatitis B virus in the Chinese population. Pediatr Infect Dis J 2014; 33(9):897–903.
49. Kubo A, Shlager L, Marks AR, et al. Prevention of vertical transmission of hep-atitis B. Ann Intern Med 2014;160(12):828.
50. Pan CQ, Duan Z, Bhamidimarri KR, et al. An algorithm for risk assessment and intervention of mother to child transmission of hepatitis B virus. Clin Gastroen-terol Hepatol 2012;10(5):452–9.

51. Zou H, Chen Y, Duan Z, et al. Virologic factors associated with failure to passive-active immunoprophylaxis in infants born to HBsAg-positive mothers. J Viral Hepat 2012;19(2):e18–25.
52. Brown RS, McMahon BJ, Lok ASF, et al. Antiviral therapy in chronic hepatitis B viral infection during pregnancy: a systematic review and meta-analysis. Hepatology 2016;63(1):319–33.
53. Antiretroviral Pregnancy Registry Steering Committee. Antiretroviral pregnancy registry interim report for 1 January 1989 through 31 January 2020. Wilmington (NC): Registry Coordinating Center; 2020. 2017. Available at: www.APRegistry.com. Accessed October 19, 2020.
54. Sarkar M, Brady CW, Fleckenstein J, et al. Reproductive health and liver disease: practice guidance by the American Association for the Study of Liver Diseases. Hepatology 2020. [Epub ahead of print].
55. Pan CQ, Duan Z, Dai E, et al. Tenofovir to prevent hepatitis B transmission in mothers with high viral load. N Engl J Med 2016;374(24):2324–34.
56. Jourdain G, Ngo-Giang-Huong N, Harrison L, et al. Tenofovir versus placebo to prevent perinatal transmission of hepatitis B. N Engl J Med 2018;378(10):911–23.
57. Terrault NA, Feld JJ, Lok ASF. Tenofovir to prevent perinatal transmission of hepatitis B. N Engl J Med 2018;378(24):2348–50.
58. Dusheiko G. A shift in thinking to reduce mother-to-infant transmission of hepatitis B. N Engl J Med 2018;378(10):952–3.
59. Lee D, Shin H-Y, Park SM. Cost-effectiveness of antiviral prophylaxis during pregnancy for the prevention of perinatal hepatitis B infection in South Korea. Cost Eff Resour Alloc 2018;16(1):6.
60. Nayeri UA, Werner EF, Han CS, et al. Antenatal lamivudine to reduce perinatal hepatitis B transmission: a cost-effectiveness analysis. Am J Obstet Gynecol 2012;207(3):231.e1-7.
61. Schillie S, Vellozzi C, Reingold A, et al. Prevention of hepatitis B virus infection in the United States: recommendations of the advisory committee on immunization practices. MMWR Recomm Rep 2018;67(1):1–31.
62. ACOG Immunization and Emerging Infections Expert Work Group. Practice advisory: hepatitis B prevention. 2018. Available at: https://www.acog.org/Clinical-Guidance-and-Publications/Practice-Advisories/Practice-Advisory-Hepatitis-B-Prevention. Accessed October 19, 2020.
63. Schillie S, Wester C, Osborne M, et al. CDC recommendations for hepatitis C screening among adults—United States, 2020. MMWR Recomm Rep 2020;69(2):1–17.
64. Owens DK, Davidson KW, Krist AH, et al. Screening for hepatitis C virus infection in adolescents and adults: US preventive services task force recommendation statement. JAMA 2020;323(10):970–5.
65. Pergam SA, Wang CC, Gardella CM, et al. Pregnancy complications associated with hepatitis C: data from a 2003-2005 Washington State Birth Cohort. Am J Obstet Gynecol 2008;199(1):38.e1-9.
66. Reddick KLB, Jhaveri R, Gandhi M, et al. Pregnancy outcomes associated with viral hepatitis. J Viral Hepat 2011;18(7):e394–8.
67. Huang Q-T, Hang L-L, Zhong M, et al. Maternal HCV infection is associated with intrauterine fetal growth disturbance: a meta-analysis of observational studies. Medicine (Baltimore) 2016;95(35):e4777.
68. Connell LE, Salihu HM, Salemi JL, et al. Maternal hepatitis B and hepatitis C carrier status and perinatal outcomes. Liver Int 2011;31(8):1163–70.

69. Wijarnpreecha K, Thongprayoon C, Sanguankeo A, et al. Hepatitis C infection and intrahepatic cholestasis of pregnancy: a systematic review and meta-analysis. Clin Res Hepatol Gastroenterol 2017;41(1):39–45.

70. Conte D, Fraquelli M, Prati D, et al. Prevalence and clinical course of chronic hepatitis C virus (HCV) infection and rate of HCV vertical transmission in a cohort of 15,250 pregnant women. Hepatology 2000;31(3):751–5.

71. Benova L, Mohamoud YA, Calvert C, et al. Vertical transmission of hepatitis C virus: systematic review and meta-analysis. Clin Infect Dis 2014;59(6):765–73.

72. Resti M, Azzari C, Mannelli F, et al. Mother to child transmission of hepatitis C virus: prospective study of risk factors and timing of infection in children born to women seronegative for HIV-1. Tuscany Study Group on Hepatitis C Virus Infection. BMJ 1998;317(7156):437–41.

73. Zanetti AR, Paccagnini S, Principi N, et al. Mother-to-infant transmission of hepatitis C virus. Lancet 1995;345(8945):289–91.

74. Gibb DM, Goodall RL, Dunn DT, et al. Mother-to-child transmission of hepatitis C virus: evidence for preventable peripartum transmission. Lancet 2000; 356(9233):904–7.

75. Yeung L, King SM, Roberts EA. Mother-to-infant transmission of hepatitis C virus. Hepatology 2001;34(2):223–9.

76. Hughes BL, Page CM, Kuller JA. Hepatitis C in pregnancy: screening, treatment, and management. Am J Obstet Gynecol 2017;217(5):B2–12.

77. AASLD-IDSA. Recommendations for testing, managing, and treating hepatitis C. Available at: www.hcvguidelines.org. Accessed October 19, 2020.

78. World Health Organization. Guidelines for the care and treatment of persons diagnosed with chronic hepatitis C infection. Geneva (Switzerland); 2018. Available at: http://www.who.int/hepatitis/publications/hepatitis-c-guidelines-2018/en/. Accessed October 19, 2020.

79. Jazwinski AB, Muir AJ. Direct-acting antiviral medications for chronic hepatitis C virus infection. Gastroenterol Hepatol (N Y) 2011;7(3):154–62.

80. El-Sayed MH, Elakel W, Elsharkawy A, et al. THU-137-DAA therapy in women of child bearing age: accidental conception during therapy and pregnancy outcome. J Hepatol 2019;70(1):e221.

81. Chappell CA, Scarsi KK, Kirby BJ, et al. Ledipasvir plus sofosbuvir in pregnant women with hepatitis C virus infection: a phase 1 pharmacokinetic study. Lancet Microbe 2020;1(5):e200–8.

82. Barritt AS, Jhaveri R. Treatment of hepatitis C during pregnancy-weighing the risks and benefits in contrast to HIV. Curr HIV/AIDS Rep 2018;15(2):155–61.

83. Centers for Disease Control and Prevention. HIV surveillance report, 2018 (Updated); vol. 31. Available at: http://www.cdc.gov/hiv/libraryreports/hiv-surveillance.html. Accessed October 21, 2020.

84. Nesheim SR, FitzHarris LF, Lampe MA, et al. Reconsidering the number of women with HIV infection who give birth annually in the United States. Public Health Rep 2018;133(6):637–43.

85. Centers for Disease Control and Prevention. Monitoring selected national HIV prevention and care objectives by using HIV surveillance data—United States and 6 dependent areas, 2018. HIV Surveillance Supplemental Report 2020;25(No. 2). Available at: http://www.cdc.gov/hiv/library/reports/hiv-surveillance.html. Accessed October 21, 2020.

86. Peters H, Francis K, Sconza R, et al. UK mother-to-child HIV transmission rates continue to decline: 2012-2014. Clin Infect Dis 2017;64(4):527–8.

87. Townsend CL, Byrne L, Cortina-Borja M, et al. Earlier initiation of ART and further decline in mother-to-child HIV transmission rates, 2000-2011. AIDS 2014;28(7): 1049–57.

88. Cooper ER, Charurat M, Mofenson L, et al. Combination antiretroviral strategies for the treatment of pregnant HIV-1-infected women and prevention of perinatal HIV-1 transmission. J Acquir Immune Defic Syndr 2002;29(5):484–94.

89. Mofenson LM, Lambert JS, Stiehm ER, et al. Risk factors for perinatal transmission of human immunodeficiency virus type 1 in women treated with zidovudine. N Engl J Med 1999;341(6):385–93.

90. Mandelbrot L, Tubiana R, Le Chenadec J, et al. No perinatal HIV-1 transmission from women with effective antiretroviral therapy starting before conception. Clin Infect Dis 2015;61(11):civ578.

91. Hoffman RM, Black V, Technau K, et al. Effects of highly active antiretroviral therapy duration and regimen on risk for mother-to-child transmission of HIV in Johannesburg, South Africa. J Acquir Immune Defic Syndr 2010;54(1):35–41.

92. Siegfried N, van der Merwe L, Brocklehurst P, et al. Antiretrovirals for reducing the risk of mother-to-child transmission of HIV infection. Cochrane Database Syst Rev 2011;(7):CD003510.

93. Fowler MG, Qin M, Fiscus SA, et al. Benefits and risks of antiretroviral therapy for perinatal HIV prevention. N Engl J Med 2016;375(18):1726–37.

94. Tubiana R, Le Chenadec J, Rouzioux C, et al. Factors associated with mother-to-child transmission of HIV-1 despite a maternal viral load <500 copies/mL at delivery: a case-control study nested in the French Perinatal Cohort (EPF-ANRS CO1). Clin Infect Dis 2010;50(4):585–96.

95. John GC, Nduati RW, Mbori-Ngacha DA, et al. Correlates of mother-to-child human immunodeficiency virus type 1 (HIV-1) transmission: association with maternal plasma HIV-1 RNA load, genital HIV-1 DNA shedding, and breast infections. J Infect Dis 2001;183(2):206–12.

96. Graham SM, Holte SE, Peshu NM, et al. Initiation of antiretroviral therapy leads to a rapid decline in cervical and vaginal HIV-1 shedding. AIDS 2007;21(4):501–7.

97. Fiore JR, Suligoi B, Saracino A, et al. Correlates of HIV-1 shedding in cervicovaginal secretions and effects of antiretroviral therapies. AIDS 2003;17(15): 2169–76.

98. King CC, Ellington SR, Davis NL, et al. Prevalence, magnitude, and correlates of HIV-1 genital shedding in women on antiretroviral therapy. J Infect Dis 2017; 216(12):1534–40.

99. Cu-Uvin S, DeLong AK, Venkatesh KK, et al. Genital tract HIV-1 RNA shedding among women with below detectable plasma viral load. AIDS 2010;24(16): 2489–97.

100. Launay O, Tod M, Tschöpe I, et al. Residual HIV-1 RNA and HIV-1 DNA production in the genital tract reservoir of women treated with HAART: the prospective ANRS EP24 GYNODYN study. Antivir Ther 2011;16(6):843–52.

101. McCormack SA, Best BM. Protecting the fetus against HIV infection: a systematic review of placental transfer of antiretrovirals. Clin Pharmacokinet 2014; 53(11):989–1004.

102. Panel on Treatment of Pregnant Women with HIV Infection and Prevention of Perinatal Transmission. Recommendations for the use of antiretroviral drugs in pregnant women with HIV infection and interventions to reduce perinatal HIV transmission in the United States. Available at: https://clinicalinfo.hiv.gov/sites/default/files/inline-files/PerinatalGL.pdf. Accessed October 21, 2020.

103. Briand N, Warszawski J, Mandelbrot L, et al. Is intrapartum intravenous zidovudine for prevention of mother-to-child HIV-1 transmission still useful in the combination antiretroviral therapy era? Clin Infect Dis 2013;57(6):903–14.

104. Zash R, Holmes L, Diseko M, et al. Neural-tube defects and antiretroviral treatment regimens in Botswana. N Engl J Med 2019;381(9):827–40.

105. Pereira G, Kim A, Jalil E, et al. No occurrences of neural tube defects among 382 women on dolutegravir at pregnancy conception in Brazil. Presented at: International AIDS Society Conference. July 21-24, 2019 Mexico City, Mexico.

106. Sibiude J, Le Chenadec J, Mandelbrot L, et al. Risk of birth defects and perinatal outcomes in HIV-infected women exposed to integrase strand inhibitors during pregnancy. AIDS 2020. [Epub ahead of print].

107. Williams PL, Yildirim C, Chadwick EG, et al. Association of maternal antiretroviral use with microcephaly in children who are HIV-exposed but uninfected (SMARTT): a prospective cohort study. Lancet HIV 2020;7(1):e49–58.

108. Williams PL, Crain MJ, Yildirim C, et al. Congenital anomalies and in utero antiretroviral exposure in human immunodeficiency virus-exposed uninfected infants. JAMA Pediatr 2015;169(1):48–55.

109. Sibiude J, Mandelbrot L, Blanche S, et al. Association between prenatal exposure to antiretroviral therapy and birth defects: an analysis of the French Perinatal Cohort Study (ANRS CO1/CO11). PLoS Med 2014;11(4):e1001635.

110. Sibiude J, Le Chenadec J, Bonnet D, et al. In utero exposure to zidovudine and heart anomalies in the ANRS French Perinatal Cohort and the nested PRIMEVA randomized trial. Clin Infect Dis 2015;61(2):270–80.

111. Rough K, Sun JW, Seage GR, et al. Zidovudine use in pregnancy and congenital malformations. AIDS 2017;31(12):1733–43.

112. Townsend C, Schulte J, Thorne C, et al. Antiretroviral therapy and preterm delivery-a pooled analysis of data from the United States and Europe. BJOG 2010;117(11):1399–410.

113. Kourtis AP, Schmid CH, Jamieson DJ, et al. Use of antiretroviral therapy in pregnant HIV-infected women and the risk of premature delivery: a meta-analysis. AIDS 2007;21(5):607–15.

114. Chagomerana MB, Miller WC, Pence BW, et al. PMTCT option B+ does not increase preterm birth risk and may prevent extreme prematurity: a retrospective cohort study in Malawi. J Acquir Immune Defic Syndr 2017;74(4):367–74.

115. Schulte J, Dominguez K, Sukalac T, et al, Pediatric Spectrum of HIV Disease Consortium. Declines in low birth weight and preterm birth among infants who were born to HIV-infected women during an era of increased use of maternal antiretroviral drugs: pediatric spectrum of HIV disease, 1989-2004. Pediatrics 2007;119(4):e900–6.

116. Mesfin YM, Kibret KT, Taye A. Is protease inhibitors based antiretroviral therapy during pregnancy associated with an increased risk of preterm birth? Systematic review and a meta-analysis. Reprod Health 2016;13(1):30.

117. Favarato G, Townsend CL, Bailey H, et al. Protease inhibitors and preterm delivery: another piece in the puzzle. AIDS 2018;32(2):243–52.

118. Ekouevi DK, Coffie PA, Becquet R, et al. Antiretroviral therapy in pregnant women with advanced HIV disease and pregnancy outcomes in Abidjan, Côte d'Ivoire. AIDS 2008;22(14):1815–20.

119. Njom Nlend AE, Nga Motazé A, Moyo Tetang S, et al. Preterm birth and low birth weight after in utero exposure to antiretrovirals initiated during pregnancy in Yaoundé, Cameroon. PLoS One 2016;11(3):e0150565.

120. Wang L, Zhao H, Cai W, et al. Risk factors associated with preterm delivery and low delivery weight among HIV-exposed neonates in China. Int J Gynaecol Obstet 2018;142(3):300–7.
121. Cotter AM, Garcia AG, Duthely ML, et al. Is antiretroviral therapy during pregnancy associated with an increased risk of preterm delivery, low birth weight, or stillbirth? J Infect Dis 2006;193(9):1195–201.
122. Briand N, Mandelbrot L, Le Chenadec J, et al. No relation between in-utero exposure to HAART and intrauterine growth retardation. AIDS 2009;23(10): 1235–43.
123. Tuomala RE, Shapiro DE, Mofenson LM, et al. Antiretroviral therapy during pregnancy and the risk of an adverse outcome. N Engl J Med 2002;346(24): 1863–70.
124. Szyld EG, Warley EM, Freimanis L, et al. Maternal antiretroviral drugs during pregnancy and infant low birth weight and preterm birth. AIDS 2006;20(18): 2345–53.
125. Wedi COO, Kirtley S, Hopewell S, et al. Perinatal outcomes associated with maternal HIV infection: a systematic review and meta-analysis. Lancet HIV 2016;3(1):e33–48.
126. Read DJS. Late postnatal transmission of HIV-1 in breast-fed children: an individual patient data meta-analysis. J Infect Dis 2004;189(12):2154–66.
127. Arikawa S, Rollins N, Jourdain G, et al. Contribution of maternal antiretroviral therapy and breastfeeding to 24-month survival in human immunodeficiency virus-exposed uninfected children: an individual pooled analysis of African and Asian studies. Clin Infect Dis 2018;66(11):1668–77.
128. Rousseau CM, Nduati RW, Richardson BA, et al. Longitudinal analysis of human immunodeficiency virus type 1 RNA in breast milk and of its relationship to infant infection and maternal disease. J Infect Dis 2003;187(5):741–7.
129. Shapiro RL, Hughes MD, Ogwu A, et al. Antiretroviral regimens in pregnancy and breast-feeding in Botswana. N Engl J Med 2010;362(24):2282–94.
130. Marazzi MC, Nielsen-Saines K, Buonomo E, et al. Increased infant human immunodeficiency virus-type one free survival at one year of age in sub-Saharan Africa with maternal use of highly active antiretroviral therapy during breast-feeding. Pediatr Infect Dis J 2009;28(6):483–7.
131. World Health Organization. Consolidated guidelines on the use of antiretroviral drugs for treating and preventing HIV infection: recommendations for a public health approach. Geneva (Switzerland): World Health Organization; 2016. Available at: http://www.who.int/hiv/pub/arv/arv-2016/en/. Accessed October 27, 2020.
132. Dong E, Du H, Gardner L. An interactive web-based dashboard to track COVID-19 in real time. Lancet Infect Dis 2020;20(5):533–4.
133. Siston AM, Rasmussen SA, Honein MA, et al. Pandemic 2009 influenza A(H1N1) virus illness among pregnant women in the United States. JAMA 2010;303(15): 1517–25.
134. Mosby LG, Rasmussen SA, Jamieson DJ. 2009 pandemic influenza A (H1N1) in pregnancy: a systematic review of the literature. Am J Obstet Gynecol 2011; 205(1):10–8.
135. Delahoy MJ, Whitaker M, Chai SJ, et al. Characteristics and maternal and birth outcomes of hospitalized pregnant women with laboratory-confirmed COVID-19–COVID-NET, 13 states, March 1-August 22, 2020. MMWR Morb Mortal Wkly Rep 2020;69(38):1347–54.

136. Panagiotakopoulos L, Myers TR, Gee J, et al. SARS-CoV-2 infection among hospitalized pregnant women: reasons for admission and pregnancy characteristics—eight U.S. Health Care Centers, March 1–May 30, 2020. MMWR Morb Mortal Wkly Rep 2020;69(38):1355–9.

137. Ellington S, Strid P, Tong VT, et al. Characteristics of women of reproductive age with laboratory-confirmed SARS-CoV-2 infection by pregnancy status—United States, January 22–June 7, 2020. MMWR Morb Mortal Wkly Rep 2020;69(25): 769–75.

138. Knight M, Bunch K, Vousden N, et al. Characteristics and outcomes of pregnant women admitted to hospital with confirmed SARS-CoV-2 infection in UK: national population based cohort study. BMJ 2020;369:m2107.

139. Amorim MMR, Soligo Takemoto ML, da Fonseca EB. Maternal deaths with coronavirus disease 2019: a different outcome from low- to middle-resource countries? Am J Obstet Gynecol 2020;223(2):298–9.

140. Huntley BJF, Huntley ES, Di Mascio D, et al. Rates of maternal and perinatal mortality and vertical transmission in pregnancies complicated by severe acute respiratory syndrome coronavirus 2 (SARS-Co-V-2) infection: a systematic review. Obstet Gynecol 2020;136(2):303–12.

141. Khoury R, Bernstein PS, Debolt C, et al. Characteristics and outcomes of 241 births to women with severe acute respiratory syndrome coronavirus 2 (SARS-CoV-2) infection at five New York City medical centers. Obstet Gynecol 2020; 136(2):273–82.

142. Juan J, Gil MM, Rong Z, et al. Effect of coronavirus disease 2019 (COVID-19) on maternal, perinatal and neonatal outcome: systematic review. Ultrasound Obstet Gynecol 2020;56(1):15–27.

143. Fenizia C, Biasin M, Cetin I, et al. Analysis of SARS-CoV-2 vertical transmission during pregnancy. Nat Commun 2020;11(1):5128.

144. Vivanti AJ, Vauloup-Fellous C, Prevot S, et al. Transplacental transmission of SARS-CoV-2 infection. Nat Commun 2020;11(1):3572.

145. Kotlyar AM, Grechukhina O, Chen A, et al. Vertical transmission of coronavirus disease 2019: a systematic review and meta-analysis. Am J Obstet Gynecol 2020. S0002-9378(20)30823-1.

146. Schwartz A, Yogev Y, Zilberman A, et al. Detection of SARS-CoV-2 in vaginal swabs of women with acute SARS-CoV-2 infection: a prospective study. BJOG 2020. 1471-0528.16556.

147. Dumitriu D, Emeruwa UN, Hanft E, et al. Outcomes of neonates born to mothers with severe acute respiratory syndrome coronavirus 2 infection at a large medical center in New York City. JAMA Pediatr 2020;e204298.

148. Kyle MH, Glassman ME, Khan A, et al. A review of newborn outcomes during the COVID-19 pandemic. Semin Perinatol 2020;151286.

149. Baroutjian A, Sanchez C, Boneva D, et al. SARS-CoV-2 pharmacologic therapies and their safety/effectiveness according to level of evidence. Am J Emerg Med 2020;38(11):2405–15.

150. RM B, SY, KE S, et al. OUP accepted manuscript. Clin Infect Dis 2020. https://doi.org/10.1093/cid/ciaa1466.

151. ACOG Committee Opinion No. 741. Obstet Gynecol 2018;131(6):e214–7.

152. Kroger AT, Duchin J, Vazquez M. Special situations. General best practice guidelines for immunization: best practices guidance of the advisory committee on immunization practices (ACIP). Available at: http://www.cdc.gov/vaccines/hcp/acip-recs/general-recs/special-situations.html. Accessed October 27, 2020.

Stroke in Pregnancy
A Multidisciplinary Approach

Erica C. Camargo, MD, MMSc, PhD, Aneesh B. Singhal, MD*

KEYWORDS

- Ischemic stroke • Hemorrhagic stroke • Pregnancy
- Hypertensive disorders of pregnancy

KEY POINTS

- Pregnancy and puerperium confer a substantially increased risk of ischemic and hemorrhagic stroke. The period of highest risk is from the third trimester until 6 weeks postpartum.
- Hemorrhagic stroke is the most common type of obstetric stroke. Common etiologies include eclampsia, reversible cerebral vasoconstriction syndrome, and rupture of arteriovenous malformations and cerebral aneurysms.
- Common risk factors for pregnancy-associated stroke include older age, African American race, congenital and acquired heart disease, preeclampsia, eclampsia, infection, diabetes, and cesarean delivery.
- Conditions associated with ischemic stroke in pregnancy include peripartum cardiomyopathy, posterior reversible encephalopathy, reversible cerebral vasoconstriction syndrome, cerebral venous sinus thrombosis, paradoxic cardioembolism across a patent foramen ovale, and cervical arterial dissection.
- Acute ischemic stroke therapies seem to be safe during pregnancy and should not be withheld.

INTRODUCTION
Incidence, Prevalence, and Temporal Trends

Pregnancy and the puerperium confer an increased risk for ischemic as well as hemorrhagic stroke, with incidence rates being 3-fold higher as compared with nonpregnant women. A meta-analysis of the epidemiologic characteristics and risk factors for stroke in pregnancy found that the mean age ranged from 22 to 33 years, and the crude incidence rate was 30 in 100,000 (95% confidence interval [CI], 18.8–49.4 in 100,000), which was nearly 3 times that of nonpregnant women of childbearing age suffering a stroke.[1] The rate of ischemic and hemorrhagic stroke was 12.2 in 100,000 pregnancies, whereas for cerebral venous sinus thrombosis (CVST) the rate

Department of Neurology, Massachusetts General Hospital, Harvard Medical School, 55 Fruit Street, WACC 729-C, Boston, MA 02114, USA
* Corresponding author.
E-mail address: asinghal@partners.org

Obstet Gynecol Clin N Am 48 (2021) 75–96
https://doi.org/10.1016/j.ogc.2020.11.004
0889-8545/21/© 2020 Elsevier Inc. All rights reserved.
obgyn.theclinics.com

was 9.1 in 100,000 pregnancies. In this meta-analysis, the rates of pregnancy-associated stroke remained unchanged from 1990 to 2017.[1] Subsequently, using hospital discharge data from the US Nationwide Inpatient Sample, Kuklina and colleagues[2] reported that the rate of stroke from 1994 to 1995 to 2006 to 2007 increased by 47% for antenatal stroke and by 83% for postnatal strokes. Changes in the prevalence of hypertensive disorders of pregnancy (HDP) and heart disease from 1994 to 1995 to 2006 to 2007 explained almost all the increase in postpartum hospitalizations. Such changes in the incidence of stroke were not replicated in other studies[2]; Furthermore, a more recent study of data from the US National Inpatient Sample reported a decrease in the incidence of stroke during the delivery period from 10 in 100,000 to 6 in 100,000 deliveries from 2004 to 2014, despite an increase in the prevalence of HDP from 8.4% to 10.9% during that timeframe.[3]

Timing

The rate of prepartum and peripartum stroke is 18.3 in 100,000 pregnancies, whereas for postpartum stroke the rate is 14.7 in 100,000. Given the short duration of the postpartum period, the daily rate of stroke is higher in the postpartum as compared with prepartum or peripartum periods.[1] Concordantly, a recent study has shown that the majority of readmissions for postpartum stroke occur in the first 10 days after hospital discharge.[4] Different rates have been reported in England: 10.7 in 100,000 person-years, antepartum, but 9-fold higher in the peripartum period (161.1 in 100,000 person-years) and 3-fold higher in the early postpartum period (47.1 in 100,000 person-years).[5] It is postulated that these differences could be due to variances in access to obstetric care between the United States and England. The postpartum period with highest risk for thrombotic events is the first 6 weeks. Although the period of 7 to 12 weeks postpartum also has an increased, albeit lower, risk of thrombotic events compared with weeks 0 to 6, there is no significant increase in stroke risk.[6]

Hemorrhage rates in pregnancy are also significantly higher during the third trimester (2.9 in 100,000 pregnancies) and in the first 12 weeks postpartum (4.4 in 100,000).[7]

RISK FACTORS
Patient Characteristics

A study of the Nationwide Inpatient Sample showed that the absolute risk of stroke increased with age: compared with patients less than 20 years of age, those age 35 to 39 years had an odds ratio (OR) for stroke of 2.0 (95% CI, 1.4–2.7; $P<.01$), and those 40 years and older had an OR of 3.1 (95% CI, 2–4.6).[8] This finding was confirmed in a later study of the Nationwide Inpatient Sample, which showed a substantially higher risk of acute stroke during pregnancy and the puerperium for women 45 years of age and older.[9] Interestingly, 1 study found that younger women, but not older women, had an increased stroke risk during pregnancy and the postpartum state.[10] Pregnancy at older age may, however, have negative implications for cerebrovascular health later in life. The risk of stroke in relation to age of prior pregnancy and delivery was analyzed in women aged 59 to 70 years from the observational cohort of the Women's Health Study. Older age at delivery (age $\geq$40 years) was associated with a small but significant increased risk of hemorrhagic stroke in multivariate analyses (OR, 1.5; 95% CI, 1.0–2.1) compared with women less than 40 years of age at delivery. Compared with younger women at the time of delivery, women 40 years and older at delivery had a higher mean systolic blood pressure and higher rates of diabetes mellitus, heart failure, atrial fibrillation, and any alcohol use later in life.[11]

Data from the Nationwide Inpatient Sample also showed that race/ethnicity influences the incidence of pregnancy-associated stroke: African American women have a higher risk of stroke than White women (OR, 1.5; 95% CI, 1.2–1.9) and Hispanic women.[8] Additionally, minority women (Black, Hispanic, Asian/Pacific Islander) with chronic hypertension and pregnancy-induced hypertension are at substantially higher risk of stroke during delivery admissions compared with White women with the same conditions.[12]

Medical Risk Factors

The presence of vascular risk factors at the time of pregnancy contribute to the risk of stroke. Medical conditions that are strongly associated with stroke include migraine (OR, 16.9; 95% CI, 9.7–29.5), thrombophilia (OR, 16.0; 95% CI, 9.4–27.2), systemic lupus erythematosus (OR, 15.2; 95% CI, 7.4–31.2), heart disease (OR, 13.2; 95% CI, 10.2–17.0), sickle cell disease (OR, 9.1; 95% CI, 3.7–22.2), hypertension (OR, 6.1; 95% CI, 4.5–8.1), thrombocytopenia (OR, 6.0; 95% CI, 1.5–24.1), and diabetes (OR, 2.5; 95% CI, 1.3–4.6). Migraine-associated stroke in pregnancy may be mediated by HDP.[13] Additionally, pregnancy-associated complications such as transfusion, postpartum infections, and any type of infection at the time of delivery admission, especially genitourinary infections and sepsis, are strong predictors of pregnancy-associated stroke.[8,14] Infection during the delivery admission was shown to be a risk factor for stroke readmission at a median of 6.7 days. This relationship was significant for readmissions owing to postpartum ischemic stroke, but not for hemorrhagic stroke.[15] A longer length of stay during the delivery hospitalization, a potential marker of increased morbidity, is an independent risk factor for maternal stroke.[4] Furthermore, smoking is highly prevalent in women who suffer strokes during pregnancy and is also an independent risk factor for maternal stroke.[4,16] Other pregnancy-specific causes, such as peripartum cardiomyopathy, choriocarcinoma, and embolization of amniotic fluid or air, are rare. It is postulated that ischemic strokes secondary to transcardiac embolism through a patent foramen ovale may occur during pregnancy because of the higher rates pregnancy-associated venous thrombosis. However, a review article showed only a small number of such cases, most of which occurred in the first and second trimesters of pregnancy.[17]

For hemorrhagic stroke during pregnancy or the puerperium, aneurysms, AVMs, HDP, advanced maternal age, Black race, coagulopathy, and smoking are the most important risk factors.[1,7] Furthermore, chronic hypertension or pregnancy-induced hypertension strongly modify the effect of race and ethnicity on the risk of hemorrhagic stroke: minority women (Black, Hispanic, or Asian/Pacific Islander) with these conditions are at substantially higher risk of hemorrhagic stroke compared with White women.[12]

Assisted Reproductive Therapies

Conflicting data have been reported regarding the risk of cardiovascular disease and stroke after hormonally assisted reproductive therapies. A meta-analysis involving 30,477 women who received fertility therapy and 1,296,734 women who did not, who were respectively followed for a median of 9.7 and 8.6 years, showed a trend toward an increased risk of stroke or transient ischemic attack in women after ovulation induction compared with women who did not receive fertility therapy (hazard ratio, 1.25; 95% CI, 0.96–1.63; $I^2 = 0\%$). It is noteworthy that the patients included in the studies were relatively young, with mean age of 28.5 to 34.0 years at the time of delivery, which could have biased the results toward a more favorable outcome.[18]

A prospective cohort study analyzed the risk of cardiovascular disease after failed assisted reproductive therapy (defined as women who did not give birth 1 year after their last cycle of assisted reproductive therapy) in 28,442 women who received fertility therapy, after a median of 8.4 years of follow-up. A total of 67% failed reproductive therapy and had a 21% increased annual risk of cardiovascular disease (95% CI, 13%–30%), an increased risk of ischemic stroke (adjusted relative rate ratio, 1.33; 95% CI, 1.22–1.46) but not hemorrhagic stroke (adjusted relative rate ratio, 0.88; 95% CI, 0.80–0.96).[19]

The mechanisms by which assisted reproduction increases the risk of cardiovascular disease are not fully understood. It is postulated that ovarian hyperstimulation activates the renin–angiotensin system, thus modifying sodium balance, blood pressure regulation, and promoting fluid shifts with intravascular volume depletion, leading to hypercoagulability.

Cesarean Delivery

In a study of data from the Healthcare Cost and Utilization Project from 1993 and 1994, risk factors for peripartum stroke and venous sinus thrombosis were assessed among 1,408,015 sampled deliveries. In that study, the risk of peripartum stroke was 34.3 in 100,000 births for women who had a cesarean birth, compared with risk of 7.1 in 100,000 births for vaginal delivery (P<.001). The risk of intracranial venous thrombosis was also increased for cesarean delivery: 26.6 in 100,000 births for cesarean birth versus 7.4 in 100,000 births for vaginal delivery (P<.001).[20] Similar findings were observed in a population-based study from Taiwan, in which the increased risk of postpartum stroke in women undergoing cesarean delivery compared with vaginal delivery persisted up to 12 months postpartum.[21] The possibility of cesarean section being a consequence of pregnancies complicated by HDP, for which the risk of stroke is higher owing to hypertension, or owing to the actual occurrence of a cerebrovascular event is a potential confounder. However, surgery itself promotes increased risk of clotting through various mechanisms, which may account for the increased stroke risk.[20]

PATHOPHYSIOLOGY OF PREGNANCY-ASSOCIATED STROKE
Hemodynamic Changes

During pregnancy, there is high metabolic demand. To account for this need, cardiovascular changes occur to allow the maternal circulation to meet new physiologic requirements. One of the initial changes is an increase in the plasmatic volume beginning early in the first trimester, secondary to an increase in renin activity as stimulated by estrogen and other circulating hormones. There is also a development of mild hemodilutional anemia and substantial increases in the heart rate and cardiac output, with an increase of up to 45% above the nonpregnancy state by 24 weeks, and even further during labor and birth.[22,23]

Systemic vascular resistance decreases in early gestation. With this, the blood pressure decreases as well, with a nadir around 20 to 32 weeks. This change promotes relative venous stasis, heightened by vena cava compression in the supine position by the progressively growing uterus, and decreased physical activity during late pregnancy and the puerperium. Therefore, the combination of hypervolemia, increased circulatory demand, decreased blood pressure, and increased venous stasis predisposes women to circulatory complications. These changes persist until 6 to 12 weeks postpartum.

Vascular and Connective Tissue Changes

Pregnancy causes remodeling of the heart and blood vessels, with increased vascular distensibility in the first trimester. In late pregnancy, however, there is a loss of distensibility owing to a decrease in collagen and elastin content in the systemic arterial walls, which persists for months after delivery.[24] It is not clear how these vascular changes promote the development of stroke. However, it is postulated that these somewhat vulnerable vessel walls could be subject to greater hemodynamic stress in the setting of increased blood volume and cardiac output during pregnancy and delivery, and hence susceptible to rupture and a resultant hemorrhagic stroke.[16,23] Recent studies indicate that the reversible cerebral vasoconstriction syndrome (RCVS) is the most frequent cause of pregnancy-associated stroke.

Changes in the Coagulation System

Gestation is a hypercoagulable state, with a 4- to 10-fold increased risk of thrombosis during pregnancy and puerperium. The increased hypercoagulability is in part due to elevations of procoagulant factors VII, IX, X, XII, and XIII; fibrinogen; and von Willebrand factor. Further, physiologic anticoagulation is partly impaired by reductions in protein S activity, decrease in antithrombin III levels (with a nadir in the third trimester), and the development of acquired activated protein C resistance in the second and third trimesters in one-third of pregnant women. Fibrinolysis is also reduced because of increases in serum plasminogen activator inhibitor type 1 and placental-derived plasminogen activator inhibitor type 2. Iron deficiency also contributes to a procoagulant state. All of these factors, combined with venous stasis, congestion, and compression of the inferior vena cava and aorta by the pregnant uterus, promote an enhanced hypercoagulable state predominantly in the third trimester and puerperium. Further contributing to the risk of thrombosis in the puerperium is the acute phase response to surgical trauma and hemorrhage of delivery.[16,23,25]

PATHOLOGIC CONDITIONS, CONDITION-SPECIFIC MANAGEMENT, AND OUTCOMES
Hypertensive Disorders of Pregnancy

HDP are a group of conditions occurring in pregnancy and puerperium with a common background of hypertension, defined as a blood pressure of 140/90 mm Hg or higher. Included in this group are gestational hypertension, preeclampsia, severe preeclampsia (eclampsia and hemolysis elevated liver enzymes and low platelets syndrome), and chronic hypertension with superimposed preeclampsia. HDP are of clinical relevance given their prevalence and the strong risk of cardiovascular disease and stroke during pregnancy and the puerperium as well as later in life, with the associated increased risk of cardiovascular mortality.[26–30] Preeclampsia is associated with a 2- to 4-fold increase in future incident heart failure and a 2-fold increased risk in coronary heart disease, stroke, and cardiovascular death.[28,29] HDP lead to a loss of women's premenopausal cardiovascular advantage, and cardiovascular disease may occur as early as the first year after a first preeclamptic pregnancy, and up to a decade earlier than expected for HDP. Owing to these important findings, HDP should be considered as a risk factor for future cardiovascular disease and should prompt earlier screening for such conditions.[29]

The prevalence of HDP, gestational hypertension, and preeclampsia is 5.2% to 8.2%, 1.8% to 4.4%, and 0.2% to 9.2%, respectively. HDP is more common in developing countries, although its prevalence has increased substantially in the United States in the past 20 years.[31,32] HDP is also more common in African Americans.[31]

Modifiable risk factors for HDP include increased body mass index, anemia, and lower education. Nonmodifiable risk factors for HDP include older and younger age (age of >35 years and < 20 years, respectively), primiparity and multiparity, previous

HDP, gestational diabetes mellitus, preexisting hypertension, preexisting type 2 diabetes mellitus, preexisting urinary tract infection, and a family history of hypertension, type 2 diabetes mellitus, and preeclampsia.[31] Additionally, coagulopathies and underlying prothrombotic conditions also increase the risk of pregnancy-associated stroke in women with preeclampsia.[33]

HDP are associated with 26% of maternal deaths in Latin America and the Caribbean and 16% of maternal deaths in developing countries. HDP also account for 10% of preterm births, and 1 in 50 stillbirths.[34]

HDP are associated with a 1.7- to 5.2-fold increase in the risk of stroke. Furthermore, preeclampsia occurs in 21% to 47% of pregnancy-associated strokes.[8,35] Importantly, the rate of stroke associated with HDP increased 103% in the United States between 1994/1995 and 2010/2011.[30]

Hypertension in pregnancy may predate the gestation or may be diagnosed de novo during pregnancy.

De novo hypertension

1. Gestational hypertension is diagnosed when hypertension develops in a woman at 20 weeks gestation or thereafter, in the absence of proteinuria or other metabolic abnormalities.[36] It may be mild, when the blood pressure ranges from 140 to 149/90 to 99 mm Hg; moderate when the blood pressure is 150 to 159/100 to 109 mm Hg; and severe when the blood pressure is 160/110 mm Hg or higher. Gestational hypertension is usually a relatively benign condition. However, 25% of women with gestational hypertension may develop preeclampsia, and those that have gestational hypertension before 34 weeks of gestation are at greatest risk.

2. Preeclampsia is a multisystem disorder of mid to late pregnancy diagnosed by the presence of de novo hypertension after 20 weeks gestation accompanied by proteinuria ($\geq$300 mg protein/24 h urine) or evidence of maternal acute kidney injury, liver dysfunction, neurologic changes (encephalopathy, seizures), hemolysis or thrombocytopenia, or fetal growth restriction. Preeclampsia may occur intrapartum and less frequently early postpartum, usually within 48 hours. Eclampsia, one of the most dreaded consequences of preeclampsia, is the development of seizures in a patient with preeclampsia. This syndrome occurs in about 0.1% of all pregnancies, and is 10 to 30 times more common in developing countries.[31,37]

The pathophysiology of preeclampsia is not fully understood. There is evidence that immune maladaptation is central to its cause. Abnormal placentation, leading to a restricted placental blood flow, may be the key factor promoting a cascade of events culminating with preeclampsia. Restricted placental blood flow leads to the development of a necrotizing spiral artery arteriopathy, coined acute atherosis, that resembles the early stages of systemic atherosclerosis. The resultant placental oxidative and endoplasmic reticulum stress leads to the release of components from the intervillous space into the maternal circulation, promoting maternal intravascular inflammatory response (increase in tumor necrosis factor alpha, IL-6, ICAM-1, C-reactive protein, IL-2), generalized endothelial dysfunction, immune and clotting activation, decreased intravascular volume, and increased vascular reactivity. Microthrombi may be seen in multiple organs.[34,38] The endothelial dysfunction may lead to disruption of the blood–brain barrier, leading to cerebral edema and hemorrhage, as well as possible disruption of vascular cerebral autoregulation.[39]

The importance of the diagnosis and early management of preeclampsia cannot be overstated. The maternal mortality rate in preeclampsia–eclampsia is 6.4 in 10,000 cases at delivery, with a nearly 20-fold increased risk of maternal mortality when preeclampsia develops before 32 weeks of gestation.[40] A recent study has shown that mortality attributed to stroke in preeclampsia occurs in approximately 60% of cases. Furthermore, the ability to modify a patient's outcome by more rapidly attending to clinical warning signs and symptoms of stroke occurred in 91%, and opportunities for improved medical management occurred in 76%.[41] The most common type of stroke occurring after preeclampsia is hemorrhagic stroke, usually present in the postpartum period.[35] Additionally, there is a clear overlap syndrome of postpartum angiopathy or the RCVS, posterior reversible encephalopathy syndrome (PRES), and preeclampsia and eclampsia.[37] The relative risk of stroke occurring later in life after preeclampsia is 1.76 (95% CI, 1.40–2.22) for nonfatal stroke, and a relative risk of 2.98 (95% CI, 1.11–7.96) for fatal stroke.[42] For women with preeclampsia, those who have severe preeclampsia or eclampsia, hypercoagulable states, chronic hypertension, peripartum infections, and coagulopathies are at greatest risk for stroke.[33]

Management

1. Delivery: The definitive treatment for preeclampsia is delivery of the baby and of the diseased placenta. For women with an onset of preeclampsia at 37 weeks or later, delivery should be performed (**Table 1**). For women with preeclampsia that begins at less than 37 weeks of gestation, they should be managed with an expectant approach (preferably with maternal fetal medicine involvement for gestational age <34 weeks), unless features of severe disease develop.[36]
2. Aspirin: Aspirin was first shown to decrease the risk of preeclampsia in women in 1979.[43] Thereafter, it has been studied in multiple clinical trials. A recent study showed that for patients at high risk of developing preeclampsia, aspirin 150 mg/ d, from weeks 11 to 14 to week 36 of gestation, was superior to placebo for the prevention of preterm preeclampsia (1.6% vs 4.3%, respectively; OR, 0.38; 95% CI, 0.20–0.74), without increasing the risk of poor neonatal outcomes.[44] This therapy has been recommended in the recently published consensus statement on HDP from the International Society for the Study of Hypertension in Pregnancy.[36]

Recent data from a prospective cohort study showed that for women less than 60 years old with a prior history of HDP, those taking aspirin had a lower risk of stroke

Table 1 Key treatment points for stroke in pregnancy and puerperium	
Pregnancy-Associated Disease	**Treatment**
Gestational hypertension	Blood pressure control to <140/85 mm Hg, preferably with oral or intravenous labetalol, hydralazine, and nicardipine.
Preeclampsia and eclampsia	Prevention of preterm preeclampsia: aspirin 150 mg daily from weeks 11–14 to week 36 of gestation. Definitive treatment: delivery of the fetus and diseased placenta.
Arterial ischemic stroke	Intravenous tissue plasminogen activator should be considered within 4.5 h after symptom onset. Mechanical thrombectomy should be offered to patients with large-vessel occlusion strokes.
Hemorrhagic stroke	Treatment involves blood pressure control. Treatment of the underlying vascular lesion as appropriate.
CVST	Treatment: unfractionated or low molecular weight heparin.

compared with nonusers of aspirin. These thought-provoking findings prompt consideration of clinical trials of aspirin use for stroke prevention in women with prior HDP.[45]

3. Calcium: Ahigh calcium intake during pregnancy has been shown to be associated with a decreased incidence of preeclampsia. The mechanism whereby calcium might mediate this effect is through a decrease in parathyroid hormone release and a decrease in intracellular calcium, leading to decreased smooth muscle contractility. Additionally, calcium supplementation could also decrease uterine smooth muscle contractility and prevent preterm labor and delivery.[46–48] Calcium supplementation at 1.2 to 2.5 g/day is also recommended, in addition to aspirin, for women at high risk of preeclampsia who have a low daily calcium intake or in whom the daily intake of calcium cannot be estimated.[36]

4. Hypertension management: For patients with severe hypertension (a blood pressure of $\geq$160/110) during pregnancy or the puerperium, blood pressure should be controlled in a monitored setting, with agents including intravenous labetalol or hydralazine, or oral nifedipine. Management recommendations for moderate hypertension vary by medical society. For example, the American College of Obstetricians and Gynecologists does not recommend the treatment of mild or moderate hypertension.[49] Conversely, a 2014 statement from the American Heart Association suggests consideration of treatment of moderate hypertension in pregnancy.[50] The divergent opinions stem from concerns regarding (a) fetal outcomes, because aggressive blood pressure control may lead to low birth weight owing to relative placental insufficiency and (b) maternal outcomes, given an increased maternal stroke risk and the risk of development of severe hypertension during gestation. A 2015 randomized, controlled clinical trial addressed this question. In that study, 987 pregnant women at 14 to 33 weeks of gestation, with nonproteinuric hypertension or gestational hypertension, were randomized to blood pressure control with target diastolic blood pressure of 100 mm Hg (control group) or target diastolic blood pressure of 85 mm Hg. The primary outcome (pregnancy loss or high-level neonatal care >48 hours in the first 28 postnatal days) occurred in 31.4% of controls and in 30.7% receiving aggressive blood pressure control (adjusted OR, 1.02; 95% CI, 0.77–1.35). There was also no significant difference in the percentage of infants with low birth weight between the 2 groups. Serious maternal complications did not differ between the study arms.[51] Since the reporting of this study's results, the International Society for the Study of Hypertension in Pregnancy has recommended treatment of any type of maternal hypertension, aiming for a target diastolic blood pressure of 85 mm Hg.[36]

5. Magnesium sulfate is recommended for women with preeclampsia who have proteinuria and severe hypertension, or hypertension with neurologic signs or symptoms.[36] The use of magnesium sulfate in preeclamptic women with severe features has been shown to decrease the rate of progression to eclampsia by 58%, as compared with placebo.[52] Magnesium sulfate is also superior to diazepam and phenytoin for the prevention of recurrent seizures in eclampsia.[53,54]

6. Regular exercise during pregnancy to maintain an appropriate body weight is recommended, because it will decrease the likelihood of hypertension.[36]

Posterior Reversible Encephalopathy

PRES refers to a syndrome of hypertensive encephalopathy characterized by reversible brain edema. This syndrome usually occurs in the setting of elevated blood pressure or relative hypertension (compared with a patient's baseline blood pressure). Patients typically presents with headache, visual symptoms referable to the occipital lobes, and seizures. The disease may be complicated by cerebral hemorrhages and ischemic strokes.

There is an overlap between PRES and severe preeclampsia and eclampsia.[55] A small, single-center, retrospective cohort study showed radiologic features suggestive of PRES in 98% of women with eclampsia.[56] Similarly, another small retrospective cohort study reported radiologic features suggestive of PRES in 92% of women with eclampsia and in 19% of women with preeclampsia.[57]

The typical radiographic appearance of PRES is that of subcortical white matter and cortical edema in the bilateral parietal and occipital lobes. In less typical PRES, there can be an extension to the frontal lobes, inferior temporal lobes, cerebellar hemispheres, brainstem, and deep white matter.[58] A diffusion-weighted MRI can also show restricted diffusion and intracranial hemorrhages. Atypical radiologic features and intracranial hemorrhages are less commonly seen in obstetric PRES.[59]

The goals of therapy are to normalize the systemic blood pressure, control seizures, and minimize vasospasm and the risks of secondary infarct and hemorrhage.

Outcomes in nonobstetric PRES may be more severe than that of patients with obstetric PRES, which may be driven by the severity of the underlying comorbidities in that population.[60]

Reversible Cerebral Vasoconstriction Syndrome

RCVS denotes a group of diseases characterized by segmental narrowing and dilatation of multiple intracranial arteries of days to weeks in duration.[61–64] RCVS is relatively rare, with a female to male ratio of 2:10 to 10:1, and mean age of 42 to 44 years.[63,65,66] RCVS may be the most common cause of pregnancy-associated stroke. The most common presenting sign is recurrent thunderclap headache over days to weeks, sometimes progressing to persistent moderate headache. Focal neurologic deficits, such as hemiparesis, aphasia, and altered mental status, occur in 8% to 43% of patients.[63,65,67] Visual changes are common, including blurriness, cortical visual loss, and Balint syndrome.[65] Generalized tonic–clonic seizures occur in 1% to 17% of cases at disease onset.

The pathophysiology is uncertain. RCVS may occur owing to spontaneous or provoked failed regulation of cerebral vascular tone, likely related to serotoninergic pathways and sympathetic overactivity.[62,68] RCVS has been associated with exposure to vasoactive drugs (antidepressants, nasal decongestants, triptans, cannabis, nicotine patches, cocaine, methamphetamine, amphetamine, and lysergic acid), catecholamine-secreting tumors, immunosuppressants, blood products, uncontrolled hypertension, head trauma, and sexual activity. This condition has been seen in the postpartum state, with or without preeclampsia or eclampsia.[62,63,65,68–76] There may be overlapping mechanisms between RCVS and posterior reversible leukoencephalopathy syndrome (PRES) given the presence of reversible cerebral edema in 8% to 38% of RCVS cases, angiographic changes in patients with PRES, and similar clinical presentation between the 2 conditions.[63,65,69,77,78]

Brain parenchymal imaging is often normal on admission, but changes may be seen over time in 81% of patients, including ischemic strokes, intraparenchymal hemorrhages (42%), and convexal nonaneurysmal subarachnoid hemorrhages.[63,65,66,77,79] Vasogenic edema suggestive of PRES is seen in 28%. Vascular imaging (computed tomographic angiography, magnetic resonance angiography, or conventional transfemoral angiography) demonstrates multifocal areas of smooth arterial tapering and alternating dilatation. Initial angiographic studies may be normal in RCVS. Angiographic findings typically resolve within 90 days.[66] RCVS can be difficult to distinguish from primary angiitis of the central nervous system. The presence of recurrent thunderclap headaches, or the presence of a single thunderclap headache combined with normal neuroimaging, border zone ischemic strokes, or vasogenic edema suggestive of PRES, are highly specific for a diagnosis of RCVS.[66] The recent RCVS2 score also has high accuracy for prediction of RCVS. In this score, the variables that predict RCVS are recurrent or single thunderclap headache, presence of a trigger for vasoconstriction (drugs, postpartum state, or orgasm), female sex, and subarachnoid hemorrhage. Involvement of the intracranial internal carotid artery is a negative predictor for RCVS.[80]

RCVS and PRES may co-occur: radiologic features of PRES have been reported in 9% of patients with RCVS.[81] Additionally, cases have been reported of women with clinicoradiologic features of RCVS overlapping with PRES. In such cases, imaging shows posterior white and often gray matter change consistent with vasogenic cerebral edema or segmental narrowing and dilation of large and medium-sized cerebral arteries, the findings typical of RCVS.[69]

RCVS is best managed conservatively, with discontinuation of the offending agent, symptomatic treatment for headache and agitation, bed rest and stool softeners to avoid the Valsalva maneuver, and avoidance of physical exertion. Antiplatelets are not recommended. The blood pressure should be allowed to autoregulate, and decreases in the blood pressure avoided. Calcium channel blockers can be used for headache relief, although they are often administered to treat the vasospasm. Logically, patients should avoid exposure to precipitants of the disease as far as possible; however, there is no evidence that reexposure precipitates RCVS.[62,68] There is no role for the use of glucocorticoids in RCVS, which can lead to worse clinical outcomes.[82]

The outcome in RCVS is favorable, with more than 90% of patients having no disability. However, fewer than 5% have an aggressive course, with progression of vasospasm, severe neurologic disability, or death. This outcome might be more common in postpartum RCVS.[74,83,84] Recurrent RCVS (thunderclap headache, but without any focal deficits) has been reported in up to 5.8% of patients; postpartum RVCS was reported to occur after a subsequent delivery in 9% of patients.[85]

Cerebral Venous Sinus Thrombosis

CVST is an uncommon cerebrovascular disease characterized by thrombosis of the dural sinuses and cerebral veins, with resultant venous congestion, focal cerebral edema, and ultimately hemorrhagic venous infarctions. CVST accounts for 0.5% to 1.0% of all strokes.[86] CVST is most commonly seen in patients younger than 50 years of age, and 75% are women.[87] The most common risk factor is oral contraceptive use (54%). Genetic and acquired thrombophilias are seen in 34% of patients. Other conditions include malignancy, hematologic disorders, pregnancy in 6.3%, puerperium in 13.8%, and infections. Forty-four percent of patients may have a combination of risk factors.[87] Obstetric CVST is most commonly associated with hypertension, cesarean delivery, and infection.[20] A recent case control study showed that the risk of gestational CVST is mostly attributable to the puerperium, with an adjusted OR for CVST of 18.7 (95% CI, 8.3–41.9) during the first 6 weeks after delivery, as opposed to an adjusted OR of 1.2 (95% CI, 0.6–2.3) during pregnancy.[88]

The most common presenting symptoms include headache (88%),[89–91] seizures (40%), papilledema (30%), visual loss, diplopia, fluctuating motor or sensory deficits, stupor, and coma.[87] The disease affects most commonly the superior sagittal sinus (62%), the transverse sinus (41%–45%), straight sinus (18%), cortical veins (17%), and deep venous system (11%).[87]

The diagnosis of CVST requires a high degree of clinical suspicion. Cerebral venous imaging is required for the diagnosis, preferably performed with computed tomography (CT) venography and MR venography. MRI susceptibility-weighted imaging is useful for the diagnosis of CVST, especially for cortical vein thrombosis.[92] Indirect parenchymal signs may be seen in CVST, which are most conspicuous on brain MRI. These signs vary from normal appearing parenchyma to focal edema, cerebral hemorrhages, and increased or decreased water diffusivity[93] (**Fig. 1**).

The mainstay of treatment of CVST is clot dissolution with anticoagulation. In the acute phase, unfractionated heparin or low-molecular-weight heparin are recommended, followed by oral anticoagulation with warfarin or dabigatran for at least 3 to 6 months.[94] The duration of anticoagulation depends on the underlying condition. Anticoagulation is considered safe in the presence of intracranial hemorrhage. However, in the peripartum period, this treatment may be complicated by a risk of bleeding

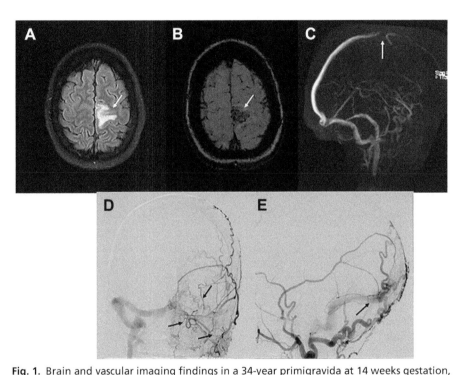

Fig. 1. Brain and vascular imaging findings in a 34-year primigravida at 14 weeks gestation, presenting with right leg weakness for hours, followed by a focal motor seizure of the right leg and arm that progressed to a generalized tonic-clonic seizure. (*A*) Brain magnetic resonance imaging (MRI, fluid-attenuated inversion recovery sequence) shows hyperintense signal in the cortical -subcortical region of the left frontal lobe (*arrow*). (*B*) Susceptibility-weighted MRI shows hemorrhage in the same region (arrow). These findings suggest hemorrhagic infarction, raising concern for venous sinus thrombosis. (*C*) Magnetic resonance venography shows thrombo-occlusion in the anterior portion of the superior sagittal sinus (*arrow*) and decreased flow-related enhancement of cortical veins overlying the left hemisphere. The patient was diagnosed with cerebral venous sinus and cortical vein thrombosis. She received therapeutic anticoagulation with low-molecular-weight heparin. (*D, E*) A subsequent digital subtraction angiogram of the brain revealed a dural arterial-venous fistula of the brain, with extensive arterial supply from the bilateral occipital arteries and middle meningeal arteries. The *arrows* depict areas of extensive fistulization between the cerebral arterial and venous circulations. Because the patient was clinically stable, treatment of the vascular malformation was postponed until after delivery..

after delivery or cesarean surgery. Because of its safety profile, warfarin and direct-acting oral anticoagulants should be avoided during pregnancy. After delivery, women may be transitioned from low-molecular-weight heparin to warfarin, even if nursing. Direct-acting oral anticoagulants are not considered safe to use while breastfeeding.[95] Thrombectomy is not routinely performed in CVST and has not shown to improve clinical outcomes when compared with medical management[96] (see **Table 1**).

CVST is usually a benign condition, whereby 87% of patients will have none to mild deficits. Death occurs in 8.3% of patients.[87,97] Recurrent CVST is uncommon (2.2%), and recurrent venous thromboembolic disease in recurrent pregnancies is infrequent.[98] Seizures can occur in 10.6% of patients. Any venous thromboembolic event can occur in 5.8% of patients, especially in the first year after CVST. Severe headaches can unfortunately persist after CVST in 14% of cases.[87]

Hemorrhagic Stroke

Pregnancy increases the risk for hemorrhagic stroke much more than for ischemic stroke, with a relative risk of 2.5 during pregnancy and 28.5 postpartum[99] (see **Table 1**). Hemorrhagic stroke is an important cause of maternal and fetal pregnancy-related mortality.[7] The major established causes of pregnancy-related cerebral hemorrhage are preeclampsia or eclampsia, followed by AVMs and aneurysms.

The risk of aneurysmal rupture increases with gestational age, peaking at 30 to 34 weeks. A recent study showed an increase in the incidence of spontaneous subarachnoid hemorrhages during pregnancy in the United States from 2002 to 2014, with the greatest increase affecting African American pregnant women.[100] Cerebral aneurysmal rupture during pregnancy is associated with high maternal (35%) and fetal (17%) mortality.[101] If a ruptured aneurysm is left unsecured surgically, there is a very high rate of recurrent hemorrhage and maternal and fetal mortality (63% and 27%, respectively). These mortalities were decreased to 11% and 5%, respectively, with early surgery.[101] Thus, if aneurysmal subarachnoid hemorrhage occurs during pregnancy, then surgical control of the aneurysm should be performed immediately during pregnancy, when possible.[102] If urgent obstetric issues prevent immediate neurosurgery, then urgent cesarean delivery is recommended, followed by surgical control of the cerebral aneurysm. There is an increased risk of aneurysmal rupture near term. Therefore, it is recommended that unruptured aneurysms at significant risk of rupture be secured before pregnancy, when possible.

Hemorrhage is the most common presenting manifestation of AVMs, followed by seizures or focal neurologic deficits. Whether AVMs bleed more during pregnancy has been debated. A study from 1990 showed an annual rate of hemorrhage of 3.5% in women with AVM and no prior hemorrhage, and 5.8% in those with prior hemorrhage, with no increase secondary to pregnancy.[103] However, when considering the daily risk of rupture, there was a several-fold increase in this risk on the day of delivery.[104,105] More recent studies have shown an increase in the rate of intracranial hemorrhage in women during pregnancy and the puerperium. A retrospective Chinese study of 264 women with AVM showed an annualized rate of AVM rupture and hemorrhage of 5.59% in pregnant women as compared with 2.52% in nonpregnant women ($P = .002$).[106] Similar results were seen in an American retrospective cohort of 270 women, showing an annual hemorrhage rate of 5.7% in pregnant women versus 1.3% in nonpregnant women ($P<.001$).[107] Further, AVM bleeding during pregnancy is associated with a higher rebleeding rate than in nonpregnant women (26% vs 6%, respectively).

Regarding the management of AVMs in pregnancy, based on the considerations discussed, expert recommendation are that (1) if a woman with known AVM anticipates pregnancy, the AVM should be treated before pregnancy, (2) if an AVM is discovered during pregnancy and has not bled during the pregnancy, then conservative observation is usually recommended with plans to proceed to definitive treatment after delivery, and (3) if an AVM bleeds during pregnancy, then consideration should be given to treatment during the pregnancy, taking into account the grade of the lesion and the expected timing of benefit in lowering the risk (immediate for low-grade lesions amenable to complete surgical excision or embolization) but delayed by 1 to 3 years for higher grade lesions requiring radiosurgery and combination therapies.[108] Cesarean delivery is usually favored over vaginal delivery owing to the higher rates of hemorrhage on the day of delivery.

Blood pressure control is key to the acute management of patients with hemorrhagic stroke, irrespective of its etiology. This strategy allows for a decrease in hematoma growth. However, this factor must be balanced against the competing concern for severe hypotension, which can promote placental hypoperfusion.[109]

Cervical Artery Dissection

It is not completely understood if gestation and delivery can be complicated by cervical artery dissection, especially for women undergoing vaginal delivery, and if cervical artery dissection can lead to pregnancy-associated stroke. To address this question, a recent case control study showed that pregnancy may be accompanied by a higher risk of cervical artery dissection (incidence risk ratio, 2.2; 95% CI, 1.3–3.5). This risk was particularly high during the postpartum period, on average 21 days after delivery, but not during the prepartum period. Of the patients developing cervical artery dissection during pregnancy, 45% had HDP.[110]

MANAGEMENT OF STROKE IN PREGNANCY
Acute Ischemic Stroke Management

For patients presenting with acute focal neurologic deficits concerning for cerebrovascular disease, neuroimaging should be obtained expeditiously (see **Table 1**). A noncontrast head CT scan, the initial imaging modality of choice, can be performed with abdominal shielding to protect the developing fetus. Noncontrast brain MRI is also considered safe during pregnancy. For vascular imaging, a CT angiogram of the head and neck and or/CT venography can be safely performed with iodinated contrast, which does not cross the placenta. Head and neck MR angiography can be performed with time-of-flight techniques, which also do not require contrast. However, gadolinium-based MR contrast should not be administered to pregnant patients because it may cross the placenta and deposit in fetal tissues.[111]

For nonpregnant patients with acute ischemic stroke, early thrombolytic therapy and endovascular clot retrieval are the recommended hyperacute therapies to improve long-term clinical outcomes. However, these therapies have not been studied in randomized trials involving pregnant women. Further, this therapy is often withheld in many women given concerns for life-threatening maternal and placental hemorrhages, including the risk of fetal demise. The most widespread used thrombolytic, tissue plasminogen activator, does not cross the placenta and, therefore, does not cause direct fetal harm. There have been numerous case reports and small case series of use of thrombolytic therapy for arterial ischemic stroke and other systemic indications, without clear evidence of harm or benefit.[112] A recent study sought to address this question. Using data from the American Heart Association Get with the Guidelines Registry, the authors compared 338 pregnant or postpartum women with 24,303 women, all acute ischemic stroke sufferers who received reperfusion therapy (intravenous thrombolytic or catheter-based thrombolysis and clot retrieval). Pregnant women were less likely to receive intravenous thrombolysis than the nonpregnant women, but the overall rates of reperfusion therapy were similar between the 2 groups. Furthermore, patients in both groups had similar rates of discharge to home. There was a nonsignificant trend of increased rates of symptomatic intracranial hemorrhage in pregnant women who received intravenous thrombolysis as compared with nonpregnant women. Fetal outcomes were not reported in this study. However, this study did show that it may be reasonable to offer reperfusion to pregnant and post-partum women who suffered an ischemic stroke. Intra-arterial therapy is an especially interesting approach to acute stroke management in this population.[113] A subsequent smaller study reported on 34 patients from the literature who received thrombolytic therapy for acute stroke: most of the cases reported favorable maternal and fetal outcomes.[114]

A multicenter case series of 7 patients with acute ischemic stroke during pregnancy who received acute endovascular therapy showed promising results, with successful revascularization in all cases, no symptomatic hemorrhages, favorable NIHSS scores at discharge, and good outcomes at 3 months.[115]

Delivery

The timing of delivery for women who have suffered a stroke during pregnancy is determined by the severity of the mother's medical condition and fetal stability. For women who suffer a stroke at less than 24 weeks of gestation, decisions regarding continuing the pregnancy versus therapeutic termination rely on the clinical state of the patient and the need for use of thrombolysis, which can increase the risk of fetal loss. For women who suffer a stroke at 24 to 32 weeks of gestation, antenatal gluco-corticoids may be given to accelerate fetal lung maturation. If the mother and fetus are clinically stable, then pregnancy may be continued, aiming for controlled induction at 34 to 39 weeks of gestation. Cesarean delivery should be avoided if possible.[112,116] In regards to antithrombotic management, heparinoids should be discontinued 24 hours before induction and labor, and may be resumed 24 hours after delivery.[117]

Secondary Stroke Prevention of Ischemic Stroke in Pregnancy and the Puerperium

The choice of antithrombotic will be determined by the stroke mechanism and patient preferences. Aspirin is by the far the most widely used antithrombotic for secondary stroke prevention. It is deemed safe for use in the second and third trimesters for the fetus and the mother. In the first trimester, however, aspirin use has been reported to have an association with an increased incidence of fetal gastroschisis and other fetal malformations.[95] Other studies and metanalyses of aspirin use for the prevention of preeclampsia even before 11 weeks do not support the same findings. A large meta-analysis of studies of antiplatelets use in women at high risk for preeclampsia showed the safety of antiplatelets without adverse fetal outcomes, an increase in fetal systemic or intracranial hemorrhages, adverse effects on fetal weight, and more favor-able maternal outcomes.[118] The safety of other antiplatelets during pregnancy has not been established in clinical trials.

Regarding anticoagulants, warfarin is contraindicated in pregnancy owing to its teratogenic effects and the risk for fetal hemorrhages. It should be avoided in early pregnancy, and if at all also throughout the entire pregnancy because it may also cause central nervous system abnormalities in the second and third trimesters. Pref-erence should be given to heparins. Unfractionated heparin and low-molecular-weight heparins do not cross the placenta, although unfractionated heparin can increase the risk of maternal thrombocytopenia and osteoporosis. The novel oral anticoagulants should not be used during pregnancy given their uncertain safety profile. After delivery, nursing mothers may continue to take low-dose aspirin, warfarin, unfractionated heparin, and low-molecular-weight heparin. However, novel oral anticoagulants are not recommended.[95,119]

Statins are often used for the secondary prevention of ischemic stroke. There are currently insufficient data to assess the safety of statins during pregnancy.[120] Furthermore, statins are classified as category X by the US Food and Drug Administration. Therefore, they should be avoided during gestation.

IMPORTANCE OF MULTIDISCIPLINARY CARE

A multidisciplinary collaboration in the care of the pregnant patient with stroke is key to success. In the emergency setting, health care providers should be well-versed in the diagnosis and management of headaches associated with cerebrovascular diseases in pregnancy. In the emergency department, systems of care should be in place and readily activated in the case of an acute stroke syndrome. For the success of such treatments, teams should include emergency medicine practitioners, neurologists, neuroradiologists, neurointerventional radiologists, and anesthesiologists, among other professionals. The guidance of high-risk obstetricians is important for management decisions regarding thrombolysis and thrombectomy for acute ischemic stroke. After a stroke, patients benefit from care in highly specialized stroke units, which have been shown to improve outcomes when compared with standard inpatient care. In such units, stroke-specific care is offered by stroke neurologists and nurses, and patients receive specialized therapy for poststroke recovery from physical and occupational therapists, as well as speech and language pathologists. Hematologists may be involved when coagulation dyscrasias are identified. Interventional cardiologists may be consulted when cardiac procedures are required to decrease the risk of subsequent stroke. After a stroke, collaborations with social workers are important to facilitate transitions into the community. In certain cases, vocational counselors may help to guide professional transitions into the community.

STROKE OUTCOMES
Morbidity and Mortality

Stroke morbidity is determined by the type of stroke, its severity, and therapies received for early management and secondary prevention. Mortality rates for stroke in pregnancy are reported at 2.7% to 20.4%.[1,9] Mortality related to an acute stroke during pregnancy was almost 385 times higher than that of pregnant women without acute stroke in 1 study.[9] Although previous studies had not shown a significant decrease in stroke-related mortality, a recent study of the National Inpatient Sample showed that the rates of in-hospital mortality for acute stroke during pregnancy and puerperium decreased from 5.5% in 2007 to 2.7% in 2015, despite unchanged rates of acute stroke during that period. Independent predictors of in-house stroke-related mortality included age 40 years or older, Black or Asian race, hemorrhagic stroke, anemia, heart failure, preeclampsia or eclampsia, gestational diabetes, and cesarean delivery.[9]

Risk of Recurrent Stroke

For women of childbearing age who have a stroke or venous sinus thrombosis, the risk of a recurrent stroke during pregnancy is not substantially high. A study of 441 women with a first ever stroke followed for 5 years showed that only 13 strokes occurred in that time; only 2 strokes occurred during pregnancy or the puerperium. The puerperium was the period of highest risk for an obstetric ischemic stroke. Therefore, having had a previous ischemic stroke should not preclude women of childbearing age to seek pregnancy.[121] A subsequent study of 252 women with pregnancy-associated stroke confirmed that the risk of recurrent stroke or venous thrombosis during a subsequent pregnancy is low (2%).[122] However, women with prior stroke who become pregnant seem to have a significantly higher risk of miscarriages, fetal loss, and pregnancy complications than pregnant women without prior stroke. These studies did not determine the cause of this association, although it is postulated that the underlying etiology of the index stroke could impact fertility, such as in patients with antiphospholipid syndrome or other hypercoagulable states.[123]

DISCLOSURES

Dr A.B. Singhal received research grant support from NIH-NINDS; consulting fees from Omniox, Deck Therapeutics, and Medicolegal firms; authorship royalty payments from UptoDate and Medlink, Inc; and his wife is an employee and owns stock in Biogen.

REFERENCES

1. Swartz RH, Cayley ML, Foley N, et al. The incidence of pregnancy-related stroke: a systematic review and meta-analysis. Int J Stroke 2017;12(7):687–97.
2. Kuklina EV, Tong X, Bansil P, et al. Trends in pregnancy hospitalizations that included a stroke in the United States from 1994 to 2007: reasons for concern? Stroke 2011;42(9):2564–70.
3. Wu P, Jordan KP, Chew-Graham CA, et al. Temporal trends in pregnancy-associated stroke and its outcomes among women with hypertensive disorders of pregnancy. J Am Heart Assoc 2020;9(15):e016182.
4. Too G, Wen T, Boehme AK, et al. Timing and risk factors of postpartum stroke. Obstet Gynecol 2018;131(1):70–8.
5. Ban L, Sprigg N, Abdul Sultan A, et al. Incidence of first stroke in pregnant and nonpregnant women of childbearing age: a population-based cohort study from England. J Am Heart Assoc 2017;6(4):e004601.
6. Kamel H, Navi BB, Sriram N, et al. Risk of a thrombotic event after the 6-week postpartum period. N Engl J Med 2014;370(14):1307–15.
7. Meeks JR, Bambhroliya AB, Alex KM, et al. Association of primary intracerebral hemorrhage with pregnancy and the postpartum period. JAMA Netw Open 2020;3(4):e202769.
8. James AH, Bushnell CD, Jamison MG, et al. Incidence and risk factors for stroke in pregnancy and the puerperium. Obstet Gynecol 2005;106(3):509–16.
9. Elgendy IY, Gad MM, Mahmoud AN, et al. Acute stroke during pregnancy and puerperium. J Am Coll Cardiol 2020;75(2):180–90.
10. Miller EC, Gatollari HJ, Too G, et al. Risk of pregnancy-associated stroke across age groups in New York State. JAMA Neurol 2016;73(12):1461–7.
11. Qureshi AI, Saeed O, Malik AA, et al. Pregnancy in advanced age and the risk of stroke in postmenopausal women: analysis of Women's Health Initiative Study. Am J Obstet Gynecol 2017;216(4):409 e401–6.
12. Miller EC, Zambrano Espinoza MD, Huang Y, et al. Maternal race/ethnicity, hypertension, and risk for stroke during delivery admission. J Am Heart Assoc 2020;9(3):e014775.
13. Bandoli G, Baer RJ, Gano D, et al. Migraines during pregnancy and the risk of maternal stroke. JAMA Neurol 2020;77(9):1177–9.

14. Miller EC, Gallo M, Kulick ER, et al. Infections and risk of peripartum stroke during delivery admissions. Stroke 2018;49(5):1129–34.
15. Miller EC, Wen T, Elkind MSV, et al. Infection during delivery hospitalization and risk of readmission for postpartum stroke. Stroke 2019;50(10):2685–91.
16. Sanders BD, Davis MG, Holley SL, et al. Pregnancy-associated stroke. J Midwifery Womens Health 2018;63(1):23–32.
17. Chen L, Deng W, Palacios I, et al. Patent foramen ovale (PFO), stroke and pregnancy. J Investig Med 2016;64(5):992–1000.
18. Dayan N, Filion KB, Okano M, et al. Cardiovascular risk following fertility therapy: systematic review and meta-analysis. J Am Coll Cardiol 2017;70(10):1203–13.
19. Udell JA, Lu H, Redelmeier DA. Failure of fertility therapy and subsequent adverse cardiovascular events. CMAJ 2017;189(10):E391–7.
20. Lanska DJ, Kryscio RJ. Risk factors for peripartum and postpartum stroke and intracranial venous thrombosis. Stroke 2000;31(6):1274–82.
21. Lin SY, Hu CJ, Lin HC. Increased risk of stroke in patients who undergo cesarean section delivery: a nationwide population-based study. Am J Obstet Gynecol 2008;198(4):391 e391–397.
22. Sanghavi M, Rutherford JD. Cardiovascular physiology of pregnancy. Circulation 2014;130(12):1003–8.
23. Feske SK, Singhal AB. Cerebrovascular disorders complicating pregnancy. Continuum (Minneap Minn) 2014;20(1 Neurology of Pregnancy):80–99.
24. Poppas A, Shroff SG, Korcarz CE, et al. Serial assessment of the cardiovascular system in normal pregnancy. Role of arterial compliance and pulsatile arterial load. Circulation 1997;95(10):2407–15.
25. Brenner B. Haemostatic changes in pregnancy. Thromb Res 2004;114(5–6):409–14.
26. Coutinho T, Lamai O, Nerenberg K. Hypertensive disorders of pregnancy and cardiovascular diseases: current knowledge and future directions. Curr Treat Options Cardiovasc Med 2018;20(7):56.
27. Ray JG, Vermeulen MJ, Schull MJ, et al. Cardiovascular health after maternal placental syndromes (CHAMPS): population-based retrospective cohort study. Lancet 2005;366(9499):1797–803.
28. Wu P, Haththotuwa R, Kwok CS, et al. Preeclampsia and future cardiovascular health: a systematic review and meta-analysis. Circ Cardiovasc Qual Outcomes 2017;10(2):e003497.
29. Leon LJ, McCarthy FP, Direk K, et al. Preeclampsia and cardiovascular disease in a large UK pregnancy cohort of linked electronic health records: a CALIBER study. Circulation 2019;140(13):1050–60.
30. Leffert LR, Clancy CR, Bateman BT, et al. Hypertensive disorders and pregnancy-related stroke: frequency, trends, risk factors, and outcomes. Obstet Gynecol 2015;125(1):124–31.
31. Umesawa M, Kobashi G. Epidemiology of hypertensive disorders in pregnancy: prevalence, risk factors, predictors and prognosis. Hypertens Res 2017;40(3):213–20.
32. Kuklina EV, Ayala C, Callaghan WM. Hypertensive disorders and severe obstetric morbidity in the United States. Obstet Gynecol 2009;113(6):1299–306.
33. Miller EC, Gatollari HJ, Too G, et al. Risk factors for pregnancy-associated stroke in women with preeclampsia. Stroke 2017;48(7):1752–9.
34. Steegers EA, von Dadelszen P, Duvekot JJ, et al. Pre-eclampsia. Lancet 2010;376(9741):631–44.

35. Bateman BT, Schumacher HC, Bushnell CD, et al. Intracerebral hemorrhage in pregnancy: frequency, risk factors, and outcome. Neurology 2006;67(3):424–9.

36. Brown MA, Magee LA, Kenny LC, et al. Hypertensive disorders of pregnancy: ISSHP classification, diagnosis, and management recommendations for international practice. Hypertension 2018;72(1):24–43.

37. Bushnell C, Chireau M. Preeclampsia and stroke: risks during and after pregnancy. Stroke Res Treat 2011;2011:858134.

38. Rodie VA, Freeman DJ, Sattar N, et al. Pre-eclampsia and cardiovascular disease: metabolic syndrome of pregnancy? Atherosclerosis 2004;175(2): 189–202.

39. Hammer ES, Cipolla MJ. Cerebrovascular dysfunction in preeclamptic pregnancies. Curr Hypertens Rep 2015;17(8):64.

40. MacKay AP, Berg CJ, Atrash HK. Pregnancy-related mortality from preeclampsia and eclampsia. Obstet Gynecol 2001;97(4):533–8.

41. Judy AE, McCain CL, Lawton ES, et al. Systolic hypertension, preeclampsia-related mortality, and stroke in California. Obstet Gynecol 2019;133(6):1151–9.

42. Bellamy L, Casas JP, Hingorani AD, et al. Pre-eclampsia and risk of cardiovascular disease and cancer in later life: systematic review and meta-analysis. BMJ 2007;335(7627):974.

43. Crandon AJ, Isherwood DM. Effect of aspirin on incidence of pre-eclampsia. Lancet 1979;1(8130):1356.

44. Rolnik DL, Wright D, Poon LC, et al. Aspirin versus placebo in pregnancies at high risk for preterm preeclampsia. N Engl J Med 2017;377(7):613–22.

45. Miller EC, Boehme AK, Chung NT, et al. Aspirin reduces long-term stroke risk in women with prior hypertensive disorders of pregnancy. Neurology 2019;92(4): e305–16.

46. Hofmeyr GJ, Lawrie TA, Atallah AN, et al. Calcium supplementation during pregnancy for preventing hypertensive disorders and related problems. Cochrane Database Syst Rev 2014;6:CD001059.

47. Bassaw B, Roopnarinesingh S, Roopnarinesingh A, et al. Prevention of hypertensive disorders of pregnancy. J Obstet Gynaecol 1998;18(2):123–6.

48. Villar J, Repke JT. Calcium supplementation during pregnancy may reduce preterm delivery in high-risk populations. Am J Obstet Gynecol 1990;163(4 Pt 1): 1124–31.

49. American College of O, Gynecologists, Task Force on Hypertension in P. Hypertension in pregnancy. Report of the American College of Obstetricians and Gynecologists' Task Force on Hypertension in Pregnancy. Obstet Gynecol 2013; 122(5):1122–31.

50. Bushnell C, McCullough LD, Awad IA, et al. Guidelines for the prevention of stroke in women: a statement for healthcare professionals from the American Heart Association/American Stroke Association. Stroke 2014;45(5):1545–88.

51. Magee LA, von Dadelszen P, Rey E, et al. Less-tight versus tight control of hypertension in pregnancy. N Engl J Med 2015;372(5):407–17.

52. Altman D, Carroli G, Duley L, et al. Do women with pre-eclampsia, and their babies, benefit from magnesium sulphate? The Magpie Trial: a randomised placebo-controlled trial. Lancet 2002;359(9321):1877–90.

53. Which anticonvulsant for women with eclampsia? Evidence from the collaborative eclampsia trial. Lancet 1995;345(8963):1455–63.

54. Lucas MJ, Leveno KJ, Cunningham FG. A comparison of magnesium sulfate with phenytoin for the prevention of eclampsia. N Engl J Med 1995;333(4): 201–5.

55. McDermott M, Miller EC, Rundek T, et al. Preeclampsia: association with posterior reversible encephalopathy syndrome and stroke. Stroke 2018;49(3):524–30.

56. Brewer J, Owens MY, Wallace K, et al. Posterior reversible encephalopathy syndrome in 46 of 47 patients with eclampsia. Am J Obstet Gynecol 2013;208(6): 468 e461–466.

57. Mayama M, Uno K, Tano S, et al. Incidence of posterior reversible encephalopathy syndrome in eclamptic and patients with preeclampsia with neurologic symptoms. Am J Obstet Gynecol 2016;215(2):239 e231–235.

58. Bartynski WS, Boardman JF. Distinct imaging patterns and lesion distribution in posterior reversible encephalopathy syndrome. AJNR Am J Neuroradiol 2007; 28(7):1320–7.

59. Liman TG, Bohner G, Heuschmann PU, et al. Clinical and radiological differences in posterior reversible encephalopathy syndrome between patients with preeclampsia-eclampsia and other predisposing diseases. Eur J Neurol 2012; 19(7):935–43.

60. Postma IR, Slager S, Kremer HP, et al. Long-term consequences of the posterior reversible encephalopathy syndrome in eclampsia and preeclampsia: a review of the obstetric and nonobstetric literature. Obstet Gynecol Surv 2014;69(5): 287–300.

61. Call GK, Fleming MC, Sealfon S, et al. Reversible cerebral segmental vasoconstriction. Stroke 1988;19(9):1159–70.

62. Calabrese LH, Dodick DW, Schwedt TJ, et al. Narrative review: reversible cerebral vasoconstriction syndromes. Ann Intern Med 2007;146(1):34–44.

63. Ducros A, Boukobza M, Porcher R, et al. The clinical and radiological spectrum of reversible cerebral vasoconstriction syndrome. A prospective series of 67 patients. Brain 2007;130(Pt 12):3091–101.

64. Singhal AB. Cerebral vasoconstriction syndromes. Top Stroke Rehabil 2004; 11(2):1–6.

65. Singhal AB, Hajj-Ali RA, Topcuoglu MA, et al. Reversible cerebral vasoconstriction syndromes: analysis of 139 cases. Arch Neurol 2011;68(8):1005–12.

66. Singhal AB, Topcuoglu MA, Fok JW, et al. RCVS and PACNS: clinical, imaging, and angiographic comparison. Ann Neurol 2016;79(6):882–94.

67. Chen SP, Fuh JL, Lirng JF, et al. Recurrent primary thunderclap headache and benign CNS angiopathy: spectra of the same disorder? Neurology 2006;67(12): 2164–9.

68. Ducros A. Reversible cerebral vasoconstriction syndrome. Lancet Neurol 2012; 11(10):906–17.

69. Singhal AB. Postpartum angiopathy with reversible posterior leukoencephalopathy. Arch Neurol 2004;61(3):411–6.

70. Singhal AB, Caviness VS, Begleiter AF, et al. Cerebral vasoconstriction and stroke after use of serotonergic drugs. Neurology 2002;58(1):130–3.

71. Nighoghossian N, Derex L, Trouillas P. Multiple intracerebral hemorrhages and vasospasm following antimigrainous drug abuse. Headache 1998;38(6): 478–80.

72. Razavi M, Bendixen B, Maley JE, et al. CNS pseudovasculitis in a patient with pheochromocytoma. Neurology 1999;52(5):1088–90.

73. Verillaud B, Ducros A, Massiou H, et al. Reversible cerebral vasoconstriction syndrome in two patients with a carotid glomus tumour. Cephalalgia 2010; 30(10):1271–5.

74. Fugate JE, Wijdicks EF, Parisi JE, et al. Fulminant postpartum cerebral vasoconstriction syndrome. Arch Neurol 2012;69(1):111–7.

75. Lee JH, Martin NA, Alsina G, et al. Hemodynamically significant cerebral vasospasm and outcome after head injury: a prospective study. J Neurosurg 1997; 87(2):221–33.

76. Wolff V, Lauer V, Rouyer O, et al. Cannabis use, ischemic stroke, and multifocal intracranial vasoconstriction: a prospective study in 48 consecutive young patients. Stroke 2011;42(6):1778–80.

77. Ducros A, Fiedler U, Porcher R, et al. Hemorrhagic manifestations of reversible cerebral vasoconstriction syndrome: frequency, features, and risk factors. Stroke 2010;41(11):2505–11.

78. Dodick DW. Reversible segmental cerebral vasoconstriction (Call-Fleming syndrome): the role of calcium antagonists. Cephalalgia 2003;23(3):163–5.

79. Kumar S, Goddeau RP Jr, Selim MH, et al. Atraumatic convexal subarachnoid hemorrhage: clinical presentation, imaging patterns, and etiologies. Neurology 2010;74(11):893–9.

80. Rocha EA, Topcuoglu MA, Silva GS, et al. RCVS2 score and diagnostic approach for reversible cerebral vasoconstriction syndrome. Neurology 2019; 92(7):e639–47.

81. Chen SP, Fuh JL, Wang SJ, et al. Magnetic resonance angiography in reversible cerebral vasoconstriction syndromes. Ann Neurol 2010;67(5):648–56.

82. Singhal AB, Topcuoglu MA. Glucocorticoid-associated worsening in reversible cerebral vasoconstriction syndrome. Neurology 2017;88(3):228–36.

83. Hajj-Ali RA, Furlan A, Abou-Chebel A, et al. Benign angiopathy of the central nervous system: cohort of 16 patients with clinical course and long-term followup. Arthritis Rheum 2002;47(6):662–9.

84. Singhal AB, Kimberly WT, Schaefer PW, et al. Case records of the Massachusetts General Hospital. Case 8-2009. A 36-year-old woman with headache, hypertension, and seizure 2 weeks post partum. N Engl J Med 2009;360(11): 1126–37.

85. Boitet R, de Gaalon S, Duflos C, et al. Long-term outcomes after reversible cerebral vasoconstriction syndrome. Stroke 2020;51(2):670–3.

86. Bousser MG, Ferro JM. Cerebral venous thrombosis: an update. Lancet Neurol 2007;6(2):162–70.

87. Ferro JM, Canhao P, Stam J, et al. Prognosis of cerebral vein and dural sinus thrombosis: results of the International study on cerebral vein and dural sinus thrombosis (ISCVT). Stroke 2004;35(3):664–70.

88. Silvis SM, Lindgren E, Hiltunen S, et al. Postpartum period is a risk factor for cerebral venous thrombosis. Stroke 2019;50(2):501–3.

89. Biousse V, Ameri A, Bousser MG. Isolated intracranial hypertension as the only sign of cerebral venous thrombosis. Neurology 1999;53(7):1537–42.

90. Ferro JM, Correia M, Pontes C, et al. Cerebral vein and dural sinus thrombosis in Portugal: 1980-1998. Cerebrovasc Dis 2001;11(3):177–82.

91. Cumurciuc R, Crassard I, Sarov M, et al. Headache as the only neurological sign of cerebral venous thrombosis: a series of 17 cases. J Neurol Neurosurg Psychiatr 2005;76(8):1084–7.

92. Idbaih A, Boukobza M, Crassard I, et al. MRI of clot in cerebral venous thrombosis: high diagnostic value of susceptibility-weighted images. Stroke 2006; 37(4):991–5.

93. Yuh WT, Simonson TM, Wang AM, et al. Venous sinus occlusive disease: MR findings. AJNR Am J Neuroradiol 1994;15(2):309–16.

94. Ferro JM, Coutinho JM, Dentali F, et al. Safety and efficacy of dabigatran etexilate vs dose-adjusted warfarin in patients with cerebral venous thrombosis: a randomized clinical trial. JAMA Neurol 2019;76(12):1457–65.

95. Caso V, Falorni A, Bushnell CD, et al. Pregnancy, hormonal treatments for infertility, contraception, and menopause in women after ischemic stroke: a consensus document. Stroke 2017;48(2):501–6.

96. Coutinho JM, Zuurbier SM, Bousser MG, et al. Effect of endovascular treatment with medical management vs standard care on severe cerebral venous thrombosis: the TO-ACT randomized clinical trial. JAMA Neurol 2020;77(8):966–73.

97. Canhao P, Ferro JM, Lindgren AG, et al. Causes and predictors of death in cerebral venous thrombosis. Stroke 2005;36(8):1720–5.

98. Aguiar de Sousa D, Canhao P, Crassard I, et al. Safety of pregnancy after cerebral venous thrombosis: results of the ISCVT (International Study on Cerebral Vein and Dural Sinus Thrombosis)-2 PREGNANCY study. Stroke 2017;48(11): 3130–3.

99. Kittner SJ, Stern BJ, Feeser BR, et al. Pregnancy and the risk of stroke. N Engl J Med 1996;335:768–74.

100. Limaye K, Patel A, Dave M, et al. Secular increases in spontaneous subarachnoid hemorrhage during pregnancy: a nationwide sample analysis. J Stroke Cerebrovasc Dis 2019;28(4):1141–8.

101. Dias MS, Sekhar LN. Intracranial hemorrhage from aneurysms and arteriovenous malformations during pregnancy and the puerperium. Neurosurgery 1990;27:855–65.

102. Meyers PM, Halbach VV, Malek AM, et al. Endovascular treatment of cerebral artery aneurysms during pregnancy: report of three cases. AJNR Am J Neuroradiol 2000;21:1306–11.

103. Horton JC, Chambers WA, Lyons SL, et al. Pregnancy and the risk of hemorrhage from cerebral arteriovenous malformations. Neurosurgery 1990;27: 867–72.

104. Parkinson D, Bachers G. Arteriovenous malformations: summary of 100 consecutive supratentorial cases. J Neurosurg 1980;53:285–99.

105. Weir B, MR L. Management of intracranial aneurysms and arteriovenous malformations during pregnancy. In: Wilkins RH, Rengachary SS, editors. Neurosurgery. New York (NY): McGraw-Hill; 1996. p. 2421–7.

106. Zhu D, Zhao P, Lv N, et al. Rupture risk of cerebral arteriovenous malformations during pregnancy and puerperium: a single-center experience and pooled data analysis. World Neurosurg 2018;111:e308–15.

107. Porras JL, Yang W, Philadelphia E, et al. Hemorrhage risk of brain arteriovenous malformations during pregnancy and puerperium in a North American cohort. Stroke 2017;48(6):1507–13.

108. Ogilvy CS, Stieg PE, Awad I, et al. Recommendations for the management of intracranial arteriovenous malformations: a statement for healthcare professionals for a special writing group of the Stroke Council, American Stroke Association. Stroke 2001;32:1458–71.

109. Toossi S, Moheet AM. Intracerebral hemorrhage in women: a review with special attention to pregnancy and the post-partum period. Neurocrit Care 2019;31(2): 390–8.

110. Salehi Omran S, Parikh NS, Poisson S, et al. Association between pregnancy and cervical artery dissection. Ann Neurol 2020. https://doi.org/10.1002/ana.25813.

111. Chansakul T, Young GS. Neuroimaging in pregnant women. Semin Neurol 2017; 37(6):712–23.
112. Shainker SA, Edlow JA, O'Brien K. Cerebrovascular emergencies in pregnancy. Best Pract Res Clin Obstet Gynaecol 2015;29(5):721–31.
113. Leffert LR, Clancy CR, Bateman BT, et al. Treatment patterns and short-term outcomes in ischemic stroke in pregnancy or postpartum period. Am J Obstet Gynecol 2016;214(6):723.e1–11.
114. Ryman KM, Pace WD, Smith S, et al. Alteplase therapy for acute ischemic stroke in pregnancy: two case reports and a systematic review of the literature. Pharmacotherapy 2019;39(7):767–74.
115. Limaye K, Van de Walle Jones A, Shaban A, et al. Endovascular management of acute large vessel occlusion stroke in pregnancy is safe and feasible. J Neurointerv Surg 2020;12(6):552–6.
116. Lee M-JH,S. Cerebrovascular disorders complicating pregnancy. In: Biller JL CJ, editor. UpToDate. Waltham (MA): UpToDate; 2018.
117. Barghouthi T, Bushnell C. Prevention and management of stroke in obstetrics and gynecology. Clin Obstet Gynecol 2018;61(2):235–42.
118. Duley L, Henderson-Smart D, Knight M, et al. Antiplatelet drugs for prevention of pre-eclampsia and its consequences: systematic review. BMJ 2001;322(7282): 329–33.
119. Bates SM, Greer IA, Middeldorp S, et al. VTE, thrombophilia, antithrombotic therapy, and pregnancy: antithrombotic therapy and prevention of thrombosis, 9th ed: American College of Chest Physicians evidence-based clinical practice guidelines. Chest 2012;141(2 Suppl):e691S–736S.
120. Karalis DG, Hill AN, Clifton S, et al. The risks of statin use in pregnancy: a systematic review. J Clin Lipidol 2016;10(5):1081–90.
121. Lamy C, Hamon JB, Coste J, et al. Ischemic stroke in young women: risk of recurrence during subsequent pregnancies. French Study Group on Stroke in Pregnancy. Neurology 2000;55(2):269–74.
122. Karjalainen L, Tikkanen M, Rantanen K, et al. Pregnancy-associated stroke -a systematic review of subsequent pregnancies and maternal health. BMC Pregnancy Childbirth 2019;19(1):187.
123. van Alebeek ME, de Vrijer M, Arntz RM, et al. Increased risk of pregnancy complications after stroke: the future study (follow-up of transient ischemic attack and stroke patients and unelucidated risk factor evaluation). Stroke 2018; 49(4):877–83.

Neuroimaging During Pregnancy and the Postpartum Period

Dara G. Jamieson, MD[a],*, Jennifer W. McVige, MA, MD[b]

KEYWORDS

- Pregnancy • Magnetic resonance imaging • Headache • Eclampsia
- Cerebral venous thrombosis • Reversible cerebral vasoconstriction syndrome
- Ischemic stroke • Intraparenchymal hemorrhage

KEY POINTS

- The new onset or the exacerbation of preexisting neurologic symptoms during pregnancy often necessitates immediate brain or spinal cord imaging.
- Although headaches early in pregnancy often have a benign etiology, the new onset of headaches in the last trimester and the postpartum period may indicate cerebrovascular disease or an expanding mass lesion, for which brain imaging is necessary.
- Magnetic resonance is the preferred modality to image the brain, cerebral vessels, and the spinal cord during pregnancy and the postpartum period. The ionizing radiation with computed tomography (CT) imaging and the contrast material with magnetic resonance or CT imaging are not known to be hazardous but should be avoided, if possible, during pregnancy.
- The continuum of vascular disorders in pregnancy, including hypertensive disorders of pregnancy (preeclampsia/eclampsia/hemolysis, elevated liver enzymes, and low platelet count syndrome) with its radiological correlate posterior reversible encephalopathy syndrome, cerebral venous thrombosis, reversible cerebral vasoconstriction syndrome/postpartum cerebral angiopathy, and both ischemic and hemorrhagic strokes, is diagnosed by brain and vessel imaging.

INTRODUCTION

During pregnancy and the postpartum period, multiple physiologic changes can exacerbate preexisting neurologic conditions or cause the onset of new neurologic disorders.[1] Neuroimaging, an extension of the neurologic examination in many central nervous system (CNS) disorders, can be crucial in order to differentiate between acute disorders that require immediate intervention and less concerning chronic or benign

The authors have no relevant disclosures.

[a] Department of Neurology, Weill Cornell Medicine, 525 East 68th Street, New York, NY 10065, USA; [b] Dent Neurologic Institute, 3980 Sheridan Drive, Amherst, NY 14226, USA
* Corresponding author.
E-mail address: dgj2001@med.cornell.edu

conditions. Neuroimaging can be problematic during pregnancy, however, because of concern for the fetus. Magnetic resonance (MR) techniques, including MR imaging (MRI), MR angiography (MRA), and MR venography (MRV), are the preferred imaging modalities, especially prior to delivery. Certain neurologic complaints and focal neurologic deficits mandate neuroimaging during pregnancy and the postpartum period. The new onset of a headache is most concerning in the third trimester and up to a couple months after delivery, often mandating brain imaging.[2] Differentiating between common, non–life-threatening headaches (primary headaches) and secondary headaches due to conditions that require neuroimaging and specific treatment is extremely important because some pregnancy-related disorders that cause headache, especially hypertensive disorders of pregnancy, can be life threatening unless treated emergently. Headache may be the initial symptom of multiple cerebrovascular disorders of pregnancy, including cerebral venous thrombosis (CVT), reversible cerebral vasoconstriction syndrome (RCVS), and hypertensive disorders of pregnancy with posterior reversible encephalopathy syndrome (PRES), as well as of expanding cerebral mass lesions.

NEUROIMAGING SAFETY IN PREGNANCY

When the clinical examination and history indicate a need for emergent neuroimaging during pregnancy and the peripartum period, the risk and benefit to mother and fetus must be examined. The potential fetal and maternal risks involving exposure to ionizing radiation, high magnetic fields, contrast dye, increased temperatures, and loud noises must be weighed against the benefits of a maternal imaging diagnosis. Therefore, deferring elective neuroimaging until after delivery may be advised, if appropriate. If neuroimaging is indicated, however, selecting the type of imaging and adapting the procedure in order to maintain the lowest possible risk are recommended.[3]

The recommendations for when to image a pregnant woman do not differ materially from those for imaging a nonpregnant woman, with the exception of routine monitoring of a known lesion that can be planned before or after pregnancy. Brain and spinal cord imaging, especially MR techniques without contrast, generally is safe, so that if imaging would have been obtained in order to evaluate a nonpregnant woman with concerns about an acute neurologic condition, then imaging should be obtained in a similarly symptomatic pregnant woman. An interdisciplinary approach with neurologic consultation is important in order to guide patient care and imaging. For example, a neurologic consultation may determine that the new onset of headache with migraine characteristics in early pregnancy does not need imaging. A consultation about the new onset of a postpartum headache, with or without blood pressure elevation, may suggest emergent brain imaging with techniques used to diagnose brain parenchymal and arterial and venous disorders. Neurologic guidance in choosing the best spinal imaging technique in a postpartum woman with bilateral leg weakness can avoid a less useful technique (eg, computed tomography [CT] scan) in favor of a technique that is able to visualize spinal cord compression or acute lesions (ie, MRI scan).

Neuroimaging with Computed Tomography

CT imaging involves risks related to ionizing radiation exposure; however, the American College of Obstetricians and Gynecologists (ACOG) committee lists the radiation dose as 0.001 mGy to 0.01 mGy (units of absorbed dose) for a head and neck CT scan, which places it in the very-low-dose examinations (<0.1-mGy) category.[3]

CT radiation is highly collimated; therefore, risk to the fetus with scanning of the head and neck is significantly lower due to increased scatter, compared with CT imaging of the chest, abdomen, and pelvis, where the beam is located closer to the uterus.[4] Shielding the abdomen during imaging of the head and neck "does not significantly reduce the minimal fetal radiation exposure but may help to alleviate maternal anxiety."[5] The risk of childhood cancer is less than 1:1000 for most radiologic procedures; however, the risk of fetal carcinogenesis increases by a factor of 2, with larger doses of fetal megagray exposure, such as with a pelvic CT, although the absolute risk is low (1:250).[6,7] Radiation exposure less than 50 mGy has not been associated with fetal injury or side effects; however, higher radiation levels can cause concern depending on the gestational age of the fetus. The mother should be counseled about these risks and benefits prior to the procedure. The ACOG committee opinion recommends that use of a CT scan should not be withheld if clinically indicated, but an MRI scan should be considered a safer alternative if it is appropriate for diagnosis and can be obtained in a timely manner.[3] With few exceptions, MR techniques are more sensitive than CT techniques in detection of parenchymal brain and spinal cord lesions.

Intravenous (IV), low-osmolality iodinated contrast dye, which is elective with a CT scan of the head but mandatory with a CT angiogram (CTA) of the head and neck vessels, can cross the human placenta to the fetus, without well-controlled studies indicating fetal risk. Hypothyroidism in newborns has been reported after receiving fat-soluble, not water-soluble, iodinated contrast in utero. In 2020 the American College of Radiology (ACR) noted, "Given that there are no available data to suggest any potential harm to the fetus from exposure to iodinated contrast medium via maternal IV or intra-arterial injection, we do not recommend routine screening for pregnancy prior to contrast media use."[8] Because an MRA without contrast can provide excellent images of head and neck vessels, however, a CTA, which must be performed with iodinated contrast, rarely is performed during pregnancy. Because of the negligible amount of iodinated contrast excreted in breast milk and then absorbed in the infant's gastrointestinal tract, breastfeeding can be continued without interruption after its use.[3]

Neuroimaging with Magnetic Resonance Imaging

The potential theoretic risks of MRI to a developing fetus include exposure to a static magnetic field (associated with possible cellular changes), pulsed radiofrequency (associated with increased heat), and varying gradient-echo electromagnetic fields (associated with increased noise) as well as to gadolinium-based contrast agents (GBCAs).[6] During the first trimester, MRI scanning may be avoided unless clinically imperative; however, inadvertent exposure does not appear harmful and there is no evidence of teratogenesis, tissue heating effect, or acoustic damage associated with MRI scanning, regardless of trimester.[3,8] Fetal exposure to MRI in the first trimester of pregnancy is not associated with an increased risk of harm to the fetus or to the growing child early in life. The ACR found no evidence that fetal exposure to MRI on a 1.5T or a 3T magnet caused harm to the fetus. Fetal MRI, including single-shot fast spin-echo T2-weighted imaging and diffusion-weighted imaging (DWI), emphasizes that an MRI can be used safely in pregnancy.[8]

Unless the risk outweighs the benefit to the fetus and mother, GBCAs should be avoided, because their use rarely is crucial in MRI studies of the brain and spine, and a GBCA is not necessary for adequate visualization of arteries and veins using MRA and MRV, respectively. In 2020, the ACR recommended, "Because it is unclear how GBCAs will affect the fetus, these agents should be administered with caution to pregnant or potentially pregnant patients. GBCAs should only be used if their usage is considered critical and the potential benefits justify the potential unknown risk to the fetus."[8] As with iodinated contrast, the amount of GBCA excreted in breast milk and absorbed in the infant's gastrointestinal tract is very low, without reports of harm, so breastfeeding should not be interrupted after administration.[3]

Two general concerns with the use GBCAs are rare nephrogenic systemic fibrosis in patients with severe renal disease and the deposition and retention of gadolinium in organs, including the brain, unrelated to any underlying disease.[9] Because nephrogenic systemic fibrosis with severe systemic fibrosis of internal organs can be life threatening, GBACs should be avoided in patients with severe acute or end-stage renal failure. Despite evidence linking MRI signal changes in deep nuclei of the brain with repeated doses of GBACs, the clinical significance of retained gadolinium is unknown, with no data showing any adverse clinical effects.[10] Of the 2 chemical structures of GBCAs, the linear GBCAs, which result in more frequent and more durable retention than do the macrocyclic GBCAs, now rarely are used.

ANESTHETIC COMPLICATIONS OF PREGNANCY: EPIDURAL HEMATOMA, POSTDURAL PUNCTURE HEADACHE, AND PNEUMOCEPHALUS

Imaging of the brain and spinal cord can diagnose anesthetic complications of pregnancy.[11] Persistent leg weakness after spinal or epidural analgesia, accompanied by back pain with bladder and bowel dysfunction, necessitates an MRI of lumbar spine to rule out blood compressing the distal spinal cord and lumbosacral nerve roots. A CT scan of the lumbar spine alone cannot rule out a lumbosacral collection of blood, although the sensitivity of a CT scan may be improved in combination with a lumbar myelogram.

A postpartum postdural puncture headache (PDPH) typically occurs when intracranial pressure decreases due to cerebrospinal fluid (CSF) leakage through an anesthesia-related dural puncture. An unintentional dural puncture occurs in 0.15% to 1.5% of cases of epidural analgesia during labor, with a 50% to 80% risk of developing a PDPH.[12] Although PDPH may be suspected based on alteration in the severity of pain with head position, imaging indicates the diagnosis and the accompanying cerebrovascular lesions. An MRI with contrast injection showing enhancement of the dura and outer layer of arachnoid (pachymeningeal enhancement) along with sagging of the cerebellar tonsils and brainstem due to decreased CSF volume confirms the diagnosis.[5] Downward traction of the brain causing rupture of draining veins may lead to unilateral or bilateral subdural hematomas (**Figs. 1** and **2**) or to thrombosis of cerebral veins with surrounding subarachnoid blood[13,14] (**Fig. 3**). Either CT myelography or MRI of the spine may localize the CSF leak; however, the investigation of a postpartum PDPH beyond head imaging generally is not indicated. Intrathecal air or anesthetic agent causing acute headache with alteration in consciousness immediately after delivery is diagnosed by pneumocephalus seen on CT or MRI of the head (**Fig. 4**).

IMAGING OF HEADACHES IN PREGNANCY
Primary Headaches

Headache accounts for half of emergency department visits of pregnant women with neurologic complaints, most of whom have normal examinations and neuroimaging[15] (**Box 1**). Brain imaging is not needed for most women early in pregnancy who have primary headaches, generally migraine and tension-type headaches, as described in the *International Classification of Headache Disorders*, 3rd edition.[16] Migraines are common in women of reproductive age and approximately 5% of pregnancies are affected by a new-onset or new vtype of headache, which most often is migraine.[17] Although both migraine and tension-type headaches are common in pregnancy and the

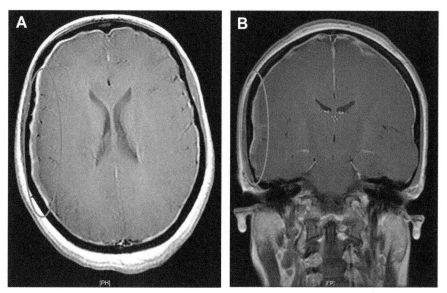

Fig. 1. PDPH. (*A*) Axial and (*B*) coronal contrasted T1 sequences on MRI show diffuse pachymenigeal enhancement and a small right hemispheric subdural hematoma (*ovals*) in a woman with a PDPH after delivery with epidural anesthesia.

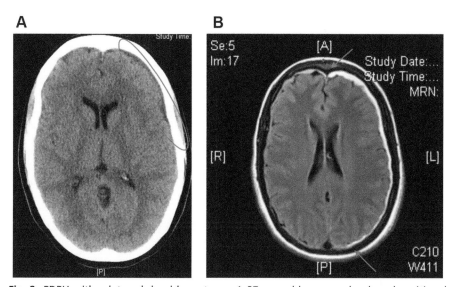

Fig. 2. PDPH with a late subdural hematoma. A 27-year-old woman developed positional headaches a day after delivery with epidural anesthesia. She was treated with an epidural blood patch, without brain imaging, but she returned a week later with persistent headaches. (*A*) An uncontrasted CT scan and (*B*) an uncontrasted MRI scan FLAIR sequence showed a thin left subdural hematoma ([*A*] [*oval*] and [*B*] [*arrows*]).

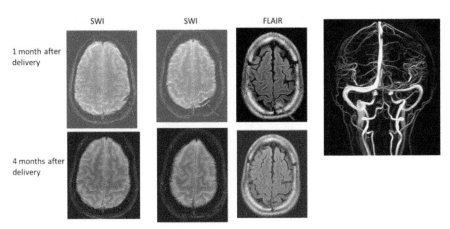

Fig. 3. CVT with surrounding subarachnoid blood. A 35-year-old woman had HELLP syndrome and intrauterine fetal demise at 30 weeks. A month later, she complained of a headache that had lasted a week. Her blood pressure was 150/100 mm Hg. An MRI showed a thrombosed left parietal cortical vein on SWI with surrounding subarachnoid blood on FLAIR sequences. An MRV was normal. After 3 months of anticoagulation, the cortical venous thrombosis had resolved.

postpartum period, the frequency and severity of migraine headaches tend to decrease during the later months of pregnancy due to the shifting ratio between maternal estrogen and progesterone.[18] Approximately 40% of postpartum women may have headaches of variable frequency and severity, often in the first weeks after delivery. Migraine headaches often resume soon after delivery, especially if the woman is not breastfeeding.

Secondary Headaches

Brain imaging, generally using MRI, MRA, and/or MRV, is advised in pregnant or postpartum women whose history and examination suggest headaches that are associated with underlying CNS or systemic disorders. Secondary headaches during pregnancy and the postpartum period can be due to life-threatening disorders for which brain imaging, as well as intracranial and extracranial vessel imaging, is essential for proper diagnosis and treatment. In a study of pregnant women receiving inpatient neurologic consultation, more than one-third of women had secondary headaches, especially women without a prior headache history. The absence of prior similar headaches and the presence of elevated blood pressure, fever, or seizures should prompt neuroimaging and blood pressure monitoring.[19] Many of the secondary headaches are caused by cerebrovascular disease, especially in the later stages of pregnancy or in the weeks immediately after delivery. Cerebrovascular disorders causing headaches, especially due to hemorrhagic and ischemic stroke, are more likely to occur in the 6 weeks immediately after delivery, than they are during pregnancy itself. In a retrospective study of neurologic consultations for acute headache in 63 postpartum women, 27.0% had a primary headache, generally migraine, and 73.0% had a secondary headache. Secondary headaches in postpartum woman were due to PDPH (46%), preeclampsia (26%), and other cerebrovascular disorders (22%), all disorders with characteristic neuroimaging abnormalities.[2]

Screening for various red flags helps indicate who should have brain imaging, usually with MR techniques. Sandoe and Lay[20] have suggested the mnemonic, PREGNANT HA (proteinuria, rapid onset, elevated blood pressure or temperature,

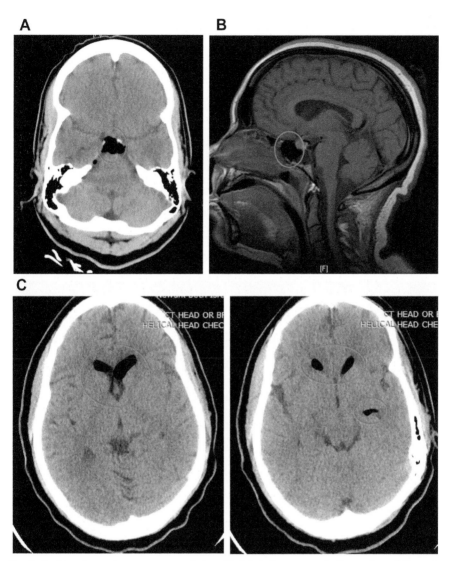

Fig. 4. Postdural puncture pneumocephalus. Air (*circles*) was seen in the region of the sella is seen on (*A*) CT and (*B*) MRI scans in a woman who became unresponsive after an emergent cesarean section with a lumbar epidural catheter. (*C*) Air (*circles*) within the lateral ventricles is seen on CT scan in a woman in labor who became bradycardic and unresponsive after insertion of a lumbar epidural catheter.

gestational age in third trimester, neurologic signs or symptoms, altered level of consciousness, no headache history or known history of a secondary headache disorder, thrombocytopenia or thrombocytosis, high liver function tests or C-reactive protein, or agonizingly severe pain), to remember the red flags for secondary causes of headache during pregnancy. The presence of a headache with elevated blood pressure; a headache different from usual headaches; a lack of significant or rapid relief with the usual effective headache treatments; new focal visual, motor, or sensory symptoms; or new

> **Box 1**
> **Headaches associated with pregnancy**
>
> Primary headaches
> - Migraine with or without aura
> - Tension-type headaches
>
> Secondary headaches caused by
> - Anesthetic complications: PDPH, pneumocephalus, subdural hematoma, CVT
> - Cerebrovascular disease
>   ○ Hypertensive disorders: preeclampsia, eclampsia, HELLP, PRES
>   ○ RCVS/postpartum cerebral angiopathy
>   ○ CVT with increased intracranial pressure, venous infarction
>   ○ Intracranial hemorrhage: subdural hematoma, IPH, SAH
>   ○ Ischemic stroke: arterial dissection, acute arterial infarction
> - Pituitary expansion: adenoma, hemorrhage, lymphocytic hypophysitis
> - Mass lesion expansion: tumor, AVM, aneurysm

abnormalities on neurologic examination, including altered mental status, should result in prompt imaging with MRI, MRA, and/or MRV studies.

Hypertensive disorders of pregnancy, CVT, PRES, and RCVS, all are heralded by a headache, with or without other neurologic complaints, and have diagnostic abnormalities on MRI, MRA, and/or MRV studies. Headache also may be prominent in arterial dissection, acute ischemic stroke, and intraparenchymal hemorrhage (IPH), all diagnoses requiring brain and vessel imaging. Pregnancy-related changes in the pituitary, both vascular and inflammatory, may be associated with a secondary headache. Even some nonvascular secondary headaches associated with pregnancy, such as PDPHs, a type of postpartum headache related to obstetric anesthesia, may have superimposed cerebrovascular conditions. Some causes of secondary headache that are particularly common in or unique to pregnancy are described later and are listed in **Box 1**.

Cerebrovascular disorders in pregnancy
Although the incidence of stroke in general has decreased over recent decades, stroke associated with pregnancy has increased[21] or remained unchanged.[22] An acute stroke occurred in 1 of every 2222 pregnancy-related hospitalizations in 2015, a rate that is unchanged compared with 2007.[22] The rate of in-hospital mortality among pregnant women with acute stroke decreased from 5.5% in 2007 to 2.7% in 2015. Risk factors for acute stroke associated with pregnancy include advanced maternal age, cardiac disease, obesity, smoking, hyperlipidemia, migraine, and gestational hypertension.[21,22]

The risk of cerebrovascular disorders in pregnancy is greatest in the 6-week period after delivery.[23] Kamel and colleagues[24] evaluated the risk of primary thrombotic events after pregnancy compared with the same period 1 year later and found that the risk was markedly higher within 6 weeks after delivery, with an absolute risk difference of 22.1 events per 100,000 deliveries, and was modestly but significant higher during the period of 7 weeks to 12 weeks after delivery, for an absolute risk difference of 3.0 events per 100,000 deliveries. An elevated risk of thrombosis persisted until at least 12 weeks after delivery, with a lower increase in risk beyond 6 weeks.[24] During this entire postpartum period, new significant neurologic complaints, both of headache and focal neurologic symptoms, should be evaluated with an MRI of the brain and with head and neck vessel imaging by MRA or CTA.

The multiple cerebrovascular disorders associated with pregnancy are interconnected with overlapping clinical presentations, pathophysiology, and imaging lesions.[25] Hypertensive disorders of pregnancy, CVT, PRES, RCVS/postpartum cerebral angiopathy, and stroke are on a continuum with hypertension, thrombosis, and vasospasm risking disabling or life-threatening maternal stroke, both ischemic and hemorrhagic. Brain and cerebral vessel imaging may reveal multiple overt and subtle imaging abnormalities apparent in the same patient indicative of sequential or simultaneous vascular disorders.

Cerebral venous thrombosis. The increased risk of CVT during later months of pregnancy and up to 8 weeks postpartum is caused by multiple pregnancy-related factors, including hypercoagulability, dehydration, infection, and iatrogenic intracranial hypotension from anesthetic dural puncture. Headache, change in mental status or alteration in level of consciousness, intracranial hypertension leading to papilledema with potential visual loss, focal or generalized seizures, and focal neurologic deficits due to venous infarcts with hemorrhage all can be due to CVT. When there is the sudden onset a neurologic deficit with concern about an ischemic or hemorrhagic stroke, emergent brain imaging, generally a CT scan of the head, is mandatory. When the presentation suggesting CVT is less apoplectic, an MRI of the head should be obtained because of improved visualization of large and small cerebral veins as well as dural sinuses.[26] MRV or CT venography image the thrombosed dural sinuses and the larger cerebral veins in CVT.

A noncontrasted CT scan of the head can reveal a hyperdense thrombus in the dural sinuses or cortical veins; however, the finding may be subtle, so an MRI scan of the head is preferred for diagnosis of CVT. With contrast injection, the CT scan can show an empty delta sign due to the lack of flow outlining a triangular filling defect caused by a clot in the superior sagittal sinus and the dural sinus torcula[27] (**Fig. 5**).

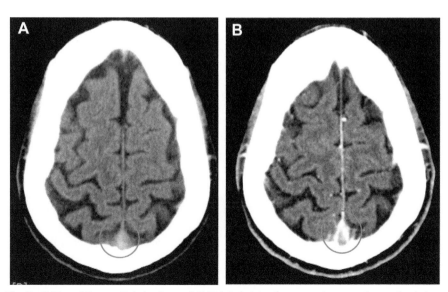

Fig. 5. CVT on CT scan. Subtle signs of CVT (*circles*) in the posterior superior sagittal sinus include (*A*) hyperdensity in the region of the thrombus on an uncontrasted CT scan and (*B*) a filling defect caused by the clot surrounded by contrast on a contrasted CT scan.

CT venography, which requires IV iodinated contrast injection, can be used in post-partum period. With intracranial hypertension due to CVT, brain imaging shows diffuse cerebral edema, posterior flattening and protrusion of the globes; enlarged subarach-noid space around the optic nerves, or an empty sella. Cases of CVT associated with PRES have been reported, indicating a continuum between the various forms of cere-brovascular disease associated with pregnancy.[28] Bleeding into a venous infarct can present as an IPH, and CVT should be considered in a peripartum woman with an IPH of unclear etiology.

MRI and MRV of the brain, without need for contrast injection, are used to evaluate pregnant women with suspected CVT; but contrast injection may increase the diag-nostic yield to evaluate suspected postpartum CVT.[29] MRV assesses flow in large draining cerebral veins and the dural sinuses; but an MRV, even with contrast, can miss thrombosis of isolated cortical veins, which is a risk for ongoing thrombosis and is better seen on susceptibility-weighted imaging (SWI) or gradient-recalled echo (GRE) sequences on MRI of the brain. MRI improves the diagnostic utility in the diagnosis of CVT, including with fluid-attenuated inversion recovery (FLAIR) se-quences showing subtle nonaneurysmal subarachnoid hemorrhage (SAH) in the areas of venous thrombosis[30] (see **Fig. 3**). Cerebral venous infarction due to CVT is associ-ated with more peri-infarct edema than with an arterial infarction and is associated with a hyperintense signal on T2 and FLAIR sequences. The localization of cerebral edema in CVT overlaps arterial territories, especially notable with involvement in bilat-eral hemispheres and both anterior and posterior arterial territories.

Hypertensive disorders of pregnancy: preeclampsia/eclampsia/hemolysis, elevated liver enzymes, and low platelet count syndrome. The cerebrovascular manifestations of hypertensive disorders of pregnancy are a major cause of maternal death. Blood pressure elevation in hypertensive disorders of pregnancy is accompanied by signs and symptoms of end-organ hypertensive damage, such as headaches, vision changes, seizures, abdominal pain, peripheral edema, and proteinuria. Other manifes-tations of end-organ damage include hemolysis, elevated liver function tests, and decreased platelets as part of the hemolysis, elevated liver enzymes, and low platelet count (HELLP) syndrome.[31] Untreated preeclampsia with acute blood pressure eleva-tion, especially a systolic blood pressure of greater than or equal to 160 mm Hg or dia-stolic blood pressure of greater than or equal to 110 mm Hg, onset from 20 weeks gestation through approximately 8 weeks postpartum, can cause ischemic and hem-orrhagic strokes. Postpartum women are particularly vulnerable to devastating neuro-logic complications of hypertensive disorders of pregnancy. Preeclampsia/eclampsia/ HELLP syndrome often is heralded by the new onset of headache later in pregnancy or after delivery. Other causes of peripartum headache, such as migraine, PDPH, and postpartum cerebral angiopathy/RCVS, are not associated with blood pressure eleva-tion, the hallmark of hypertensive disorders of pregnancy. The neurologic manifesta-tions of hypertensive disorders of pregnancy are caused by disordered cerebral vascular autoregulation, with endothelial damage and capillary leakage causing cere-bral edema. Biomarkers in the maternal circulation that regulate blood vessel growth can predict or diagnosis pregnancy pathologies and may reflect the severity of outcome of hypertensive disorders of pregnancy.[32] In the earliest stages of hyperten-sive disorders of pregnancy associated with headache, there may be no pathogno-monic findings on either MRI or CT, and a diagnosis should be made on clinical suspicion alone. Nevertheless, a noncontrast brain MRI should be performed to look for other conditions, in particular stroke, CVT, and PRES.[33,34] The continuum of overlapping cerebrovascular complications of pregnancy are variably associated

CT

MRI

FLAIR   FLAIR   DWI

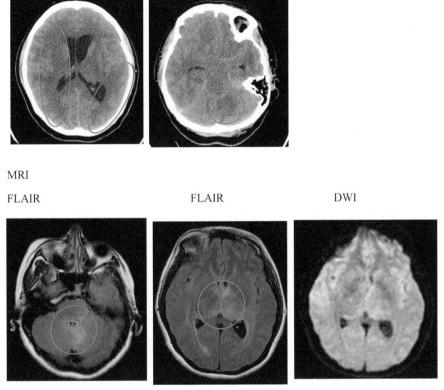

Fig. 6. PRES without elevated blood pressure. A 28-year-old normotensive woman developed a headache and dizziness 4 weeks after delivery. The CT and MRI scans showed PRES (*circles*).

with elevated blood pressure. Acute elevation in blood pressure generally, but not always, is seen with the imaging diagnosis of PRES (**Fig. 6**). Untreated, preeclampsia/eclampsia/HELLP syndrome can result in both ischemic and hemorrhagic strokes and progression to imaging showing PRES and/or RCVS (**Fig. 7**). Unlike hypertensive disorders of pregnancy and the imaging correlate PRES, isolated RCVS that is not caused by untreated elevated blood pressure generally is not associated with elevated blood pressure. Rarely, RCVS can lead to ischemic or hemorrhagic stroke in the absence of hypertension. Hypertension as a complication of pregnancy increases a woman's risk of ischemic stroke in her future, unrelated to future pregnancies.[35]

Posterior reversible encephalopathy syndrome. PRES is a characteristic neuroimaging syndrome that can present clinically with a headache, encephalopathy, visual changes, and seizures. Patchy parieto-occipital or diffuse hemispheric hyperintensities on T2 and FLAIR sequences and T1 sequence hypointensities are imaging characteristics; however, PRES can involve all areas of the brain and, in rare cases, the brainstem and spinal cord. A CT of the head may be normal or reveal patchy posterior or diffuse hypodensities in the bilateral cerebral hemispheres (**Fig. 8**). These changes do not follow a particular arterial distribution, differentiating them from cerebral arterial

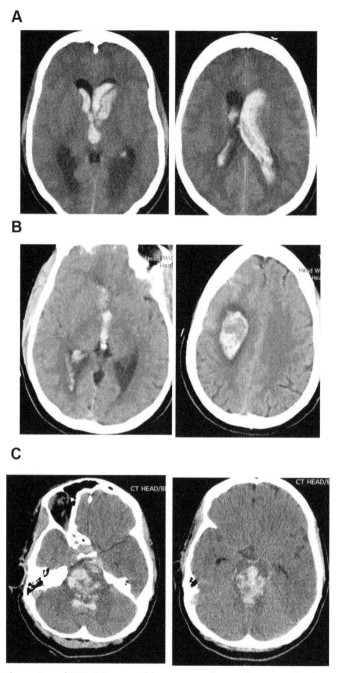

Fig. 7. Preeclampsia and IPH. IPHs caused by untreated acute hypertension in preeclampsia can originate in multiple anatomic locations, including in (A) the subcortical nuclei, (B) the cerebral cortex, and (C) the brainstem. (A) A 42-year-old woman developed elevated blood pressures a week after an uneventful delivery. After a day with a severe headache, she became unresponsive. A CT scan showed a basal ganglia hemorrhage extending into the ventricles. No underlying lesion was found on autopsy. (B) A 35-year-old woman developed

infarction but potentially confusing them with venous infarction associated with CVT. Recognition of the clinical symptoms and the significance of the elevated blood pressure as a cause of PRES should lead to immediate blood pressure lowering, with the resolution of symptoms and imaging findings. Imaging consistent with PRES often is found in women with preeclampsia/eclampsia/HELLP syndrome as well as with a multitude of other conditions, some of which are not associated with elevated blood pressure. Pregnancy-related PRES usually is a complication of untreated preeclampsia/eclampsia/HELLP syndrome but rarely can be found in normotensive peripartum women[36] (see **Fig. 6**). The underlying pathophysiology of this spectrum of disorders with the radiological presentation of PRES is thought to be due to loss of cerebral autoregulation, with increased capillary leakage resulting in vasogenic edema predominantly in the parietal and occipital lobes. Imaging changes, however, can be anywhere in the CNS.[37] Brain imaging is crucial, preferably with a noncontrast brain MRI, in pregnant women with symptoms of headache and blurred vision suspicious for a PRES-related disorder (**Fig. 9**). Untreated PRES, associated with or separate from preeclampsia/eclampsia/HELLP syndrome, can lead to strokes, both ischemic and hemorrhagic. As with the hypertensive disorders of pregnancy, there is an overlap in physiologic mechanisms of PRES and RCVS, and cases of concurrent conditions are reported.[33,38–40] The presence of vasospasm in patients with PRES has been documented by catheter angiography and MRA, again emphasizing the overlap between the various types of cerebrovascular syndromes in pregnancy.[41]

Reversible cerebral vasoconstriction syndrome/postpartum cerebral angiopathy. RCVS is a clinical and radiographic syndrome, of multiple etiologies, that is associated with a headache of generally abrupt onset, with vessel imaging showing reversible multifocal vasoconstriction in large and medium size arteries.[42–44] The vasospastic disorders of postpartum cerebral angiopathy, Call-Fleming syndrome, drug-induced cerebral vasospasm, and benign cerebral angiopathy parts of an RCVS spectrum.[45] The presence of circulating angiogenic factors may explain the increased risk of RCVS in the postpartum period.[46] In uncomplicated cases of RCVS, not associated with progression to an ischemic or hemorrhagic stroke, a CT or MRI scan of the brain generally is unrevealing. Vasospasm, with beading, may be seen on MRA of the head, CTA of the head, or cerebral catheter angiography; although, MRA of the head without contrast, the preferred vessel imaging modality in pregnant women, may reveal only subtle or nonspecific changes. Catheter angiography shows vasospasm, which may appear similar to the beaded and tapered vessels, with cutoff and ballooning, seen with CNS vasculitis (**Fig. 10**). Follow-up vascular imaging, generally MRA or CTA, may show resolution of cerebral vasospasm.

Postpartum RCVS, although generally associated with a favorable outcome, can be complicated by ischemic stroke, IPH, or nonaneurysmal SAH (**Fig. 11**). An approximately 2% mortality due to IPH and ischemic stroke has been associated with RCVS.[45] Subtle SAH associated with RCVS without an underlying cerebral aneurysm is a benign finding.[47] As with CVT, the small volume of subarachnoid blood associated

---

acute hypertension and a headache an hour after an uncomplicated cesarean section. Six hours later, after continued elevated blood pressures, she became left hemiplegic. A CT scan showed a right frontal lobar hemorrhage. No underlying lesion was found on catheter angiography. (*C*) A 30-year-old woman with elevated blood pressure, proteinuria and ankle swelling as an outpatient was found at home unresponsive at 32 weeks of pregnancy. A CT scan showed an extensive brainstem hemorrhage, originating in the pons.

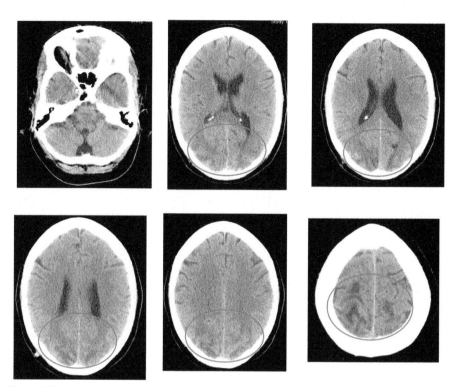

Fig. 8. Eclampsia with PRES on CT scan. A 45-year-old woman, 36 weeks pregnant in active labor, had a blood pressure of 182/88, with a headache and blurred vision. She had a generalized tonic-clonic seizure. A CT scan of the brain showed posterior hypoattenuation consistent with PRES (*circled*). A healthy baby was delivered by emergent sectioning and blood pressure was controlled with IV nicardipine. She was discharged to home on antihypertensive medication.

with RCVS usually is pericortical, as opposed to intracisternal, and the area surrounding the hemorrhage should be evaluated for a thrombosed cortical vein. Isolated RCVS usually is benign, with headache the only symptom, without blood pressure elevation, but RCVS can be caused by hypertensive disorders of pregnancy, with imaging showing PRES. An RCVS-related headache may be treated with calcium channel blockers, but the removal of the precipitating agent, including the causative elevated blood pressure, generally leads to clinical and imaging resolution. Although RCVS generally is a postpartum cerebral angiopathy, it has been reported to occur antepartum, in combination with hypertensive disorders of pregnancy and PRES.[48,49]

Intracranial hemorrhage. Intracranial hemorrhage, both IPH and aneurysmal SAH (as distinct from CVT or RCVS-associated SAH), although rare during pregnancy, constitutes the third leading cause of non–obstetric-related mortality in pregnant and postpartum women, with risk especially prominent in the postpartum period. The causes of hemorrhages in pregnancy are different from those in the general population and largely are related to physiologic changes in pregnancy, such as increased blood volume and cardiac output, elevation of blood pressure, loss of cerebral vascular autoregulation, and vascular wall remodeling. Hypertensive disorders of pregnancy are the

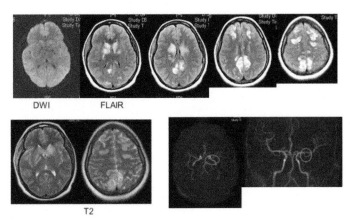

DWI   FLAIR

T2

An MRI about a week later showed resolution of the lesions.

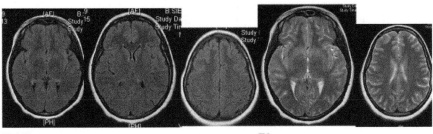

FLAIR   T2

Fig. 9. Eclampsia with PRES on MRI. A 19-year-old woman, 31 weeks pregnant with elevated blood pressure, seized. A placental abruption with fetal demise was diagnosed. Her blood pressure and seizures were controlled, and a stillborn fetus was delivered. A CT scan (not shown) revealed bilateral parietal medial hypodensities and bilateral internal capsule hypo-densities. An MRI showed multifocal changes of PRES on FLAIR and T2 imaging with vaso-spasm (*circle*) on MRA consistent with RCVS. There was a tiny area of infarction (*circle*) on DWI. HELLP syndrome was diagnosed. About a week later, there was clinical and imaging resolution.

major preventable cause of IPH during pregnancy (**Fig. 12**) and the postpartum period, but underlying structural lesions also can bleed, associated with pregnancy.

Cerebrovascular lesions present prior to pregnancy, such as arteriovenous malformations (AVMs), cavernous malformations, and cerebral aneurysms, can cause IPH.[50] Bleeding of an AVM causes parenchymal and/or intraventricular hemorrhage.[51] The risk of cavernous malformation–related symptomatic hemorrhages during pregnancy is not increased.[52] The risk of aneurysmal SAH during pregnancy and delivery is lower than in nonpregnant women.[53] Although there may be an increase in aneurysmal size with the hemodynamic changes in pregnancy, the risk of hemorrhagic cerebrovascular disease, presenting with the apoplectic onset of a severe headache, is increased immediately after delivery, with a majority of pregnancy-related aneurysmal SAHs occurring after delivery[54] (**Fig. 13**). In a pregnant or postpartum woman with the sudden onset of a severe headache, a noncontrasted CT scan of the head has high sensitivity and specificity for detecting acute intracranial blood, including in the intraventricular and subarachnoid spaces, and should be an emergency screening study prior to a more detailed imaging evaluation of the brain (**Fig. 14**). Although

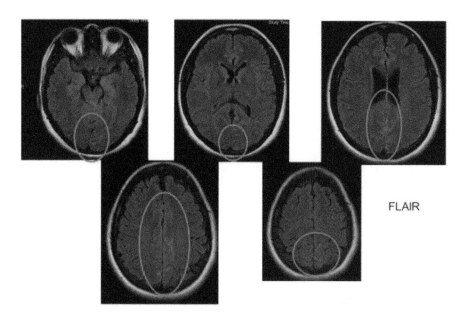

FLAIR

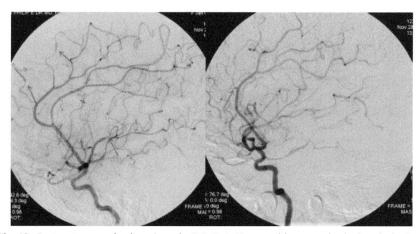

Fig. 10. Postpartum cerebral angiopathy/RCVS. A 40-year-old woman had a headache immediately prior to delivery that persisted to postpartum day 7. Her blood pressure was normal. An MRI showed subtle abnormal FLAIR signal posteriorly (*circles*) and the MRA of the head was nondiagnostic. Multifocal areas of arterial spasm (*arrows*) were seen on catheter angiography consistent with postpartum cerebral angiopathy/RCVS.

cerebral catheter angiography provides the most detailed description of a cerebral aneurysm, a CTA of the head has very high sensitivity and specificity, especially for larger aneurysms that are at high risk of bleeding.[55] Prior to delivery, an MRA of the head without contrast can be used to screen for aneurysms that are large enough to be at increased risk of bleeding. With both noninvasive imaging modalities, however, small and/or distal aneurysms, including those with some risk of bleeding, may be missed.

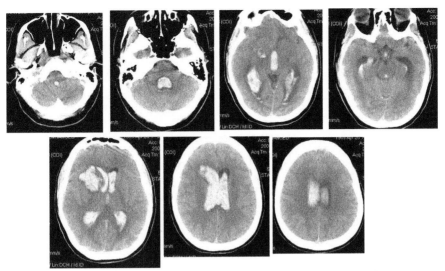

Fig. 11. Postpartum cerebral angiopathy causing an IPH. A 43-year-old woman complained of a moderate headache the day after an uneventful vaginal delivery. Her blood pressures were normal. The next day she complained of a suddenly severe headache with marked blood pressure elevation. She immediately became unresponsive. A CT scan showed a right basal ganglia IPH with intraventricular extension. No underlying brain lesion was found on autopsy. Postpartum cerebral angiopathy (RCVS) was suspected as a cause of the headache in the setting of normal blood pressures.

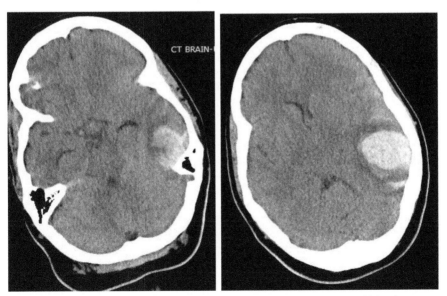

Fig. 12. HELLP and IPH. A 40-year-old woman, who had 2 days of elevated blood pressure, headache and blurred vision in the thirty-second week of her pregnancy, became confused. A CT scan showed a right posterior tempoparietal lobar IPH. HELLP syndrome was diagnosed.

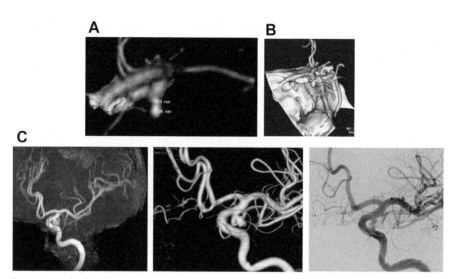

Fig. 13. Cerebral aneurysm during pregnancy. (*A*) A 40-year-old woman had a small incidental left posterior communication artery aneurysm measuring 3.6 mm × 2.4 mm on CTA of the head. (*B*) Two years later, a follow-up CTA study showed that the aneurysm, measured at 3.5 cm × 2.6 cm, essentially was unchanged in size. (*C*) At age 44 years, she became pregnant with twins. An MRA of the head at 31 weeks showed that the bilobed and irregular aneurysm had enlarged to 5 cm × 3.5 cm.

Arterial ischemic stroke. The risk of arterial ischemic stroke is increased around the time of delivery and for up to 8 weeks after delivery. In the postpartum period, acute ischemic stroke is less common than IPH. Pregnancy-specific arterial ischemic stroke risk factors include estrogen-induced hypercoagulability, cardioembolism due to pregnancy-related cardiomyopathies, hypertensive disorders of pregnancy, RCVS, and cervical arterial dissection. Paradoxic cerebral embolization occurs as embolic material, such as amniotic fluid, air, trophoblastic material, and venous clots, and crosses from the draining venous to the cerebral arterial circulations in the setting of a right-to-left cardiac shunt. Although headaches are not typical for patients with arterial ischemic stroke, they are not uncommon in pregnant patients with ischemic stroke and may be the initial reason for obtaining brain imaging.[56] Otherwise, clinical presentations of ischemic stroke in pregnancy do not differ from the usual focal neurologic deficits, change in mental status, and, less commonly, seizures, seen in the nonpregnant population. A CT scan of the head may show no abnormality early after an acute ischemic stroke, but within hours the CT scan may show loss of gray-white differentiation, sulcal effacement, and hypoattenuation of the infarcted area. Chronic infarcts appear hypodense with associated volume loss. An MRI of the brain reveals hyperintense lesions on DWI with correlating hypointense areas on apparent diffusion coefficient sequences (eg, restricted diffusion), noticeable generally minutes from symptom onset. Later ischemic changes are associated with hyperintensities on T2 and FLAIR sequences that eventually are hypointense on the T1-weighted sequence. Ruling out hemorrhage with brain imaging, generally an emergent CT scan, is imperative for appropriate acute management that should focus on preservation of maternal neurologic functioning. Pregnancy is only a relative contraindication to treatment with IV thrombolysis, which should be offered when indicated within the appropriate treatment time window. Endovascular intervention, even with its radiation and contrast exposure, could be considered if MRA of the head shows a large vessel occlusion.[57,58] A cerebellar infarct with evolving edema and hydrocephalus risks potentially fatal brainstem compression if surgical posterior fossa decompression is delayed. A CT (**Fig. 15**) or MRI (**Fig. 16**) scan of the head may help to prognosticate after postpartum cardiac arrest results in maternal hypoxic-ischemic encephalopathy.

Postpartum arterial dissection occurs with tearing of the endothelial lining of extracranial and intracranial arterial vessels, producing headache or neck pain, and local (eg, Horner syndrome and lower cranial nerve deficits) or cerebral (eg, transient ischemic attack and ischemic stroke) symptoms and signs. Ischemic stroke usually is caused by distal clot embolization from a dissection flap, with a hemodynamic cause from an occlusive dissection being less common. Postpartum arterial dissection appears to be unrelated to delivery type and can involve single or multiple, posterior, and/or anterior circulation vessels as well as cardiac and renal arteries. The reason for this postpartum vulnerability is unknown and appears to be unrelated to an underlying connective tissue disorder.[59,60] Dissection is visualized best during pregnancy by an uncontrasted MRA of head and neck; an MRA of the neck with contrast or a CTA can be obtained after delivery. Vessel imaging may show a characteristic flame-like tapering of a dissection to occlusion in the internal carotid artery (**Fig. 17**). Cross-sectional T1 imaging with fat suppression may show a characteristic crescent-shaped deformity in the wall of the dissected internal carotid artery.

CENTRAL NERVOUS SYSTEM MASS LESIONS
Cerebral Neoplasms in Pregnancy

Brain cancer is a rare malignancy during pregnancy at 1.3% (3 out of 227 pregnant cancer patients), according to a survey in Japan.[61] An intracranial mass lesion can expand or hemorrhage due to hormonal and vascular changes during pregnancy. Primary brain tumors and metastases can become symptomatic or recur or progress during pregnancy, and pathology can transition from a low-grade to a more aggressive form.[62] Neuroimaging by MRI should be used to investigate focal brain or spinal cord symptoms, because treatment of brain tumors during pregnancy may lead to a favorable outcome without apparent congenital malformations.[63] Symptomatic tumor expansion is most likely to occur with a rise in cardiac output and intravascular volume during the last trimester, causing growth in tumor vascularity and hemorrhage risk. Headaches can be due to increased intracranial pressure from accelerated tumor expansion from changes in circulating hormones (eg, progesterone, estrogen, and prostacyclins) or in tumor estrogen and progesterone receptors or from tumor hemorrhage.[64] Brain imaging prior to spinal/epidural anesthesia or vaginal delivery can evaluate for hydrocephalus with increased intracranial pressure in women who have a CNS mass lesions.

Primary brain or metastatic tumors with a significant vascular component are particularly susceptible to hemorrhage-related headaches during pregnancy. Placental derived choriocarcinomas are rare but can metastasize to the CNS, presenting with an acute headache and focal neurologic deficits in the setting of tumor hemorrhage.[65] Even benign vascular mass lesions, such as CNS hemangioblastomas, can become acutely symptomatic during pregnancy because of expansion or hemorrhage presenting as IPH.[66,67]

Meningiomas account for 35% of all primary brain tumors and are twice as common in women as in men, with incidence increasing with age.[68] They express progesterone (70%) and estrogen (30%) receptors, but the mechanism of pregnancy-related

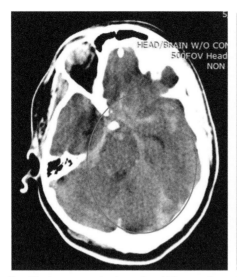
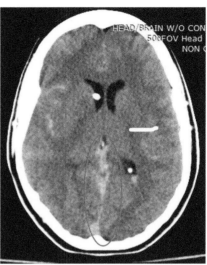

Fig. 14. Aneurysmal subarachnoid hemorrhage in woman with preeclampsia. A 25-year-old woman had headaches and elevated blood pressures at 37 weeks of pregnancy. At 38 weeks, proteinuria was detected, and she was delivered by sectioning. Two days later, still with elevated blood pressures, she had sudden worsening of her headache and she seized. A CT scan of the head showed diffuse SAH (*circled*) due to a previously undetected cerebral aneurysm.

expansion likely is vascular rather than endocrinological.[69] Meningiomas, especially the more vascular (angiomatous) ones, tend to grow rapidly during pregnancy and may become symptomatic due to mass effect, edema, hypervascularity and intratumoral hemorrhage, and/or necrosis.[70] In addition, hormones in pregnancy can act on the steroid receptors expressed by meningiomas and cause accelerated growth and vascularity.[71] Meningiomas on T1-weighted and T2-weighted MRI sequences are isointense, extraparenchymal mass lesions with a broad dural attachment and adjacent hyperostosis. A dural tail may not be seen on an unenhanced scan obtained

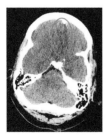
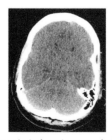
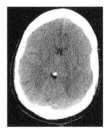
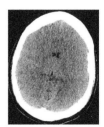

Fig. 15. Postpartum hypoxic-ischemic encephalopathy. A 35-year-old woman underwent an uncomplicated cesarean section for a full-term delivery. Approximately 6 hours after delivery she was found apneic and pulseless. She was resuscitated but unresponsive. A CT scan showed diffuse sulcal effacement with decreased ventricular size and effaced temporal horns (*arrows*) and basilar cisterns. Diffuse loss of gray-white differentiation was seen with focal hypodensity within the frontal lobes in the anterior cerebral artery distribution consistent with infarcts (*circle*).

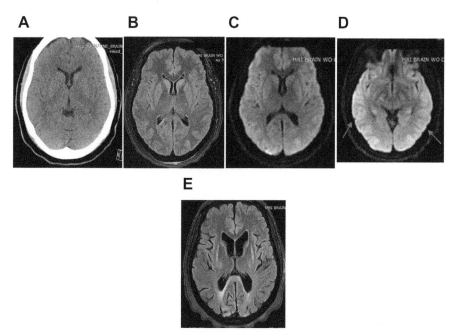

Fig. 16. Postpartum hypoxic-ischemic damage on MRI scan. A 40-year-old woman, 38 weeks pregnant, developed acute severe pulmonary edema after 2 days of severe elevation of blood pressure with proteinuria. Immediately after her baby was delivered emergently by sectioning, she had a cardiopulmonary arrest with return of spontaneous circulation in about 5 minutes. (*A*) An immediate CT scan was unremarkable, but an MRI scan obtained 4 days later showed subtle abnormal signal in the basal ganglia on (*B*) FLAIR (*circle*) and (*C*) DWI sequences as well as restricted diffusion in the cortex (*arrows*) on (*D*) DWI sequence. (*E*) An MRI scan 2 years later showed marked atrophy on the FLAIR sequence.

during pregnancy. Parasellar meningiomas may present in the later months of pregnancy with headaches due to the expanding mass effect of hydrocephalus caused by elevated intracranial pressure, distortion of the diaphragm sella, or parasellar dura irritation. Skull-based meningiomas that produce visual complaints and cranial nerve palsies during pregnancy require surgical resection.[70] The tumor mass effect in the parafalcine area can distort dural venous sinuses, as seen on MRI and MRV (**Fig. 18**).

Gliomas (grades I–IV) are the most common malignant primary brain tumor, with glioblastoma (grade IV) accounting for 16% of all primary brain tumors.[68] Gliomas grades II and III, but not grade I, grow in size during pregnancy, attributed to their increased tumor vascularity and angiogenesis.[72] In a small retrospective series, 4 pregnant women with treated gliomas delivered healthy babies.[73] MRI scanning of the brain, even without contrast injection, can suggest a glioma diagnosis prior to a biopsy for a tissue diagnosis.

Pituitary Lesions in Pregnancy

During pregnancy, the normal pituitary enlarges due to hormonal and vascular changes. Women with known prolactin-secreting pituitary adenomas should be monitored with MRI scans of the sellar region, visual field testing, and blood work because

A

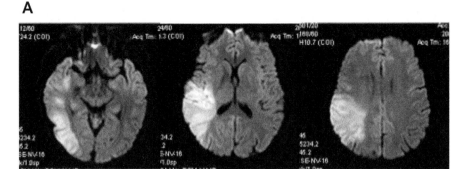

B

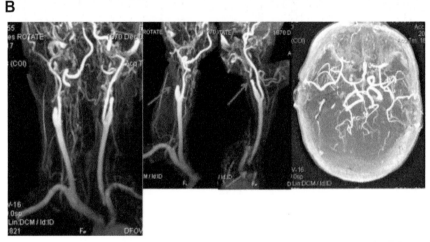

Fig. 17. Postpartum arterial dissections. Several days after delivery, a woman had the sudden onset of left-sided weakness with an acute right middle cerebral infarct on the DWI sequence on (A) MRI and (B) multiple dissections (on MRA of neck [*arrows*]), including bilateral internal carotid artery dissections on MRA. The right middle cerebral artery branch was occluded (*arrow*) on the MRA of the head.

enlargement during pregnancy occurs in 18% of macroadenomas and 2.5% of microadenomas.[74] Pituitary enlargement during pregnancy risks mass effect, hemorrhage, and infarction. The onset of headache and temporal visual loss with pituitary hemorrhage usually is apoplectic[75] (**Fig. 19**). Symptoms of panhypopituitarism in Sheehan syndrome generally occur insidiously after a pituitary infarct due to hypotension or extreme blood loss associated with delivery. MRI may show an enlarged pituitary with central hypointensity on T1-weighted images and hyperintensity on T2-weighted images with irregular enhancement. With time, the pituitary atrophies and a residual empty sella are noted.[76]

Lymphocytic hypophysitis is an inflammatory autoimmune disease of the pituitary gland of peripartum women with characteristic imaging of a nonhemorrhagic, perisellar expansion of the adenohypophysis, neurohypophysis, or infundibulum, with isodense or hypodense signals on T1-weighted images on MRI[77] (**Fig. 20**). Symptoms include headache, nausea, and vomiting and a bitemporal visual field deficit due to the compression of the enlarged pituitary on the optic chiasm. Although empiric

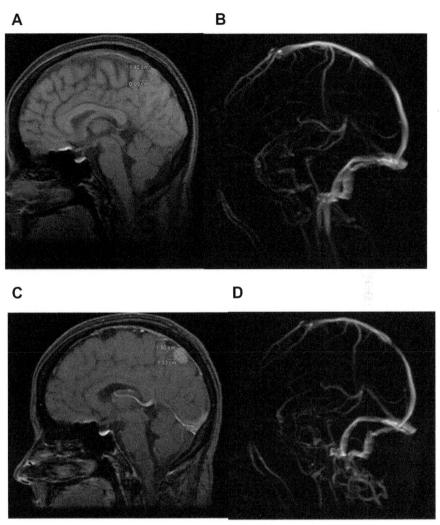

Fig. 18. Meningioma expansion with pregnancy. A 28-year-old, 9 weeks pregnant woman complained of visual blurring and a severe headache. (*A*) An MRI brain showed a rounded, extra-axial parafalcine mass on T1-weighted images. (*B*) An MRV showed focal narrowing of the superior sagittal sinus. (*C*) A contrasted MRI scan after delivery showed that the hyperintense lesion on T1 weighted images had increased in size, (*D*) with stable narrowing of the superior sagittal sinus on MRV.

steroid treatment could be considered, a diagnosis usually is made on pathologic examination of a frozen pituitary biopsy specimen, so as not to remove a functioning pituitary gland. Steroid treatment generally leads to return of the pituitary to its usual size and normal function.[78]

Central Nervous System Inflammation and Demyelination

During pregnancy, hormonal changes alter maternal anti-inflammatory responses in order to protect against fetal rejection. These changes can cause the onset of a new disease state or exacerbate a preexisting condition. With an increase in maternal

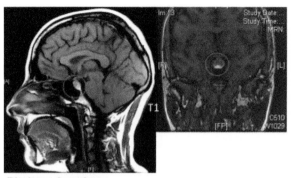
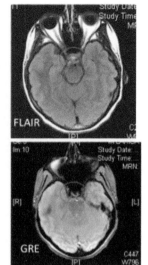

Pituitary Apoplexy
Sxs: headache, VF deficit, ophthalmoplegia, decreased
consciousness, pituitary dysfunction
Causes: pregnancy, tumor, XRT, head trauma, blood pressure
alterations, cardiac surgery, anticoagulation, dopamine
agonists

Fig. 19. Pituitary hemorrhage during pregnancy. A 33-year-old woman, 31 weeks pregnant, developed headaches without visual changes. An MRI showed hemorrhage into her pituitary gland on sagittal and coronal T1, axial FLAIR, and axial GRE sequences (*circles*). No pituitary lesion was found on follow-up imaging after delivery. The boxes are labeled as T1, FLAIR, GRE. XRT, radiation therapy; VF, visual field.

hormones, immune responses to support and protect fetal development increase, and regulatory cells that affect T-cell–mediated responses decrease.[79] Although the severity of some immune-mediated, inflammatory diseases, however, such as multiple sclerosis (MS) may be reduced, other diseases, such as neuromyelitis optica spectrum disorder (NMOSD), may worsen with pregnancy.

Multiple Sclerosis and Other Demyelinating Disorders

Demyelinating disorders, including MS, clinically isolated syndrome, NMOSD, and acute disseminated encephalomyelitis (ADEM), may present de novo or may become acutely symptomatic during pregnancy.[80] MS is an autoimmune disease, with inflammatory responses involving demyelination and axonal damage, that preferentially affects women with onset most frequently during reproductive years. NMSOD also occurs predominantly in woman of childbearing age and is associated with inflammatory and demyelinating lesions of the brain, spinal cord, and optic nerve as well as seropositivity for antibodies targeting aquaporin-4 (immunoglobulin G).

Fertility does not seem to be impaired in women with MS or NMOSD, although decisions about getting pregnant may be complicated for women with these chronic disorders that are associated with a wide range of disability. Results of studies of fertility biomarkers are variable, but a study of levels of antimüllerian hormone (AMH), an ovarian peptide hormone that is considered to be a marker for ovarian reserve, did not find a significant difference in mean serum AMH levels in women with relapsing-remitting MS and NMOSD compared with healthy controls.[81,82] Once pregnancy is achieved, hormone-mediated immune responses are believed to alter relapse rates. Pregnancy may decrease the natural history of MS relapses, with a possible increase in relapse risk in the postpartum period; pregnancy itself does not appear to be harmful for long-term prognosis of MS.[82] The use of effective disease-modifying therapies

A

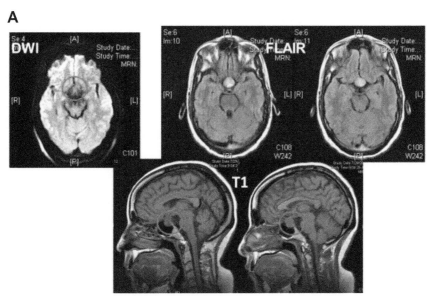

B

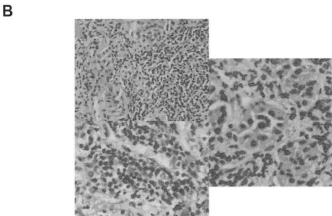

C

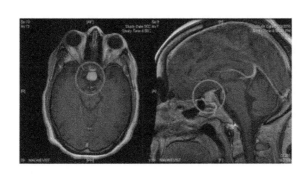

(DMTs), however, prior to pregnancy may alter the pattern of untreated disease. The rate of MS relapses during pregnancy in women on DMTs prior to pregnancy was higher in those with long washout periods prior to conception, indicating that a prolonged interruption of the use of effective DMTs was associated with an increased risk of relapses during pregnancy. For 99 pregnancies in 87 patients, the relapse rates during pregnancy and the postpartum period were 17.2% and 13.7%, respectively, with most of the relapses occurring during the first and third trimesters. Postpartum relapse occurrence in women who had been on DMTs was similar to the previously reported natural history.[83] In an administrative database study, women with MS were at increased risk for infections and preterm delivery but not other adverse pregnancy outcomes, including cerebrovascular disease of pregnancy. Disease activity before delivery was not a strong predictor of outcomes.[84] Pregnancy and breastfeeding after a diagnosis of a clinically isolated syndrome do not increase the risk of developing clinically definite MS.[85]

Neuroimaging findings of MS in pregnancy resemble those in nonpregnant patients. An MRI scan is superior to a CT scan for lesion detection in both the brain and the spinal cord (**Fig. 21**). Typical MRI findings in the brain include radiating periventricular/pericallosal, ovoid subcortical, and juxtacortical lesions, which are hyperintense on T2-weighted imaging. Demyelinating lesions on FLAIR sequences in the brain are hyperintense, and, if the demyelination is acute, the inflammatory lesions generally are associated with transient gadolinium enhancement or can appear as signal abnormalities on DWI sequences (**Fig. 22**). A minority of these acute enhancing lesions, in areas of relatively severe focal injury, may evolve through a progressive reparative process into chronic T1-hypointense lesions (T1 black holes) with irreversible demyelination and axon loss.[86] Cortical pathology, however, is more extensive than is seen on imaging, even with high-field magnets. Optic nerves can be hyperintense on T2-weighted or proton-dense sequences, with fat-suppression and CSF-suppression sequences correlating with symptoms of optic neuritis.[87] Although GBCAs are used routinely in the diagnosis and follow-up of patients with MS, their use during pregnancy should be avoided, if possible. The lack of a contrasted study, however, does not significantly hamper the accuracy of diagnosis and follow-up in MS.[88] Although MS generally is quiescent during pregnancy, this period is associated with an increase in T2 and T1 cerebral lesion load, without whole-brain or cortical atrophy. For the short term, pregnancy protects against the brain volume loss, despite an increased lesion load.[86]

Brain lesions in NMOSD generally are diencephalic surrounding the third ventricle and cerebral aqueduct, in contrast to the cortical brain lesions in MS.[87] The clinical course of NMOSD generally is more aggressive than MS, and pregnant women appear to have a worse clinical outcome with NMOSD than with MS. The relapse rate can increase during pregnancy and the first 3 months after delivery. Pregnancy can contribute to disease onset, worsen NMOSD activity, and increase the risk of disability. The risk of adverse pregnancy outcomes, such as miscarriage and

---

Fig. 20. Lymphocytic hypophysitis in pregnancy. A 34-year-old woman had headaches and bitemporal vision loss at 32 weeks of pregnancy. (*A*) An MRI of the brain showed a pituitary lesion (*circles*) that was diagnosed as (*B*) lymphocytic hypophysitis on biopsy. Her vision improved with steroids (hematoxylin-eosin, original magnification ×100, ×400, ×400). (*C*) A contrast-enhanced study after delivery showed a T1-enhancing pituitary lesion (*circles*) characteristic of lymphocytic hypophysitis.

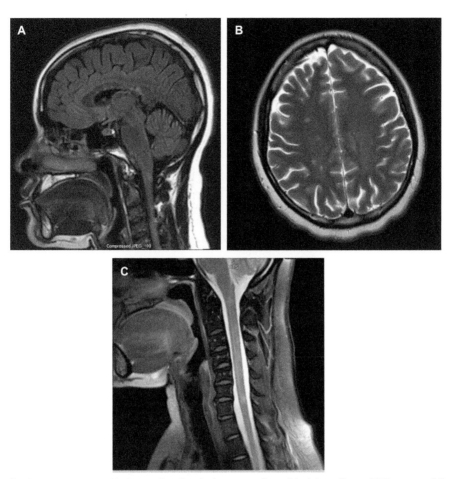

Fig. 21. Postpartum MS. Demyelinating lesions were found incidentally on MRI scan on (*A*) sagittal FLAIR and (*B*) axial T2-weighted images after a fall in 37-year-old asymptomatic pregnant woman. Two months postpartum, she developed weakness, vision changes, and increased falls. Subsequent MRI showed an increase in spinal cord lesions on (*C*) sagittal STIR (short TI inversion recovery) images.

preeclampsia, is increased in women with NMOSD.[89] Because the prognosis and treatment of NMOSD differ from those of MS, MRI scanning of the entire CNS (eg, brain, spinal cord, and optic nerves) is necessary during pregnancy if the diagnosis is suspected, in order to assess the extent of disease.[80] The comorbidity of NMSOD with multiple other immunologic diseases and the potential teratogenicity of some of its treatments may have an adverse impact on the outcome in pregnant women with NMSOD, apart from its natural history.[89]

ADEM is a monophasic episode of acute immune-mediated demyelination of the brain and/or spinal cord, usually triggered by an acute infection or vaccination. The rare case reports of pregnant women with ADEM[90,91] or acute hemorrhagic leukoencephalitis[92] do not indicate any increased vulnerability to a single episode of aggressive demyelination during pregnancy. The MRIs generally show a single large

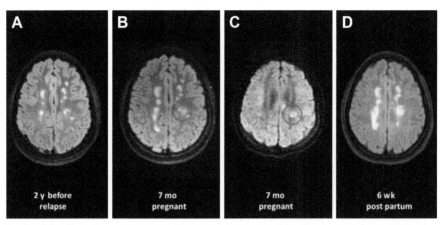

Fig. 22. MS relapse in pregnancy. A 31-year-old woman with relapsing-remitting MS had an acute relapse with right-sided weakness during her third trimester. (*B*) The MRI of the brain showed enlargement of a FLAIR lesion (*circle*), with (*C*) an associated abnormal DWI signal (*circle*) that was present but smaller on (*A*) a FLAIR sequence 2 years prior. The lesion was present 6 weeks after delivery (*D*), however, without contrast enhancement or associated DWI signal abnormality. She was treated with steroids and symptoms resolved by 4 weeks after delivery.

(tumefactive) lesion or multiple bilateral, asymmetric, patchy and poorly marginated hyperintense lesions on T2-weighted and FLAIR images in the subcortical and central white matter, cortical gray-white matter junction, thalami, basal ganglia, cerebellum, brainstem, and spinal cord.[93]

SUMMARY

Most pregnancies progress through the postpartum period without any neurologic symptomatology or need for brain or spinal cord imaging. When new-onset neurologic symptoms necessitate imaging, however, MR techniques without contrast injection are safe during any stage of pregnancy and should be obtained if a neurologic diagnosis or procedure is necessary for the health of the mother. A new-onset headache is concerning in a pregnant woman and an MRI of the brain and/or an MRA of the head and neck and/or MRV of the head should be obtained expeditiously, especially when a new-onset headache occurs in the peripartum period with focal neurologic symptoms and/or elevated blood pressure. Appropriate brain imaging of women with headache in the later stages of pregnancy and after delivery can diagnose potentially life-threatening vascular disease. Many of the cerebrovascular complications of pregnancy are preventable or easily treated. Elevated blood pressure in this peripartum period of risk for preeclampsia/eclampsia/HELLP syndrome should be treated immediately and appropriately in order to avoid the ischemic and hemorrhagic stroke complications of these hypertensive disorders of pregnancy. Mass lesions, both neoplastic and vascular, may enlarge aggressively later in pregnancy, and an MRI of the brain or spine should be used to follow these lesions and to determine the appropriate intervention. The effect of pregnancy on inflammatory demyelination disorders is variable, protecting against MS and worsening NMOSD; MRI scanning of the brain and spinal cord is used to monitor both diseases during pregnancy.

CLINICS CARE POINTS

- Neuroimaging, generally using uncontrasted magnetic resonance techniques, can be safely used to evaluate headaches and other neurological symptoms occurring pregnancy.
- Most pathological headaches for which brain imaging is indicated occur in the peri & post-partum periods.
- Hypertensive disorders of pregnancy and post-partum cerebral angiopathy are on a continuum but have distinctive neuroimaging characteristics.
- Hypertensive disorders of pregnancy and post-partum cerebral angiopathy can lead to intraparechymal hemorrhages or cerebral infarcts.

REFERENCES

1. Toscano M, Thornburg LL. Neurological diseases in pregnancy. Curr Opin Obstet Gynecol 2019;31(2):97–109.
2. Vgontzas A, Robbins MS. A hospital based retrospective study of acute post-partum headache. Headache 2018;58(6):845–51.
3. Practice CoO. Committee opinion no. 723: guidelines for diagnostic imaging during pregnancy and lactation. Obstet Gynecol 2017;130(4):e210–6.
4. Chansakul T, Young GS. Neuroimaging in pregnant women. Semin Neurol 2017; 37(6):712–23.
5. Bove RM, Klein JP. Neuroradiology in women of childbearing age. Continuum (Minneap Minn) 2014;20(1 Neurology of Pregnancy):23–41.
6. Tremblay E, Thérasse E, Thomassin-Naggara I, et al. Quality initiatives: guidelines for use of medical imaging during pregnancy and lactation. Radiographics 2012; 32(3):897–911.
7. Chen MM, Coakley FV, Kaimal A, et al. Guidelines for computed tomography and magnetic resonance imaging use during pregnancy and lactation. Obstet Gynecol 2008;112(2 Pt 1):333–40.
8. Media ACoRCoDaC. American College of Radiology manual on contrast media. American College of Radiology; 2020. p. 1–131. Available at: https://www.acr.org/Clinical-Resources/Contrast-Manual.
9. Lersy F, Boulouis G, Clément O, et al. Consensus Guidelines of the French Society of Neuroradiology (SFNR) on the use of Gadolinium-Based Contrast agents (GBCAs) and related MRI protocols in Neuroradiology. J Neuroradiol 2020. https://doi.org/10.1016/j.neurad.2020.05.008.
10. Gulani V, Calamante F, Shellock FG, et al. Gadolinium deposition in the brain: summary of evidence and recommendations. Lancet Neurol 2017;16(7):564–70.
11. Hoefnagel A, Yu A, Kaminski A. Anesthetic complications in pregnancy. Crit Care Clin 2016;32(1):1–28.
12. Buddeberg BS, Bandschapp O, Girard T. Post-dural puncture headache. Minerva Anestesiol 2019;85(5):543–53.
13. Sachs A, Smiley R. Post-dural puncture headache: the worst common complication in obstetric anesthesia. Semin Perinatol 2014;38(6):386–94.
14. Sinha A, Petkov S, Meldrum D. Unrecognised dural puncture resulting in subdural hygroma and cortical vein thrombosis. Anaesthesia 2010;65(1):70–3.
15. Bilello LA, Greige T, Singleton JM, et al. Retrospective review of pregnant patients presenting for evaluation of acute neurologic complaints. Ann Emerg Med 2020. https://doi.org/10.1016/j.annemergmed.2020.02.014.

16. Headache Classification Committee of the International Headache Society (IHS) The International Classification of Headache Disorders, 3rd edition. Cephalalgia 2018;38(1):1–211.
17. Spierings EL, Sabin TD. De Novo headache during pregnancy and puerperium. Neurologist 2016;21(1):1–7.
18. Wells RE, Turner DP, Lee M, et al. Managing migraine during pregnancy and lactation. Curr Neurol Neurosci Rep 2016;16(4):40.
19. Robbins MS, Farmakidis C, Dayal AK, et al. Acute headache diagnosis in pregnant women: a hospital-based study. Neurology 2015;85(12):1024–30.
20. Sandoe CH, Lay C. Secondary headaches during pregnancy: when to worry. Curr Neurol Neurosci Rep 2019;19(6):27.
21. Kuklina EV, Tong X, Bansil P, et al. Trends in pregnancy hospitalizations that included a stroke in the United States from 1994 to 2007: reasons for concern? Stroke 2011;42(9):2564–70.
22. Elgendy IY, Gad MM, Mahmoud AN, et al. Acute stroke during pregnancy and puerperium. J Am Coll Cardiol 2020;75(2):180–90.
23. Hovsepian DA, Sriram N, Kamel H, et al. Acute cerebrovascular disease occurring after hospital discharge for labor and delivery. Stroke 2014;45(7):1947–50.
24. Kamel H, Navi BB, Sriram N, et al. Risk of a thrombotic event after the 6-week postpartum period. N Engl J Med 2014;370(14):1307–15.
25. McDermott M, Miller EC, Rundek T, et al. Preeclampsia: association with posterior reversible encephalopathy syndrome and stroke. Stroke 2018;49(3):524–30.
26. Fam D, Saposnik G, Group SORCW. Critical care management of cerebral venous thrombosis. Curr Opin Crit Care 2016;22(2):113–9.
27. Ghoneim A, Straiton J, Pollard C, et al. Imaging of cerebral venous thrombosis. Clin Radiol 2020;75(4):254–64.
28. Petrovic BD, Nemeth AJ, McComb EN, et al. Posterior reversible encephalopathy syndrome and venous thrombosis. Radiol Clin North Am 2011;49(1):63–80.
29. van Dam LF, van Walderveen MAA, Kroft LJM, et al. Current imaging modalities for diagnosing cerebral vein thrombosis - A critical review. Thromb Res 2020;189: 132–9.
30. Sadigh G, Mullins ME, Saindane AM. Diagnostic Performance of MRI Sequences for Evaluation of Dural Venous Sinus Thrombosis. AJR Am J Roentgenol 2016;1–9. https://doi.org/10.2214/AJR.15.15719.
31. Gestational Hypertension and Preeclampsia: ACOG Practice Bulletin, Number 222. Obstet Gynecol 2020;135(6):e237–60.
32. Umapathy A, Chamley LW, James JL. Reconciling the distinct roles of angiogenic/anti-angiogenic factors in the placenta and maternal circulation of normal and pathological pregnancies. Angiogenesis 2020;23(2):105–17.
33. Fletcher JJ, Kramer AH, Bleck TP, et al. Overlapping features of eclampsia and postpartum angiopathy. Neurocrit Care 2009;11(2):199–209.
34. Fugate JE, Ameriso SF, Ortiz G, et al. Variable presentations of postpartum angiopathy. Stroke 2012;43(3):670–6.
35. Zoet GA, Linstra KM, Bernsen MLE, et al. Stroke after pregnancy disorders. Eur J Obstet Gynecol Reprod Biol 2017;215:264–6.
36. Acar H, Acar K. Posterior reversible encephalopathy syndrome in a pregnant patient without eclampsia or preeclampsia. Am J Emerg Med 2018;36(9): 1721.e3-e4.
37. McKinney AM, Short J, Truwit CL, et al. Posterior reversible encephalopathy syndrome: incidence of atypical regions of involvement and imaging findings. AJR Am J Roentgenol 2007;189(4):904–12.

38. Pop A, Carbonnel M, Wang A, et al. Posterior reversible encephalopathy syndrome associated with reversible cerebral vasoconstriction syndrome in a patient presenting with postpartum eclampsia: A case report. J Gynecol Obstet Hum Reprod 2019;48(6):431–4.
39. Singhal AB. Postpartum angiopathy with reversible posterior leukoencephalopathy. Arch Neurol 2004;61(3):411–6.
40. Fugate JE, Wijdicks EF, Parisi JE, et al. Fulminant postpartum cerebral vasoconstriction syndrome. Arch Neurol 2012;69(1):111–7.
41. Garg RK, Malhotra HS, Patil TB, et al. Cerebral-autoregulatory dysfunction syndrome. BMJ Case Rep 2013;2013doi. https://doi.org/10.1136/bcr-2013-201592.
42. Miller TR, Shivashankar R, Mossa-Basha M, et al. Reversible cerebral vasoconstriction syndrome, part 1: epidemiology, pathogenesis, and clinical course. AJNR Am J Neuroradiol 2015;36(8):1392–9.
43. Miller TR, Shivashankar R, Mossa-Basha M, et al. Reversible cerebral vasoconstriction syndrome, part 2: diagnostic work-up, imaging evaluation, and differential diagnosis. AJNR Am J Neuroradiol 2015;36(9):1580–8.
44. Ducros A, Wolff V. The typical thunderclap headache of reversible cerebral vasoconstriction syndrome and its various triggers. Headache 2016. https://doi.org/10.1111/head.12797.
45. Ducros A. Reversible cerebral vasoconstriction syndrome. Handb Clin Neurol 2014;121:1725–41. https://doi.org/10.1016/B978-0-7020-4088-7.00111-5.
46. Sheikh HU, Mathew PG. Reversible cerebral vasoconstriction syndrome: updates and new perspectives. Curr Pain Headache Rep 2014;18(5):414.
47. Ducros A, Fiedler U, Porcher R, et al. Hemorrhagic manifestations of reversible cerebral vasoconstriction syndrome: frequency, features, and risk factors. Stroke 2010;41(11):2505–11.
48. Ueno S, Takeda J, Maruyama Y, et al. Antepartum eclampsia with reversible cerebral vasoconstriction and posterior reversible encephalopathy syndromes. J Obstet Gynaecol Res 2020. https://doi.org/10.1111/jog.14410.
49. Tanaka K, Matsushima M, Matsuzawa Y, et al. Antepartum reversible cerebral vasoconstriction syndrome with pre-eclampsia and reversible posterior leukoencephalopathy. J Obstet Gynaecol Res 2015;41(11):1843–7.
50. Hacein-Bey L, Varelas PN, Ulmer JL, et al. Imaging of Cerebrovascular Disease in Pregnancy and the Puerperium. AJR Am J Roentgenol 2016;206(1):26–38.
51. Mohr JP, Kejda-Scharler J, Pile-Spellman J. Diagnosis and treatment of arteriovenous malformations. Curr Neurol Neurosci Rep 2013;13(2):324.
52. Kalani MY, Zabramski JM. Risk for symptomatic hemorrhage of cerebral cavernous malformations during pregnancy. J Neurosurg 2013;118(1):50–5.
53. Kim YW, Neal D, Hoh BL. Cerebral aneurysms in pregnancy and delivery: pregnancy and delivery do not increase the risk of aneurysm rupture. Neurosurgery 2013;72(2):143–9 [discussion: 150].
54. Bateman BT, Olbrecht VA, Berman MF, et al. Peripartum subarachnoid hemorrhage: nationwide data and institutional experience. Anesthesiology 2012;116(2):324–33.
55. Hacein-Bey L, Provenzale JM. Current imaging assessment and treatment of intracranial aneurysms. AJR Am J Roentgenol 2011;196(1):32–44.
56. Jamieson DG, Cheng NT, Skliut M. Headache and acute stroke. Curr Pain Headache Rep 2014;18(9):444.
57. Blythe R, Ismail A, Naqvi A. Mechanical Thrombectomy for Acute Ischemic Stroke in Pregnancy. J Stroke Cerebrovasc Dis 2019. https://doi.org/10.1016/j.jstrokecerebrovasdis.2019.02.015.

58. Watanabe TT, Ichijo M, Kamata T. Uneventful pregnancy and delivery after thrombolysis plus thrombectomy for acute ischemic stroke: case study and literature review. J Stroke Cerebrovasc Dis 2019;28(1):70–5.
59. Kelly JC, Safain MG, Roguski M, et al. Postpartum internal carotid and vertebral arterial dissections. Obstet Gynecol 2014;123(4):848–56.
60. Salehi Omran S, Parikh NS, Poisson S, et al. Association between Pregnancy and Cervical Artery Dissection. Ann Neurol 2020. https://doi.org/10.1002/ana.25813.
61. Sekine M, Kobayashi Y, Tabata T, et al. Malignancy during pregnancy in Japan: an exceptional opportunity for early diagnosis. BMC Pregnancy Childbirth 2018;18(1):50.
62. Bonfield CM, Engh JA. Pregnancy and brain tumors. Neurol Clin 2012;30(3):937–46.
63. Verheecke M, Halaska MJ, Lok CA, et al. Primary brain tumours, meningiomas and brain metastases in pregnancy: report on 27 cases and review of literature. Eur J Cancer 2014;50(8):1462–71.
64. Taylan E, Akdemir A, Zeybek B, et al. Recurrent brain tumor with hydrocephalus in pregnancy. J Obstet Gynaecol Res 2015;41(3):464–7.
65. Mandong BM, Emmanuel I, Vandi KB, et al. Secondary brain choriocarcinoma: a case report. Niger J Med 2015;24(1):81–3.
66. Hallsworth D, Thompson J, Wilkinson D, et al. Intracranial pressure monitoring and caesarean section in a patient with von Hippel-Lindau disease and symptomatic cerebellar haemangioblastomas. Int J Obstet Anesth 2015;24(1):73–7.
67. Capone F, Profice P, Pilato F, et al. Spinal hemangioblastoma presenting with low back pain in pregnancy. Spine J 2013;13(12):e27–9.
68. Dolecek TA, Propp JM, Stroup NE, et al. CBTRUS statistical report: primary brain and central nervous system tumors diagnosed in the United States in 2005-2009. Neuro Oncol 2012;14(Suppl 5):v1–49.
69. Kurdoglu Z, Cetin O, Gulsen I, et al. Intracranial meningioma diagnosed during pregnancy caused maternal death. Case Rep Med 2014;2014:158326.
70. Lusis EA, Scheithauer BW, Yachnis AT, et al. Meningiomas in pregnancy: a clinicopathologic study of 17 cases. Neurosurgery 2012;71(5):951–61.
71. Stevenson CB, Thompson RC. The clinical management of intracranial neoplasms in pregnancy. Clin Obstet Gynecol 2005;48(1):24–37.
72. Yust-Katz S, de Groot JF, Liu D, et al. Pregnancy and glial brain tumors. Neuro Oncol 2014;16(9):1289–94.
73. Singh P, Mantilla E, Sewell J, et al. Occurrence of Glioma in Pregnant Patients: An Institutional Case Series and Review of the Literature. Anticancer Res 2020;40(6):3453–7.
74. Huang W, Molitch ME. Pituitary tumors in pregnancy. Endocrinol Metab Clin North Am 2019;48(3):569–81.
75. Woodmansee WW. Pituitary disorders in pregnancy. Neurol Clin 2019;37(1):63–83.
76. Kaplun J, Fratila C, Ferenczi A, et al. Sequential pituitary MR imaging in Sheehan syndrome: report of 2 cases. AJNR Am J Neuroradiol 2008;29(5):941–3.
77. Wada Y, Hamamoto Y, Nakamura Y, et al. Lymphocytic panhypophysitis: its clinical features in Japanese cases. Jpn Clin Med 2011;2:15–20.
78. Guo S, Wang C, Zhang J, et al. Diagnosis and management of tumor-like hypophysitis: A retrospective case series. Oncol Lett 2016;11(2):1315–20.
79. Robinson DP, Klein SL. Pregnancy and pregnancy-associated hormones alter immune responses and disease pathogenesis. Horm Behav 2012;62(3):263–71.

80. Kaplan TB. Management of demyelinating disorders in pregnancy. Neurol Clin 2019;37(1):17–30.
81. Sadeghpour N, Mirmosayyeb O, Bjørklund G, et al. Is fertility affected in women of childbearing age with multiple sclerosis or neuromyelitis optica spectrum disorder? J Mol Neurosci 2020. https://doi.org/10.1007/s12031-020-01576-x.
82. Krysko KM, Graves JS, Dobson R, et al. Sex effects across the lifespan in women with multiple sclerosis. Ther Adv Neurol Disord 2020;13. 1756286420936166.
83. Alroughani R, Alowayesh MS, Ahmed SF, et al. Relapse occurrence in women with multiple sclerosis during pregnancy in the new treatment era. Neurology 2018;90(10):e840–6.
84. MacDonald SC, McElrath TF, Hernández-Díaz S. Pregnancy outcomes in women with multiple sclerosis. Am J Epidemiol 2019;188(1):57–66.
85. Zuluaga MI, Otero-Romero S, Rovira A, et al. Menarche, pregnancies, and breastfeeding do not modify long-term prognosis in multiple sclerosis. Neurology 2019;92(13):e1507–16.
86. Khalid F, Healy BC, Dupuy SL, et al. Quantitative MRI analysis of cerebral lesions and atrophy in post-partum patients with multiple sclerosis. J Neurol Sci 2018; 392:94–9.
87. Kuchling J, Paul F. Visualizing the central nervous system: imaging tools for multiple sclerosis and neuromyelitis optica spectrum disorders. Front Neurol 2020; 11:450.
88. Eichinger P, Schön S, Pongratz V, et al. Accuracy of Unenhanced MRI in the detection of new brain lesions in multiple sclerosis. Radiology 2019;181568. https://doi.org/10.1148/radiol.2019181568.
89. Mao-Draayer Y, Thiel S, Mills EA, et al. Neuromyelitis optica spectrum disorders and pregnancy: therapeutic considerations. Nat Rev Neurol 2020;16(3):154–70.
90. Qiu K, He Q, Chen X, et al. Pregnancy-related immune changes and demyelinating diseases of the central nervous system. Front Neurol 2019;10:1070.
91. Zeb Q, Alegria A. Acute disseminated encephalomyelitis (ADEM) following a H3N3 parainfluenza virus infection in a pregnant asthmatic woman with respiratory failure. BMJ Case Rep 2014;2014doi. https://doi.org/10.1136/bcr-2013-201072.
92. George IC, Youn TS, Marcolini EG, et al. Clinical Reasoning: Acute onset facial droop in a 36-year-old pregnant woman. Neurology 2017;88(24):e240–4.
93. Pohl D, Alper G, Van Haren K, et al. Acute disseminated encephalomyelitis: Updates on an inflammatory CNS syndrome. Neurology 2016;87(9 Suppl 2):S38–45.

Psychiatric Medication Use in Pregnancy and Breastfeeding

Jennifer L. Payne, MD

KEYWORDS

- Pregnancy • Breastfeeding • Antidepressants • Mood stabilizers
- Postpartum depression

KEY POINTS

- Many psychiatric medications can be taken safely during pregnancy and breastfeeding.
- There are significant risks associated with untreated psychiatric illness during pregnancy and postpartum.
- Many studies examining infant outcomes with exposure to psychotropic medications during pregnancy are confounded by illnesses, behaviors, and other risk factors associated with psychiatric illness.
- The obstetrician-gynecologist plays a key role in identifying and treating psychiatric illness during the peripartum time period.

INTRODUCTION: THE PROBLEM

Pregnant women with psychiatric illness have higher rates of adverse pregnancy outcomes including pre-eclampsia, C-section and gestational diabetes.[1] Antepartum depression has been associated with low maternal weight gain; increased rates of preterm birth[2,3]; low birth weight[1]; increased rates of cigarette, alcohol, and other substance use[4]; increased ambivalence about the pregnancy; and overall worse health status.[5] Children exposed to peripartum depression have higher cortisol levels than those of mothers not depressed,[6] and this continues through adolescence.[6] Maternal treatment of depression during pregnancy may help normalize infant cortisol levels.[7] Although the long-term effects of elevated cortisol are unclear, these findings may partially explain the mechanism for an increased vulnerability to psychopathology in children of antepartum depressed mothers.[6]

In turn, untreated antepartum depression is one of the strongest risk factors for postpartum depression (PPD),[8] and PPD has potentially devastating consequences, including suicide and infanticide. Suicides account for up to 20% of all postpartum

Johns Hopkins Women's Mood Disorders Center, Johns Hopkins School of Medicine, 550 North Broadway, Suite 305, Baltimore, MD 21025, USA
E-mail address: Jpayne5@jhmi.edu

Obstet Gynecol Clin N Am 48 (2021) 131–149
https://doi.org/10.1016/j.ogc.2020.11.006
0889-8545/21/© 2020 Elsevier Inc. All rights reserved.
obgyn.theclinics.com

deaths and represent one of the leading causes of peripartum mortality.[9] PPD has been associated with increased rates of infantile colic and impaired maternal-infant bonding.[10] PPD also interferes with parenting behavior, leading to less adequate infant safety and less healthy child development practices,[11] such as an increased use of harsh discipline.[12] Finally, PPD has significant negative effects on infant development, including IQ, language, and behavior.[13]

Discontinuation of psychiatric medications for pregnancy also is associated with a high relapse rate of both major depressive disorder (MDD) and bipolar disorder (BD) and likely other, less studied psychiatric illnesses. Discontinuation of antidepressants in pregnant women with a history of MDD has been linked to relapse in 60% to 70% of women.[14] In women with BD, studies demonstrated a recurrence risk of 80% to 100% in pregnant women who discontinue mood stabilizers, whereas women who continued mood stabilizer treatment had a much lower risk of 29% to 37%.[15,16] Many women with psychiatric disorders experience relapse during pregnancy, both on and off medication. In 1 study, approximately 50% of women with a mood disorder reported significant mood symptoms during and/or after pregnancy.[17] Relapse then exposes the developing infant to the effects of psychiatric illness, which leads to adverse consequences for the woman, infant, and family.[2,6]

CONTROVERSIES AND LIMITATIONS OF THE LITERATURE

The treatment of psychiatric disorders during pregnancy is complicated by the fact that few studies have been conducted to determine which medications are efficacious, how changes in body weight and metabolism may affect dosing, and what alternatives to medications are available that successfully treat psychiatric illness during pregnancy. Thus, treatment decisions must be made with few hard data.

It also is important to understand that the use of psychotropic medications during pregnancy essentially is a marker for a population of women with risk factors different from those of the general population of pregnant women. These risk factors, including health-related behaviors, associated illnesses, and other characteristics, may influence the outcomes of studies attempting to examine the risks of in utero exposure of a psychotropic medication to a child. For example, diabetes, obesity, smoking, and substance use are more common in patients with psychiatric illness than in the general population. Studies that have not controlled for the underlying psychiatric illness and its confounding behaviors and characteristics may find associations between psychotropic medications and outcomes that are directly caused not by exposure to the medication itself but by characteristics and behaviors that are more highly prevalent in the population of patients who take psychotropic medications during pregnancy.

US FOOD AND DRUG ADMINISTRATION PREGNANCY CATEGORIES AND THE PREGNANCY AND LACTATION LABELING RULE

In 2014, the US Food and Drug Administration (FDA) published the Pregnancy and Lactation Labeling Rule, mandating changes to the content and format of prescription drug labeling, detailing use during pregnancy and breastfeeding. The labeling changes went into effect in 2015 for all new products and are being phased in over time for older medications and products. The new labeling attempts to summarize all currently available information to help clinicians weigh the risks and benefits of prescribing a drug during pregnancy or breastfeeding.

Because the new labeling is phased in over time, it still is important to understand the meaning of the former FDA pregnancy categories. Categories include A, B, C,

D, and X, and classification is based on the amount of evidence for safety in animal and human studies. Many clinicians assume that there is an increasing level of risk from category A to category X, which is inaccurate. For example, medications that are category B simply have not been studied adequately in humans to warrant placing them into category A as safe or in category C, category D, or category X, depending on the level of risk in humans. Most medications new to the market, therefore, are placed in category B and should not necessarily be prescribed over older medications that are classified in category C or category D, which at least has data regarding safety in pregnancy.

SCREENING

Following the 2016 US Preventative Services Task Force recommendation for routine screening for depression, including in the perinatal population,[18] current American College of Obstetricians and Gynecologists recommendations include screening for psychiatric illness, including depression and anxiety, at least once during the perinatal period, and, if a patient is screened during pregnancy, screening should be repeated at the comprehensive postpartum visit.[19] Furthermore, the Women's Preventative Services Initiative recently recommended screening all adolescents (age 13 and older) and women for anxiety disorders, including pregnant and postpartum women.[20] Several standardized, self-rated screening tools are listed in **Box 1**. Although no official organization has yet recommended screening for BD, the Mood Disorder Questionnaire,[21] which screens for BD, is included, because many patients who have BD present with depression or anxiety symptoms, and the treatment of BD requires mood-stabilizing agents and is best not treated with antidepressants without a mood stabilizer.

CLINICAL CARE PLANNING FOR PSYCHIATRIC MEDICATION MANAGEMENT DURING PREGNANCY
Prepregnancy Planning

The ideal situation is to begin planning for pregnancy prior to pregnancy (**Box 2**). Ideally, the obstetrician-gynecologist (ob-gyn) treatment provider should assume that every woman of childbearing age will get pregnant and discuss whether her prescribed medications can be used safely during pregnancy prior to pregnancy. If a woman is taking a psychiatric medication that should not be used during pregnancy unless absolutely necessary, such as valproic acid, a discussion should be held

---

Box 1
Screening tools for psychiatric disorders

Name	Number of Items	Comments
Edinburgh Postnatal Depression Scale[22]	10	Standard tool for screening for depression during and after pregnancy
Patient Health Questionnaire-9[23]	9	Screens for depression
Patient Health Questionnaire-4[24]	4	Brief screen for both depression and anxiety
Hospital Anxiety and Depression Scale[25]	14	Screens for both depression and anxiety
Mood Disorder Questionnaire[21]	15	Screens for BD

Data from Refs.[21–25]

Box 2
Planning ahead: pregnancy in women with psychiatric disorders

Encourage the patient to have regular psychiatric care during and after pregnancy.

All medication changes should be done before pregnancy if possible.

All medication changes should be done in consultation with the psychiatric treatment provider.

Ideally, the patient should be stable psychiatrically before attempting pregnancy.

Use medications for which there are data: older is usually (but not always) better.

Minimize the number of exposures for the baby, including exposure to psychiatric illness (do not undertreat).

Consider breastfeeding when planning for pregnancy.

If a baby was exposed to a medication during pregnancy, it may not make sense to discontinue the medication (or alternatively not breastfeed) for breastfeeding.

Use a team approach—communicate with the family and other involved treatment providers frequently.

Be supportive if the patient does not take your recommendations.

FDA category B can mean there are not data in pregnancy in humans—category B is not necessarily safer than category C or category D.

---

with the woman and, if possible, her partner to discuss this fact and to plan what should be done in case of accidental pregnancy. The ob-gyn also should consider discussing the patient's case with the psychiatric treatment provider so that he or she can understand whether or not that particular medication is critical for the patient. Ultimately, prepregnancy medication changes should be made by the treating psychiatrist, in consultation with the ob-gyn. Because as many as 45% of pregnancies continue to be unplanned in the United States,[26] discussing contingency plans for an unplanned pregnancy ahead of time minimizes the chances that psychiatric medications are discontinued abruptly and the patient relapses.

Prepregnancy medication changes ideally should be done 6 months to 12 months before attempting pregnancy so that there is enough time to make changes and ensure stability before pregnancy (see **Box 2**). Ideally, the psychiatric and ob-gyn providers work together during the prepregnancy planning phase. Prepregnancy planning should consider the patient's

- Past psychiatric history
- Severity of illness
- Medication response history
- Wishes and worries about treatment during pregnancy

Every case should be considered individually, and, ultimately, there are no right answers—just the weighing of risks and benefits of the various options.

The patient and her partner's wishes regarding medication use during pregnancy also should be considered when designing a treatment plan. If one or the other is strongly against medication use during pregnancy, it is best for the treatment provider to make sure they understand the risks of no treatment (**Box 3**) and the rates of relapse and to outline a course of close psychiatric follow-up during and after pregnancy, rather than insist on the use of medication during pregnancy. A partnership with good communication is important to maintain so that if there is a relapse of illness, the patient remains safe and is more likely to seek care and treatment.

Box 3
Adverse pregnancy outcomes associated with antenatal depression and anxiety

Preterm birth[27]

Low birth weight[27]

Cesarean section[1]

Gestational diabetes[1]

Preeclampsia[1]

Decreased intention to breastfeed[27]

PPD[27]

Data from Refs.[1,27]

Most important, the primary goal of treatment in pregnancy is to minimize the number of exposures. The goal not only is to minimize the number of medications but also to limit exposure to psychiatric illness. If a woman is planning her pregnancy well in advance and she is on a newer, less-studied psychiatric medication, she and her providers can attempt to switch to a medication about which more safety data are available before pregnancy—but only if she does not have a history of nonresponse to that medication.

Unplanned Pregnancy

Given the high rate of unplanned pregnancies, most practitioners have the experience at some point in their career of having a patient on psychiatric medications get pregnant unexpectedly. The principles, discussed previously, for prepregnancy planning also apply in cases of an unplanned pregnancy. **Box 4** offers some additional tips on dos and don'ts in this situation. The most important principle to remember is, Do not stop all psychiatric medications precipitously in a knee-jerk reaction in response to the news of an unplanned pregnancy. This reaction can

- Cause great stress and anxiety for the patient
- Precipitate discontinuation symptoms or withdrawal
- Precipitate a relapse of mental illness

Box 4
Managing an unplanned pregnancy in women with psychiatric disorders

See or talk to the patient as soon as possible.

Discuss the case with the psychiatric treatment provider as soon as possible.

Do not stop all psychiatric medications immediately—most can be continued.

If a decision is made to discontinue a medication, taper whenever possible.

Consider stopping medications that are known to be teratogenic.

As in prepregnancy planning, try to minimize the number of medications the patient is taking, but do so taking the patient's history into account, and remember that exposure to psychiatric illness counts as an exposure to the child.

If the patient is psychiatrically ill, make a plan that includes treating the illness.

The best approach is to review the medication list based on the principles, discussed previously, for prepregnancy planning and discuss a plan of action with the psychiatric treatment provider as soon as possible. Keep in mind that the baby already is exposed, and, although stopping some medications may be necessary, doing so in a controlled and logical fashion is ideal. One common scenario is for a pregnant woman on a newer medication to receive the recommendation to switch to an older medication that has more evidence for safety during pregnancy. Although this might have made sense before pregnancy, this plan actually increases exposures for the baby to the following:

- The original medication
- The second medication
- Potential relapse

Thus, continuing on the current but newer medication limits the exposures to one exposure, while switching increases the number of exposures to at least 2 and possibly 3 or more if the woman relapses with her illness.

If a decision is made to stop a medication, the medication should be tapered if at all possible. Tapering eliminates the risk of withdrawal or discontinuation symptoms, thus maximizing outcomes for both mother and baby. It also is important to make a plan for treatment if the patient is psychiatrically ill. Many patients and practitioners overlook the fact that the patient may need more, not less, treatment in the excitement of an unplanned pregnancy.

General Recommendations for Breastfeeding

The benefits of breastfeeding for the baby are well documented, and the American Academy of Pediatrics advocates breastfeeding through the first 6 months of life. All psychotropic medications pass readily into breast milk. If an infant was exposed in utero to a psychiatric medication, it does not make sense to switch to another for breastfeeding. Exceptions include the following:

- The mother's psychiatric illness has relapsed and the current medication regimen is not working.
- The mother is on a medication that has a risk of severe side effects with continued exposure for the infant (eg, clozapine).
- The infant appears to be having side effects or medical complications related to the medication exposure during breastfeeding.

If the medication regimen needs to be changed during breastfeeding (due to recurrent illness or intolerance), the patient and her treatment team should consider whether continued breastfeeding is worth the risks of increasing the number of exposures to medications for the infant.

It is important to involve the pediatrician in the decision-making process and to help monitor the baby for potential side effects. If the baby is being exposed to a medication that can be monitored via blood levels, then blood levels should be monitored in the baby intermittently and as needed. A common side effect for many psychiatric medications is sedation, and the baby should be monitored for excessive sleepiness and decreased feeding, particularly during the feeding after the mother takes the medication. If the baby is exposed to an antipsychotic medication, the baby also should be monitored for stiffness, cogwheeling, and extrapyramidal side effects, although these side effects are uncommon. At times, it can be difficult to distinguish potential medication side effects from what simply is a fussy baby. When in doubt, the wisest choice is to do what makes the parents the most comfortable.

CLASSES OF PSYCHIATRIC MEDICATIONS
Antidepressants

Antidepressants are the most commonly prescribed psychotropic medication during pregnancy.[28] The literature examining infant outcomes associated with antidepressant use during pregnancy is large and exemplifies the problem of confounding by indication found throughout this literature: several possible negative outcomes have been identified over the past several years by studies that did not control for the underlying psychiatric illness. Subsequent, more properly controlled studies, however, generally have demonstrated either no or a very slight increased risk of adverse outcomes.

Major organ malformations

Overall, antidepressant use during pregnancy appears to be relatively safe and not associated with major organ malformations. A small increase in the absolute risk of rare defects with selective serotonin reuptake inhibitor (SSRI) exposure was reported in 1 study,[29] but 4 meta-analyses examining the risk of major malformations with first-trimester SSRI exposure found no statistically significant increased risk.[30–33] Compared with the SSRIs, there are few data for other types of antidepressants. Most studies examining the risk of tricyclic antidepressant exposure have found no increased risk of malformations,[34–38] although 1 large epidemiologic study found a significant increase in severe malformations (odds ratio 1.36; 95% CI, 1.07 - 1.72.[39] Several studies of bupropion have found no association with major malformations.[40–42] The data available for other types of antidepressants are small but reassuring.[43,44]

Cardiac defects

The evolving literature examining in utero antidepressant exposure and infant cardiac defects is a good example of the importance of controlling for confounding factors in psychiatric clinical research. Some but not all previous studies demonstrated a possible association between in utero antidepressant (in particular, SSRI) exposure and heart defects (reviewed by Chisolm and Payne[45]). Most of these studies, however, compared psychiatric population outcomes with the general population and did not control for risk factors and behaviors associated with MDD. More recent studies have done a better job of comparing apples to apples and have not found an association between antidepressant exposure and heart defects. For example, a more recent study,[46] with a sample size of more than 900,000 women, did not find an association between first-trimester antidepressant exposure and cardiac malformations when the statistical analyses controlled for MDD by comparing the outcomes of women with MDD who took antidepressants to outcomes of women with MDD who did not take antidepressants. Another study[47] performed a meta-analysis of prospective cohort studies and found no association between SSRI use in the first trimester and heart defects when comparing women with MDD who took SSRIs in the first trimester with women with MDD who did not take antidepressants in pregnancy. Thus, the previously identified association between in utero antidepressant exposure and heart defects likely is associated with other risk factors and behaviors that are prevalent in the population of women with MDD.

Persistent pulmonary hypertension

Another possibly associated outcome with in utero antidepressant exposure is persistent pulmonary hypertension in the newborn (PPHN). PPHN is a failure of the pulmonary vasculature to decrease resistance at birth, resulting in breathing difficulties for the infant, leading to hypoxia and often intubation, and carries a 10% to 20%

mortality.[48] An association between SSRI exposure and PPHN first was noted in 2006[49] and led to an FDA alert and label change. Since this first study, 8 additional studies cohort or case-control studies with mixed results. Two meta-analyses,[50,51] the most recent including all 9 previously conducted cohort and case-control studies, have concluded that there appears to be a significant, although very small, increase in the odds of developing PPHN in antidepressant exposed newborns. Overall, 99% of exposed babies do not develop PPHN if the association is accurate. Both studies concluded that the risks of untreated maternal psychiatric illness were far larger and the risk of PPHN "might not warrant the recommendation to withdraw antidepressant therapy."[51] The story is complicated by the fact that several known risk factors for PPHN, including obesity, smoking, and cesarean section, are more common in the psychiatric population. This fact is highlighted by 1 study that found that a history of psychiatric hospitalization significantly increased the risk for PPHN even when women did not take antidepressants in pregnancy.[52]

Autism

In utero antidepressant exposure also has been associated in a few studies with autism in exposed children. Again, however, studies that control for underlying confounds associated with psychiatric illness, in general, are negative. A recent systematic review and meta-analysis found that maternal psychiatric illness is a "major confounding factor" in the association between SSRI exposure and autism and that there was not an increased risk for autism when analyses controlled for maternal psychiatric illness.[53]

Spontaneous abortion

Although the studies in this area also are plagued with lack of controlling for the underlying psychiatric illness and associated risk factors, the overall results suggest that the use of antidepressants in early pregnancy may be associated with a modestly increased risk of spontaneous abortion, with odds ratios in the range of 1.4 to 1.6.[44,54–56]

Preterm birth and low birth weight

Antidepressant use in pregnancy has been associated repeatedly with preterm birth and low birth weight in exposed infants. Recent work indicates, however, that these outcomes instead may be, at least in part, associated with the underlying psychiatric illness. For example, a recent meta-analysis examined neonatal outcomes in women with MDD receiving no treatment and compared them with outcomes in women without MDD.[57] This study found that untreated depression was associated with significantly increased risks of preterm birth and low birth weight, indicating that exposure to the illness, MDD, affected infant outcomes.

Poor neonatal adaptation syndrome

One other outcome that appears to be associated with in utero antidepressant exposure is poor neonatal adaptation syndrome (PNAS), a transient cluster of symptoms seen in newborns. The first report of withdrawal symptoms in babies exposed to antidepressants occurred in 1973.[58] It is unclear if PNAS is actually a result of withdrawal from the antidepressant or is due to toxicity or even a combination of both. There are several limitations in the available literature, including inconsistent definitions, no standardized measurement tool, a lack of blinded ratings, and a lack of studies investigating treatment or prevention of the syndrome as well as long-term outcomes. The FDA instituted a class labeling change in 2004 for both SSRIs and serotonin-norepinephrine reuptake inhibitors antidepressants, warning that third-trimester exposure may be associated with PNAS. According to the label change, "reported clinical findings have included respiratory distress, cyanosis, apnea, seizures, temperature instability, feeding difficulty, vomiting, hypoglycemia, hypotonia, hypertonia, hyperreflexia, tremor, jitteriness, irritability, and constant crying." (See for example ref#[59]) Most cases of the PNAS appear to be mild and self-limited and have not been associated with lasting repercussions.[60] Available data suggest that approximately one-third of exposed infants have at least mild symptoms consistent with the syndrome, and this risk increases when multiple agents, in particular, benzodiazepines, are used.[61] Clearly, larger, more rigorous studies of the syndrome as well as strategies to minimize the risk of PNAS are needed.

Breastfeeding

In general, antidepressant use during breastfeeding is considered safe, with most studies demonstrating low or undetectable blood levels.[62] Infants should be monitored for sedation, difficulty feeding, and difficulty sleeping, although these side effects are uncommon.

Mood Stabilizers

In general, valproic acid and carbamazepine should not be used during pregnancy because of high rates of malformation associated with these medications. Valproic acid is associated with as much as a 10% rate of malformations with first-trimester exposure, including neural tube defects, effects on cognition and brain volume, craniofacial anomalies, cardiac defects, cleft palate, and hypospadias,[56] and may be linked to autism.[63,64] Carbamazepine also carries an increased risk of malformations, primarily of spina bifida, as well as other neural tube defects, facial abnormalities, skeletal abnormalities, hypospadias, and diaphragmatic hernia.[56] Carbamazepine also is a competitive inhibitor of prothrombin precursors and may increase the risk of neonatal hemorrhage. Providers should encourage pregnant women who elect to continue any anticonvulsant to take high-dose folate (4 mg per day) for the theoretic benefit of reducing the risk of neural tube defects and to undergo a second-trimester ultrasound to screen for major congenital anomalies. In contrast to pregnancy, both valproic acid and carbamazepine are considered safe during breastfeeding.[62]

There appears to be no increased risk of congenital defects above the baseline risk with lamotrigine monotherapy.[65] An early study found a possible increased risk of cleft palate defects.[66] A more recent and larger study, however, using a population-based case-control design using data from the EUROCAT congenital malformation registries, which included data on 3.9 million births, did not find an increased risk of cleft palate.[67] Lamotrigine levels may decrease over the course of pregnancy and thus should be followed and adjusted if needed.[68] Lamotrigine also is considered safe in breastfeeding.[62]

Lithium use during the first trimester has been associated with an increased risk of a serious congenital heart defect, known as Ebstein anomaly. The risk for Ebstein anomaly with first-trimester exposure originally was thought to be much higher (400 times higher than baseline), but a pooled analysis of lithium-exposed pregnancies found that this defect occurs in only less than 1% of exposed children.[69] Lithium also has been associated with perinatal toxicity, including case reports of hypotonia, cyanosis, neonatal goiter, and diabetes insipidus.[45,56] For women with severe BD, the risk of recurrence during pregnancy may overshadow the relatively small risk of Ebstein anomaly. On the other hand, for women with significant periods of euthymia and few past mood episodes, slowly tapering off lithium and reintroducing lithium after the first trimester may help reduce the risk of relapse. There are few data on the long-term outcomes of children exposed in utero, but a follow-up of children up to age 5 demonstrated no evidence of cognitive or behavioral issues in a small sample of children.[70] Lithium levels should be followed closely during pregnancy, and the dose should be held with the initiation of labor. Hydration during delivery should be maintained and the dosage reduced to prepregnancy levels (if increased during pregnancy) with close monitoring of serum levels.[56] Breastfeeding while taking lithium can be tricky due to the risk of elevated lithium levels in a dehydrated baby. A recent systematic review demonstrated relatively low levels of lithium in breastfeeding infants—3 reports of adverse events that were confounded by other factors—and concluded that the decision to breastfeed while taking lithium should be an individualized decision "and should not be contraindicated for all."[71] If a woman breastfeeds while taking lithium, levels should be monitored periodically in the baby, and there should be a low threshold for taking the infant to the emergency room in the setting of dehydration (such as a gastrointestinal illness).

Antipsychotics

Overall, it appears that antipsychotics are, for the most part, relatively safe to use in pregnancy and that not using these medications when indicated for serious mental illness poses a much greater risk, including suicide and infanticide.[72] For example, a study that examined birth outcomes in a matched cohort of women who used antipsychotics in pregnancy (n = 1021) and women with psychiatric illness who did not (n = 1021) and in an unmatched cohort of women who used antipsychotics in pregnancy (n = 1200) and who did not (n = 40,000) revealed an increased risk of adverse outcomes in the unmatched cohort only, indicating that the psychiatric illness itself, not the use of antipsychotics, increased the risk of adverse outcomes for the infant.[73] Furthermore, a recent large Medicaid-based study found that antipsychotics (as a group) used early in pregnancy did not increase the risk for congenital malformations or cardiac malformations when analyses were controlled for confounding factors, although there was a small increased risk for congenital malformations for risperidone.[74] Quetiapine, risperidone, haloperidol, and olanzapine exhibit the lowest placental transfer from mother to fetus.[75]

Normal metabolic changes in pregnancy may increase the risk for gestational diabetes in conjunction with the use of antipsychotics.[76] Many antipsychotics are associated with excessive maternal weight gain, increased infant birth weight, and increased risk of gestational diabetes.[75,77] Routine ultrasound monitoring of fetal size in late pregnancy for women taking these medications is warranted.[77,78] Several studies suggest increased risk of hyperglycemia associated with the use of atypical antipsychotics in pregnancy.[76] This may, however, be due to higher baseline rates of diabetes in women prescribed antipsychotics,[79] reinforcing the need for a thorough evaluation and appropriate glucose monitoring for women prescribed these medications.

There is a lack of evidence regarding late pregnancy exposure to antipsychotics, including little on longer-term developmental outcomes, so the risks remain unclear. Behaviors observed in infants exposed to antipsychotics in utero include motor restlessness, dystonia, hypertonia, and tremor.[80,81] In 2011, the FDA issued a drug safety communication for all antipsychotics regarding the potential risks of abnormal muscle movements and withdrawal symptoms in exposed infants.[82] The few studies examining the relationship between in utero exposure to older typical antipsychotics and neurodevelopment have shown no difference in IQ or behavioral functioning at 5 years.[83–85] In contrast, studies of the newer atypical antipsychotics have shown associated neurodevelopmental delays at 6 months of age[86,87] that no longer are evident at 12 months.[56,86]

Antipsychotic levels in breast milk generally have been found to be low, but there is a significant lack of data on long-term outcomes and potential side effects, including effects on development and extrapyramidal side effects.[88] Women should be counseled regarding this lack of data, and exposed infants should be monitored carefully by their pediatrician.

Antianxiety Agents

Studies of benzodiazepine use during pregnancy have been contradictory. Benzodiazepine use during pregnancy has been associated with case reports of perinatal toxicity, including temperature dysregulation, apnea, depressed Apgar (appearance, pulse, grimace, activity, and respiration) scores, hypotonia, and poor feeding.[89] In addition, early studies revealed an elevated risk of oral cleft palate defects. More recent studies, however, have shown that the overall risk of cleft lip and palate with benzodiazepine use in pregnancy likely is quite low.[89] A recent study also found an increased risk of spontaneous abortion with both long-acting and short-acting benzodiazepines taken early in pregnancy, although the study was not able to completely control for several potentially important confounders, such as smoking and alcohol use.[90] Infants exposed to an SSRI in combination with a benzodiazepine may have a higher incidence of congenital heart defects, even when controlling for maternal illness characteristics,[91] and are more likely to display symptoms of PNAS when combined with an antidepressant.[61] Shorter-acting agents are preferred for breastfeeding to limit sedating side effects in the infant.[62]

A recent study found that benzodiazepine use before conception increased the risk of an ectopic pregnancy slightly, although the study also found evidence that the underlying psychiatric conditions may contribute to this increased risk.[92]

In general, although not approved for the treatment of anxiety, gabapentin is considered a safe alternative for the management of anxiety symptoms during pregnancy. Several studies have indicated that there is no increased risk of major congenital malformations with gabapentin,[93,94] although 2 recent studies found higher rates of preterm birth, low birth weight, and need for neonatal intensive care admission.[95,96] Like gabapentin, pregabalin is not approved for the treatment of anxiety but clinically has some utility in decreasing anxiety symptoms. It is less studied than gabapentin, and a recent review concluded that there was no "clear signal" that pregabalin use in pregnancy is associated with major organ malformations or adverse neonatal outcomes, but that the data were sparse and underpowered.[97]

Buspirone also is useful for anxiety; animal studies have not demonstrated evidence of teratogenesis, but there is no available evidence in humans.

In considering the risks and benefits of antianxiety agents use during pregnancy, clinicians also should consider the risks of untreated insomnia and anxiety in pregnancy, which may lead to physiologic effects as well as diminished self-care, worsening mood, and impaired functioning. Given the consequences of untreated psychiatric symptoms to both women and children and the limited risks associated with antianxiety agent use, some women with overwhelming anxiety symptoms or sleep disturbance may find that the benefits outweigh any theoretic risks.

Stimulants

The data regarding stimulant exposure in pregnancy and lactation are sparse and plagued by small numbers and polypharmacy. For many women, the lack of knowledge about safety in pregnancy and lactation supports discontinuation of stimulants, which typically are prescribed for attention-deficit/hyperactivity disorder or as an adjunctive medication. To date, there is no evidence of increased organ malformations,[98,99] although there may be an increased risk of spontaneous abortion.[98,100] The long-term neurobehavioral effects on children exposed to stimulants in pregnancy and/or breastfeeding are unknown.[99]

Box 5 describes general approaches for management of different classes of psychiatric medications during pregnancy.

Brexanolone: A New Treatment of Postpartum Depression

Brexanolone is a synthetic version of the natural neurosteroid and progesterone metabolite, allopregnanolone. Allopregnanolone levels, like estrogen and progesterone, drop precipitously in the immediate postpartum time period, and some research suggests that women with lower levels of allopregnanolone during pregnancy have an increased risk for PPD. Currently, Brexanolone is not recommended for use during

Box 5 General recommendations by psychiatric medication type		
Class of Psychiatric Medication	**General Comments: Pregnancy**	**General Comments: Lactation**
Antidepressants	Generally considered safe Use older medications over newer one if possible. Risks: small risk of PPHN, moderate risk of PNAS, preterm birth May increase risk of spontaneous abortion	Generally considered safe
Mood-stabilizing medications	Do not use valproic acid or carbamazepine. Lithium has a <1% chance of Ebstein anomaly and can be used.	Valproic acid and carbamazepine can be used safely in lactation. Use lithium with caution in breastfeeding.
Antipsychotics	No major organ malformations associated Mild developmental delay can be seen at 6 mo, which resolves.	Little is known about long-term exposure in breastfeeding.
Benzodiazepine	No major organ malformations Can cause neonatal toxicity and withdrawal Generally, try to limit to as needed use, particularly in third trimester. May increase risk of spontaneous abortion	Can cause sedation in the infant
Other antianxiety agents	Gabapentin generally is considered safe with no major organ malformation. Pregabalin has few data but so far appears to have no major organ malformations. Buspirone has no human data.	Gabapentin generally is considered safe. Pregabalin has fewer data. Both may cause sedation in the breastfeeding infant. Buspirone has few data.
Stimulants	No major organ malformations Generally, discontinue if possible.	Unknown long-term neurobehavioral outcomes with prolonged exposure

pregnancy or lactation, but ob-gyns should be aware of its existence because many hospitals are administering it on ob-gyn wards because patients require constant pulse oximetry monitoring, making it difficult to administer on psychiatry units. Brexanolone has been studied in 2 multicenter, randomized, placebo-controlled trials[101]; is infused intravenously over 60 hours; and can produce rapid (12–24 hours) results in moderate to severe perinatal depression. Common adverse effects included somnolence, dizziness, and headache. A small number of patients required cessation of the infusion due to excessive sedation or loss of consciousness. A Risk Evaluation and Mitigation Strategy program is in place to minimize adverse events, and inpatient admission with 24-hour pulse oximetry monitoring is required.

SUMMARY

Although growing, the data regarding the safety of psychiatric medications during pregnancy and lactation continue to be limited, primarily by studies that have not properly controlled for the risk factors and behaviors that are more common in the psychiatric population that may influence pregnancy outcomes. Most well-controlled studies are reassuring to date, especially for antidepressants. Areas that need further research include the safety of antipsychotics in pregnancy and breast-feeding and long-term outcomes for children exposed to psychiatric medications. The area also will benefit from studies that examine the issue of dosing of psychiatric medications in pregnancy and prevention of recurrent illness both in and after pregnancy. One fact that is clear from the available literature is that psychiatric illness is associated with negative outcomes for both mother and child and should be actively clinically managed despite the lack of data.

CLINICAL CARE POINTS

- Ideally, make a plan for psychiatric management prior to pregnancy.
- Communicate directly with the treating psychiatrist/provider prior to making or recommending medication changes.
- Most but not all psychiatric medications can be used during pregnancy and lactation, and the risk of not treating psychiatric illness is high to both mother and child.
- Try to minimize the number of exposures for the child, including number of medications, as well as exposure to psychiatric illness.
- Screening for a history of psychiatric illness or new-onset illness prior to pregnancy and during pregnancy and postpartum is ideal in the ob-gyn setting.
- Do not undertreat psychiatric illness during pregnancy and lactation.

DISCLOSURE

Dr J.L. Payne has a patent for Epigenetic Biomarkers of Postpartum Depression and in the past year has served on advisory boards for Janssen Pharmaceuticals and for Sage Therapeutics.

REFERENCES

1. Steinig J, Nagl M, Linde K, et al. Antenatal and postnatal depression in women with obesity: a systematic review. Arch Womens Ment Health 2017;20(4): 569–85.

2. Yonkers KA, Wisner KL, Stewart DE, et al. The management of depression during pregnancy: a report from the american psychiatric association and the american college of obstetricians and gynecologists. Gen Hosp Psychiatry 2009;31(5):403–13.

3. Li D, Liu L, Odouli R. Presence of depressive symptoms during early pregnancy and the risk of preterm delivery: a prospective cohort study. Hum Reprod 2009; 24(1):146–53.

4. Zuckerman B, Amaro H, Bauchner H, et al. Depressive symptoms during pregnancy: relationship to poor health behaviors. Am J Obstet Gynecol 1989;160(5): 1107.

5. Orr ST, Blazer DG, James SA, et al. Depressive symptoms and indicators of maternal health status during pregnancy. J Womens Health (Larchmt) 2007; 16(4):535–42.

6. Osborne S, Biaggi A, Chua TE, et al. Antenatal depression programs cortisol stress reactivity in offspring through increased maternal inflammation and cortisol in pregnancy: the psychiatry research and motherhood - depression (PRAM-D) study. Psychoneuroendocrinology 2018;98:211–21.

7. Brennan PA, Pargas R, Walker EF, et al. Maternal depression and infant cortisol: Influences of timing, comorbidity and treatment. J Child Psychol Psychiatry 2008;49(10):1099–107.

8. Robertson E, Grace S, Wallington T, et al. Antenatal risk factors for postpartum depression: a synthesis of recent literature. Gen Hosp Psychiatry 2004;26(4): 289–95.

9. Lindahl V, Pearson JL, Colpe L. Prevalence of suicidality during pregnancy and the postpartum. Arch Womens Ment Health 2005;8(2):77–87.

10. Akman I, Kuşçu K, Ozdemir N, et al. Mothers' postpartum psychological adjustment and infantile colic. Arch Dis Child 2006;91(5):417–9.

11. Flynn HA, Davis M, Marcus SM, et al. Rates of maternal depression in pediatric emergency department and relationship to child service utilization. Gen Hosp Psychiatry 2004;26(4):316–22.

12. McLearn KT, Minkovitz CS, Strobino DM, et al. The timing of maternal depressive symptoms and mothers' parenting practices with young children: Implications for pediatric practice. Pediatrics 2006;118(1):174.

13. Grace SL, Evindar A, Stewart DE. The effect of postpartum depression on child cognitive development and behavior: A review and critical analysis of the literature. Arch Womens Ment Health 2003;6(4):263–74.

14. Cohen LS, Altshuler LL, Harlow BL, et al. Relapse of major depression during pregnancy in women who maintain or discontinue antidepressant treatment. J Am Med Assoc 2006;295(5):499–507.

15. Viguera AC, Whitfield T, Baldessarini RJ, et al. Risk of recurrence in women with bipolar disorder during pregnancy: prospective study of mood stabilizer discontinuation. Am J Psychiatry 2007;164(12):1817–24 [quiz 1923].

16. Newport DJ, Stowe ZN, Viguera AC, et al. Lamotrigine in bipolar disorder: efficacy during pregnancy. Bipolar Disord 2008;10(3):432–6.

17. Payne JL, Roy PS, Murphy-Eberenz K, et al. Reproductive cycle-associated mood symptoms in women with major depression and bipolar disorder. J Affect Disord 2007;99(1–3):221–9.

18. Siu AL, US Preventive Services Task Force (USPSTF), Bibbins-Domingo K, et al. Screening for depression in adults: US preventive services task force recommendation statement. JAMA 2016;315(4):380–7.

19. ACOG committee opinion no. 757 summary: Screening for perinatal depression. Obstet Gynecol 2018;132(5):1314–6. Available at: https://journals.lww.com/greenjournal/Fulltext/2018/11000/ACOG_Committee_Opinion_No__757_Summary__Screening.37.aspx.
20. Gregory KD, Chelmow D, Nelson HD, et al. Screening for anxiety in adolescent and adult women: a recommendation from the women's preventive services initiative. Ann Intern Med 2020;173(1):48–56.
21. Hirschfeld RM. The mood disorder questionnaire: a simple, patient-rated screening instrument for bipolar disorder. Prim Care Companion J Clin Psychiatry 2002;4(1):9–11.
22. Cox JL, Chapman G, Murray D, et al. Validation of the edinburgh postnatal depression scale (EPDS) in non-postnatal women. J Affect Disord 1996;39(3): 185–9.
23. Spitzer RL, Kroenke K, Williams JB. Validation and utility of a self-report version of PRIME-MD: The PHQ primary care study. primary care evaluation of mental disorders. patient health questionnaire. JAMA 1999;282(18):1737–44.
24. Kroenke K, Spitzer RL, Williams JB, et al. An ultra-brief screening scale for anxiety and depression: The PHQ-4. Psychosomatics 2009;50(6):613–21.
25. Zigmond AS, Snaith RP. The hospital anxiety and depression scale. Acta Psychiatr Scand 1983;67(6):361–70.
26. Finer LB, Zolna MR. Declines in unintended pregnancy in the united states, 2008-2011. N Engl J Med 2016;374(9):843–52.
27. Pearlstein T. Depression during pregnancy. Best Pract Res Clin Obstet Gynaecol 2015;29(5):754–64.
28. Hanley GE, Oberlander TF. The effect of perinatal exposures on the infant: antidepressants and depression. Best Pract Res Clin Obstet Gynaecol 2014;28: 37–48.
29. Alwan S, Reefhuis J, Rasmussen SA, et al, National Birth Defects Prevention Study. Patterns of antidepressant medication use among pregnant women in a united states population. J Clin Pharmacol 2011;51(2):264–70.
30. Rahimi R, Nikfar S, Abdollahi M. Pregnancy outcomes following exposure to serotonin reuptake inhibitors: a meta-analysis of clinical trials. Reprod Toxicol 2006;22(4):571–5.
31. Addis A, Koren G. Safety of fluoxetine during the first trimester of pregnancy: a meta-analytical review of epidemiological studies. Psychol Med 2000;30(1): 89–94.
32. Einarson TR, Einarson A. Newer antidepressants in pregnancy and rates of major malformations: a meta-analysis of prospective comparative studies. Pharmacoepidemiol Drug Saf 2005;14:823–7.
33. O'Brien L, Einarson TR, Sarkar M, et al. Does paroxetine cause cardiac malformations? J Obstet Gynaecol Can 2008;30(8):696–701.
34. Davis RL, Rubanowice D, McPhillips H, et al. Risks of congenital malformations and perinatal events among infants exposed to antidepressant medications during pregnancy. Pharmacoepidemiol Drug Saf 2007;16:1086–94.
35. Nulman I, Barrera M, Pulver A, et al. Neurodevelopment of children exposed in utero to venlafaxine: preliminary results. Birth Defects Res A Clin Mol Teratol 2010;88(5):363.
36. Pastuszak A, Schick-Boschetto B, Zuber C, et al. Pregnancy outcome following first-trimester exposure to fluoxetine (prozac). JAMA 1993;269(17):2246–8.
37. Simon GE, Cunningham ML, Davis RL. Outcomes of prenatal antidepressant exposure. Am J Psychiatry 2002;159(12):2055–61.

38. Ramos E, St-Andre M, Rey E, et al. Duration of antidepressant use during pregnancy and risk of major congenital malformations. Br J Psychiatry 2008;192(5): 344–50.

39. Reis M, Kallen B. Delivery outcome after maternal use of antidepressant drugs in pregnancy: an update using swedish data. Psychol Med 2010;40(10): 1723–33.

40. Chun-Fai-Chan B, Koren G, Fayez I, et al. Pregnancy outcome of women exposed to bupropion during pregnancy: a prospective comparative study. Am J Obstet Gynecol 2005;192(3):932–6.

41. Cole JA, Modell JG, Haight BR, et al. Bupropion in pregnancy and the prevalence of congenital malformations. Pharmacoepidemiol Drug Saf 2007;16(5): 474–84.

42. Alwan S, Reefhuis J, Botto LD, et al. Maternal use of bupropion and risk for congenital heart defects. Am J Obstet Gynecol 2010;203(1):52.e1–6.

43. Byatt N, Deligiannidis KM, Freeman MP. Antidepressant use in pregnancy: a critical review focused on risks and controversies. Acta Psychiatr Scand 2013;127:94–114.

44. Yonkers KA, Blackwell KA, Glover J, et al. Antidepressant use in pregnant and postpartum women. Annu Rev Clin Psychol 2014;10(1):369–92. Available at: https://search.datacite.org/works/10.1146/annurev-clinpsy-032813-153626.

45. Chisolm MS, Payne JL. Management of psychotropic drugs during pregnancy. BMJ 2016;532:h5918.

46. Huybrechts KF, Palmsten K, Avorn J, et al. Antidepressant use in pregnancy and the risk of cardiac defects. N Engl J Med 2014;370(25):2397.

47. Wang S, Yang L, Wang L, et al. Selective serotonin reuptake inhibitors (SSRIs) and the risk of congenital heart defects: A meta-analysis of prospective cohort studies. J Am Heart Assoc 2015;4(5). https://doi.org/10.1161/JAHA.114. 001681.

48. Walsh-Sukys MC, Tyson JE, Wright LL, et al. Persistent pulmonary hypertension of the newborn in the era before nitric oxide: practice variation and outcomes. Pediatrics 2000;105(1 Pt 1):14–20.

49. Chambers CD, Hernandez-Diaz S, Van Marter LJ, et al. Selective serotonin-reuptake inhibitors and risk of persistent pulmonary hypertension of the newborn. N Engl J Med 2006;354(6):579–87.

50. Grigoriadis S, Vonderporten EH, Mamisashvili L, et al. Prenatal exposure to antidepressants and persistent pulmonary hypertension of the newborn: systematic review and meta-analysis. BMJ 2014;348:f6932.

51. Ng QX, Venkatanarayanan N, Ho CYX, et al. Selective serotonin reuptake inhibitors and persistent pulmonary hypertension of the newborn: an update meta-analysis. J Womens Health (Larchmt) 2019;28(3):331–8.

52. Kieler H, Artama M, Engeland A, et al. Selective serotonin reuptake inhibitors during pregnancy and risk of persistent pulmonary hypertension in the newborn: population based cohort study from the five nordic countries. BMJ 2012; 344(7842):1.

53. Kobayashi T, Matsuyama T, Takeuchi M, et al. Autism spectrum disorder and prenatal exposure to selective serotonin reuptake inhibitors: a systematic review and meta-analysis. Reprod Toxicol 2016;65:170–8.

54. Ross LE, Grigoriadis S, Mamisashvili L, et al. Selected pregnancy and delivery outcomes after exposure to antidepressant medication: a systematic review and meta-analysis. JAMA Psychiatry 2013;70(4):436–43.

55. Nakhai-Pour HR, Broy P, Berard A. Use of antidepressants during pregnancy and the risk of spontaneous abortion. CMAJ 2010;182(10):1031–7.
56. Pearlstein T. Use of psychotropic medication during pregnancy and the postpartum period. Womens Health (Lond) 2013;9:605–15.
57. Jarde A, Morais M, Kingston D, et al. Neonatal outcomes in women with untreated antenatal depression compared with women without depression: a systematic review and meta-analysis. JAMA Psychiatry 2016;73(8):826–37.
58. Webster PA. Withdrawal symptoms in neonates associated with maternal antidepressant therapy. Lancet 1973;2(7824):318–9.
59. GlaxoSmithKline. Paroxetine [package insert]. Research Triangle Park (NC); 2011.
60. Moses-Kolko E, Bogen D, Perel J, et al. Neonatal signs after late in utero exposure to serotonin reuptake inhibitors: literature review and implications for clinical applications. JAMA 2005;293(19):2372.
61. Oberlander TF, Misri S, Fitzgerald CE, et al. Pharmacologic factors associated with transient neonatal symptoms following prenatal psychotropic medication exposure. J Clin Psychiatry 2004;65(2):230–7.
62. Moretti ME. Psychotropic drugs in lactation–motherisk update 2008. Can J Clin Pharmacol 2009;16:49.
63. Bromley RL, Mawer GE, Briggs M, et al. The prevalence of neurodevelopmental disorders in children prenatally exposed to antiepileptic drugs. J Neurol Neurosurg Psychiatr 2013;84(6):637–43.
64. Christensen J, Gronborg TK, Sorensen MJ, et al. Prenatal valproate exposure and risk of autism spectrum disorders and childhood autism. JAMA 2013; 309(16):1696–703.
65. Cunnington M, Tennis P, International Lamotrigine Pregnancy Registry Scientific Advisory Committee. Lamotrigine and the risk of malformations in pregnancy. Neurology 2005;64(6):955–60.
66. Holmes LB, Baldwin EJ, Smith CR, et al. Increased frequency of isolated cleft palate in infants exposed to lamotrigine during pregnancy. Neurology 2008; 70(22 Pt 2):2152–8.
67. Dolk H, Jentink J, Loane M, et al. EUROCAT antiepileptic drug working group. does lamotrigine use in pregnancy increase orofacial cleft risk relative to other malformations? Neurology 2008;71(10):714–22.
68. Clark CT, Klein AM, Perel JM, et al. Lamotrigine dosing for pregnant patients with bipolar disorder. Am J Psychiatry 2013;170(11):1240–7.
69. Cohen LS, Friedman JM, Jefferson JW, et al. A reevaluation of risk of in utero exposure to lithium. JAMA 1994;271(2):146–50.
70. Jacobson SJ, Jones K, Johnson K, et al. Prospective multicentre study of pregnancy outcome after lithium exposure during first trimester. Lancet 1992; 339(8792):530–3.
71. Newmark RL, Bogen DL, Wisner KL, et al. Risk-benefit assessment of infant exposure to lithium through breast milk: a systematic review of the literature. Int Rev Psychiatry 2019;31(3):295–304.
72. Robinson GE. Treatment of schizophrenia in pregnancy and postpartum. J Popul Ther Clin Pharmacol 2012;19:380.
73. Vigod SN, Gomes T, Wilton AS, et al. Antipsychotic drug use in pregnancy: high dimensional, propensity matched, population based cohort study. BMJ 2015; 350:h2298.

74. Huybrechts KF, Hernández-Díaz S, Patorno E, et al. Antipsychotic use in pregnancy and the risk for congenital malformations. JAMA Psychiatry 2016;73(9):938–46.

75. Newport DJ, Calamaras MR, DeVane CL, et al. Atypical antipsychotic administration during late pregnancy: placental passage and obstetrical outcomes. Am J Psychiatry 2007;164(8):1214–20.

76. McCauley-Elsom K, Gurvich C, Elsom SJ, et al. Antipsychotics in pregnancy. J Psychiatr Ment Health Nurs 2010;17:97–104.

77. Newham JJ, Thomas SH, MacRitchie K, et al. Birth weight of infants after maternal exposure to typical and atypical antipsychotics: Prospective comparison study. Br J Psychiatry 2008;192(5):333–7.

78. Paton C. Prescribing in pregnancy. Br J Psychiatry 2008;192(5):321–2.

79. Khalifeh H, Dolman C, Howard LM. Safety of psychotropic drugs in pregnancy. BMJ 2015;350:h2260.

80. Gentile S. Antipsychotic therapy during early and late pregnancy. A systematic review. Schizophr Bull 2010;36:518–44.

81. Coppola D, Russo LJ, Kwarta RF J, et al. Evaluating the postmarketing experience of risperidone use during pregnancy: pregnancy and neonatal outcomes. Drug Saf 2007;30:247–64.

82. US Food and Drug Administration. US food and drug administration drug safety communication: antipsychotic drug labels updated on use during pregnancy and risk of abnormal muscle movements and withdrawal symptoms in newborns. 2011. Available at: https://www.fda.gov/drugs/drug-safety-and-availability/fda-drug-safety-communication-antipsychotic-drug-labels-updated-use-during-pregnancy-and-risk. Accessed September 23, 2020.

83. Barnes TR. Schizophrenia Consensus Group of British Association for Psychopharmacology. Evidence-based guidelines for the pharmacological treatment of schizophrenia: Recommendations from the british association for psychopharmacology. J Psychopharmacol 2011;25(5):567–620.

84. Altshuler LL, Cohen L, Szuba MP, et al. Pharmacologic management of psychiatric illness during pregnancy: dilemmas and guidelines. Am J Psychiatry 1996;153(5):592.

85. Thiels C. Pharmacotherapy of psychiatric disorder in pregnancy and during breastfeeding: a review. Pharmacopsychiatry 1987;20(4):133–46.

86. Peng M, Gao K, Ding Y, et al. Effects of prenatal exposure to atypical antipsychotics on postnatal development and growth of infants: a case-controlled, prospective study. Psychopharmacology (Berl) 2013;228(4):577.

87. Johnson KC, LaPrairie JL, Brennan PA, et al. Prenatal antipsychotic exposure and neuromotor performance during infancy. Arch Gen Psychiatry 2012;69(8):787–94.

88. Klinger G, Stahl B, Fusar-Poli P, et al. Antipsychotic drugs and breastfeeding. Pediatr Endocrinol Rev 2013;10(3):308–17.

89. Shyken JM, Babbar S, Babbar S, et al. Benzodiazepines in pregnancy. Clin Obstet Gynecol 2019;62(1):156–67.

90. Sheehy O, Zhao JP, Bérard A. Association between incident exposure to benzodiazepines in early pregnancy and risk of spontaneous abortion. JAMA Psychiatry 2019;76(9):948–57.

91. Oberlander TF, Warburton W, Misri S, et al. Major congenital malformations following prenatal exposure to serotonin reuptake inhibitors and benzodiazepines using population-based health data. Birth Defects Res B Dev Reprod Toxicol 2008;83(1):68–76.

92. Wall-Wieler E, Robakis TK, Lyell DJ, et al. Benzodiazepine use before conception and risk of ectopic pregnancy. Hum Reprod 2020;35(7):1685–92.
93. Holmes LB, Hernandez-Diaz S. Newer anticonvulsants: lamotrigine, topiramate and gabapentin. Birth Defects Res A Clin Mol Teratol. 2012;94(8):599–606.
94. Molgaard-Nielsen D, Hviid A. Newer-generation antiepileptic drugs and the risk of major birth defects. JAMA 2011;305(19):1996–2002.
95. Fujii Y. Prevention of nausea and vomiting during termination of pregnancy. Int J Gynaecol Obstet 2010;111:3–7.
96. Patorno E, Hernandez-Diaz S, Huybrechts KF, et al. Gabapentin in pregnancy and the risk of adverse neonatal and maternal outcomes: a population-based cohort study nested in the US medicaid analytic eXtract dataset. PLoS Med 2020;17(9):e1003322.
97. Andrade C. Safety of pregabalin in pregnancy. J Clin Psychiatry 2018;79(5):18f12568.
98. Pottegard A, Hallas J, Andersen JT, et al. First-trimester exposure to methylphenidate: a population-based cohort study. J Clin Psychiatry 2014;75(1):88.
99. Ornoy A. Pharmacological treatment of attention deficit hyperactivity disorder during pregnancy and lactation. Pharm Res 2018;35(3):46-z.
100. Bro SP, Kjaersgaard MI, Parner ET, et al. Adverse pregnancy outcomes after exposure to methylphenidate or atomoxetine during pregnancy. Clin Epidemiol 2015;7:139–47.
101. Meltzer-Brody S, Colquhoun H, Riesenberg R, et al. Brexanolone injection in post-partum depression: two multicentre, double-blind, randomised, placebo-controlled, phase 3 trials. Lancet 2018;392(10152):1058–70.

Goals for Collaborative Management of Obstetric Hemorrhage

Suzanne McMurtry Baird, DNP, RN[a],*, Stephanie Martin, DO[a],
Margaret (Betsy) Babb Kennedy, PhD, RN, CNE[b]

KEYWORDS

- Obstetric hemorrhage • Transfusion • Hypovolemic shock
- Maternal morbidity and mortality

KEY POINTS

- Obstetric hemorrhage is a leading preventable cause of perinatal morbidity and mortality requiring a rapid, planned, and coordinated interprofessional response to management in order to promote optimal outcomes.
- Although blood loss is anticipated at birth, early recognition of excessive blood loss and initiation of pharmacotherapy, medical, and surgical interventions offer progressive management options.
- Goals of management include recognition and management of bleeding, maintaining tissue oxygenation and perfusion, and ongoing monitoring for coagulopathies and complications.

INTRODUCTION

Despite significant state and national initiatives to promote prevention and recognition, as well as rapidly evolving treatment modalities, obstetric hemorrhage remains a leading, preventable cause of maternal morbidity and mortality in the United States and the world.[1–4] When analyzing data from US state-led maternal mortality review committees, pregnancy-related death from hemorrhage was judged to be preventable in 70% of cases.[2] Further review outlined contributing factors leading to hemorrhage deaths, which included systems of care (36%), provider factors (31%), and patient/family factors (26%). Common themes in the systems of care category included inadequate training, unavailable personnel, absence of policies/procedures, and lack of coordination. Provider factors included issues with assessment, delays in diagnosis

[a] Clinical Concepts in Obstetrics, 101 Creekside Crossing, Suite 1700-136, Brentwood, TN 37027, USA; [b] Non-Tenure Track Faculty Affairs and Advancement, Vanderbilt University School of Nursing, 461 21st Avenue South, Nashville, TN 37240, USA
* Corresponding author.
E-mail address: suzannebaird@clinicalconceptsinob.com

Obstet Gynecol Clin N Am 48 (2021) 151–171
https://doi.org/10.1016/j.ogc.2020.11.001
0889-8545/21/© 2020 Elsevier Inc. All rights reserved.

obgyn.theclinics.com

and effective treatment, missed diagnosis, and infective treatments. Patient/family factors highlighted a lack of knowledge regarding warning signs and the need to seek care.[2]

In addition to mortality, obstetric hemorrhage is the most common indicator of severe maternal morbidity, including blood transfusion, disseminated intravascular coagulation (DIC), and hysterectomy. The need for blood transfusion during delivery hospitalization has increased 54% from 2006 to 2015 and is identified in 78% of all cases of severe maternal morbidity.[5] In a national representative sample of delivery discharges, obstetric hemorrhage is the second leading cause of severe morbidity.[6] In patients who hemorrhage and progress to hypovolemic shock, one-third require hysterectomy.[5] Racial disparities in maternal mortality and morbidity as a result of obstetric hemorrhage mirror those of overall maternal mortalities, with non-Hispanic black women being disproportionately affected.[7,8]

Definition

Obstetric hemorrhage is generally defined using blood loss and the state of cardiovascular decompensation, but specific parameters vary. Generally accepted definitions of obstetric hemorrhage include a cumulative estimated blood loss of greater than 1000 mL for either vaginal or cesarean birth, and blood loss associated with maternal signs and symptoms of hypovolemia. In addition, The American College of Obstetricians and Gynecologists (ACOG) recommends that blood loss greater than 500 mL after vaginal birth should trigger increased surveillance while simultaneously investigating the cause.[9] Further, significant physiologic changes during pregnancy may delay recognition of typical early warning signs of hypovolemia and shock, such as hypotension and tachycardia. Therefore, careful observation and preparation for rapid intervention should be implemented with blood loss greater than 500 mL to 1000 mL even in the absence of maternal symptoms.

COLLABORATIVE MANAGEMENT OF OBSTETRIC HEMORRHAGE

Caring for a patient with hemorrhage requires an interprofessional approach to management in order to optimize maternal and fetal outcomes.

There are 4 overarching goals for treatment:

1. Monitor for signs and symptoms of hemorrhage and shock
2. Manage the bleeding
3. Maintain tissue oxygenation and perfusion
4. Monitor for coagulopathy and complications.

Goal 1: Monitor for Signs and Symptoms of Hemorrhage and Shock

Physiologic changes that occur during pregnancy create reserve for anticipated blood loss at birth. As a result, the expected clinically observed signs of compromise may be more difficult to recognize in a hemorrhaging obstetric patient. The hematologic and hemostatic adaptations in pregnancy are summarized in **Table 1**.

Cardiovascular hemodynamic changes in pregnancy primarily consist of increased blood volume and increased heart rate, resulting in increased maternal cardiac output of 30% to 50% (6–10 L/min at rest in term gestation).[10] Hormonally mediated changes result in decreasing systemic vascular resistance concurrent with cardiac output increases, thus creating a high-flow, low-resistance state of pregnancy. The protective physiologic adaptations of pregnancy also create the potential for significant blood loss before manifestations of maternal symptoms. When 10% of circulating blood

Table 1
Hematologic and hemostatic adaptations in pregnancy

Alterations	Results
Blood volume to 6–7 L	• Hypercoagulable state
Plasma volume 40%–50%	○ Increased efficiency of clotting
Plasma renin activity	○ Decreased fibrinolysis
Atrial natriuretic peptide levels	• Decrease in hematocrit
Erythropoietin levels	• Leukocytosis (up to 12,200/mm^3)
Red blood cell mass	• Neutrophilia
Factors II, VII, VIII, X, XII, XIII	• Mild thrombocytopenia
von Willebrand factor	• Decreased oxygen affinity for maternal RBCs
Fibrinogen	• Platelet counts decrease slightly in third trimester,
Factors XI, XIII	but remain in normal range
= Factors V, IX	
= Protein C	
Thrombin activatable fibrinolytic inhibitor, PA-1, and PA-2	
Fibrin D-dimer, fibrin monomers, fibrinopeptides A and B	
Plasminogen activator, tissue-type plasminogen activator	
RBCs 2,3-bisphosphoglycerate	
Neutrophils	
Granulocytes	
Platelet count	

Abbreviations: PA, plasminogen activator inhibitor; RBC, red blood cell; =, no change; , increase; , decrease.

Data from Antony K.M., Racusin D.A., Aagaard K., Dildy G.A. Maternal physiology. In: Landon M.B., Galan H., Jauniaux E., et al (Eds.) Gabbe's Obstetrics: Normal and Problem Pregnancies, 8th edition. Amsterdam: Elsevier; 2021. And Kennedy BB, Baird SM. Collaborative strategies for management of obstetric hemorrhage. In: O'Malley P., Foster J. (Eds). Critical Care Nurs Clin North Am 2017;29(3):315-330.

volume is lost, compensatory vasoconstriction occurs to compensate, which maintains blood pressure in the normal range. With continued hemorrhage and a 20% loss in blood volume, progressive tachycardia occurs as a compensatory response to increase cardiac output. Hypotension is a late sign and does not occur until greater than 20% blood volume is lost. Once an average-term patient becomes hypotensive and tachycardiac, at least 2 L of blood have been lost.[11]

Early recognition, communication, and activation of appropriate team members to the bedside are key management strategies for control of hemorrhage, treatment of hypovolemia, and prevention of shock. Sustained clinical triggers for intervention and correction of hypovolemia are (1) heart rate greater than or equal to 110 beats/min, (2) blood pressure less than or equal to 85/45 mm Hg (>15% decrease), and (3) oxygen saturation less than 95%.[12]

In pregnant or postpartum patients with bleeding, physical assessments provide clues to recognition and parameters for ongoing monitoring of compromise. Increased frequency of assessments focused on defined physiologic parameters alert the clinician to potential maternal compromise. Once abnormal assessment parameters are evident, early communication and activation of appropriate response team members for management are crucial. Each institution should establish thresholds for abnormal assessment parameters and outline required actions and response to abnormal parameters (partnership for mat safety). Physical assessment parameters that reflect intravascular volume depletion, decreased cardiac output, and shock are outlined in **Table 2**.

Recognition of hypovolemic shock

Hypovolemic shock occurs when volume of blood lost exceeds the patient's ability to compensate, leading to cardiovascular compromise, tissue hypoxia, and metabolic acidosis. The initial response to loss of circulating volume is an increase in heart rate and vasoconstriction to try to maintain cardiac output and blood pressure, as shown in **Fig. 1**.

As preload decreases, vasoconstriction occurs peripherally and centrally. Peripheral vasoconstriction leads to cool extremities and weaker pulses with decreased pulse pressure, among other findings. Capillary bed vasoconstriction and autotransfusion to the central circulation temporarily increase circulating blood volume. Preferential shunting of circulating blood volume is directed to the heart, brain, and lungs, and away from nonessential organ systems, including the kidneys and uterus. When volume is not adequately restored, compensatory mechanisms ultimately fail, and progression to metabolic acidosis, end-organ dysfunction, and death can occur.[13]

Maternal hemorrhage can be classified by volume of blood loss or in a staged approach. **Table 3** outlines the 4 classes of acute blood loss and the associated noninvasive assessment changes.

Quantitative assessment of blood loss

Attempts to accurately assess blood loss are essential in the event of hemorrhage. Visual estimates of blood loss are unreliable and inaccurate, potentially delaying timely recognition and management of obstetric hemorrhage.[14] Data show that more accurate and objective blood loss assessment is achieved with quantified blood loss (QBL) measurement.[15–17] Although QBL offers increased accuracy in measurement and estimation of blood loss compared with visual methods, improved clinical outcomes have not yet been shown.[14,18–20]

Techniques for measuring QBL include weighing blood-saturated items, and use of collection devices, such as calibrated underbuttocks draping. However, the presence of amniotic fluid, urine, feces, and irrigation solution can complicate accurate determination of blood loss. One technique to improve accuracy is to stop after birth and before delivery of the placenta, assess the collected volume lost, and determine a baseline. Additional blood volume lost may then be more easily assessed. To quantify blood volume loss by weight, subtract the dry weight of the pads, sponges, or other absorbing materials from the weight of blood-containing materials using a 1 g per 1 mL conversion. Therefore, a sponge soaked with blood that weighs 100 g after subtracting the dry weight of the sponge would account for 100 mL of blood loss. Adoption of cumulative QBL procedures is recommended to standardize processes at all births, rather than implementation after significant blood loss is noted or the patient becomes symptomatic.[14,18]

Goal 2: Manage Hemorrhage

Management of obstetric hemorrhage while simultaneously determining the cause of hemorrhage is necessary to improve outcomes. If a woman is still pregnant at a viable gestational age when hemorrhage occurs, continuous electronic fetal monitoring is ongoing to determine fetal status.

Medication

Most cases of postpartum hemorrhage are caused by uterine atony. As a result, uterotonic medications to manage atony are used simultaneously or secondarily to

Table 2
Assessment of hypovolemia and shock

Parameter	Assessment	Rationale
Heart rate	Tachycardia; heart rate >110 beats/min and trending upward	Compensatory to maintain cardiac output; caused by catecholamine release; monitor for dysrhythmia
Respiratory rate	Tachypnea; respiratory rate >24 breaths/min and trending upward	Influence of stress, catecholamine release, hypoxia, and metabolic acidosis caused by decreased tissue perfusion
Blood pressure	Initially increased; decreases with reduced cardiac output	Initial increase is compensatory vasoconstriction caused by catecholamine release as an attempt to maintain cardiac output; hypotension is a late sign and associated with shock
Pulse pressure (systolic/diastolic)	Narrowing	Reflects a decrease in stroke volume; <30 mm Hg consider shock
SpO_2	Decreased to <96%	Reflects increased oxygen use and decreased perfusion; inability to monitor waveform as peripheral pulses weaken
Capillary refill	Prolonged capillary refill >4 s	Vasoconstriction occurs because of decreased intravascular volume, leading to decreased perfusion
Peripheral pulse quality	Weak, thready, progressing to absent	Decreased cardiac preload and decreased perfusion
Urine output	Oliguria <30 mL/h for 2 consecutive hours	Decreased kidney perfusion, vasoconstriction, and hypoxia
Skin temperature of extremities	Cool to touch	Peripheral vasoconstriction
Skin color	Pallor	Peripheral vasoconstriction; limited in patients with dark skin color
Skin appearance	Mottled	Low cardiac output state, decreased perfusion
Mucous membranes	Dry, pale; increased thirst	Decreased intravascular volume
Level of consciousness	Initial anxiety and confusion; progression to unconscious state	Decreased cerebral perfusion leading to cerebral hypoxia and acidosis; late sign
Cardiac arrest	Pulseless electrical activity	Caused by critical organ failure secondary to blood/fluid loss, hypoxia, dysrhythmia, decreased perfusion, and acidosis

Data from Kennedy BB, Baird SM. Collaborative strategies for management of obstetric hemorrhage. In: O'Malley P., Foster J. (Eds). Critical Care Nurs Clin North Am 2017;29(3):315-330. And Dell'Anna AM., Torrini F, Antonelli M. Shock: Definition and Recognition. In: Pinsky M., Teboul JL., Vincent JL. (eds). Hemodynamic Monitoring. Lessons from the ICU (Under the Auspices of the European Society of Intensive Care Medicine). Springer, Cham. 2019.

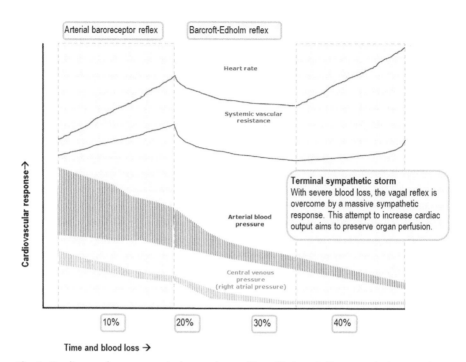

Fig. 1. Cardiovascular response to hemorrhage. (*From* Yartsev A. Response to haemorrhage: the loss of 1L of blood. Deranged Physiology: A free online resource for Intensive Care Medicine. Available at: https://derangedphysiology.com/main/cicm-primary-exam/required-reading/body-fluids-and-electrolytes/manipulation-fluids-and-electrolytes/Chapter%20118/response-haemorrhage-loss-1l-blood With permission.)

manipulation measures and should be readily available for immediate administration.[11] Oxytocin administration is recommended at birth of the fetus or after delivery of the placenta for active management of the third stage of labor to decrease the risk of hemorrhage.[21] No single uterotonic has been shown to be superior to another.[22] It is common for multiple agents to be used in attempts to control hemorrhage. If the patient fails to respond, rapid escalation to more aggressive interventions is necessary.[9]

Tranexamic acid (TXA) has shown promise as an adjunct therapy in the management of hemorrhaging patients. It works by inhibiting enzymatic breakdown of fibrin. The World Maternal Antifibrinolytic (WOMAN) trial showed a 31% reduction in maternal death caused by hemorrhage, with no adverse effects.[23] TXA 1 g may be given orally or intravenously and must be administered within 3 hours of the onset of bleeding. Data are insufficient to recommend use of TXA prophylactically or as first-line treatment of postpartum hemorrhage.[9]

Off-label administration of recombinant factor VIIa (rFVIIa) for obstetric hemorrhage is controversial but may be considered as an adjunctive hemostatic agent in the treatment of severe, uncontrolled obstetric hemorrhage despite massive transfusion and other interventions.[24–26] The major risk of rFVIIa is thrombosis, which occurs in 2% to 9% of patients.[22] Ideal obstetric dosing of rFVIIa is not defined, but starting doses of 40-90 mcg/kg as a single bolus injection over a few minutes every 2 hours until hemostasis is achieved has been reported.[26,27] In order for rFVIIa to be effective, several physiologic parameters should be met before administration, including:[28]

Table 3
Acute hemorrhage classification

	Class I	Class II	Class III	Class IV
Blood Loss (mL)	1000	1500	2000	>2500
Blood Loss (% of blood volume)	10–15	20–25	30–35	35–40
Heart Rate (beats/min)	<100	>100	>120	>140
Blood Pressure	Normal or slight increase	Normal or slight increase; orthostatic hypotension	Hypotension	Hypotension
Pulse Pressure	Normal	Narrowed	Narrowed	Narrowed
Capillary Refill	Normal	Normal	Delayed	Delayed
Respiratory Rate (Breaths/min)	14–20	20–30	30–40	>35
Urine Output (mL/h)	Normal >30 mL	20–30	5–15	Anuria
Other	Dizziness, palpitations	Sweating, weakness	Restlessness, pallor, cool extremities	Shock, air hunger, absent peripheral pulses

Adapted from Francois KE, Foley MR. (2021) Antepartum and postpartum hemorrhage. In: Landon MB., Galan H, Jauniaux E, et al (Eds.) Gabbe's Obstetrics: Normal and Problem Pregnancies, 8th edition. Amsterdam: Elsevier; 2020. p.343-374. And American College of Surgeons. Advanced Trauma Life Support (Student Manual). American College of Surgeons 1997.

- Fibrinogen (>50 to 100 mg/dL)
- Platelets (>50,000/L)
- pH greater than 7.2
- Absence of hypothermia
- Absence of hypocalcemia

Table 4 provides information regarding dosing and administration of agents used for management of postpartum hemorrhage.

Manipulation

Manipulative measures for uterine atony, including fundal massage and emptying the bladder, are the first 2 steps to improving uterine contractility. Bimanual uterine massage is performed by placing 1 hand in the vagina and placing the fist into the anterior fornix while the uterus is compressed and massaged between this fist and the other hand on the abdomen. If this is not successful in managing the hemorrhage, interventions should be escalated rapidly to include medications for atony.[9]

Uterine tamponade balloon

When pharmacologic and manipulative interventions fail to control postpartum hemorrhage because of uterine atony, placement of a uterine balloon for tamponade is a minimally invasive, effective adjunct therapy.[9,29] Balloon tamponade devices can be placed after cesarean or vaginal birth following examination to eliminate lacerations or retained placental fragments as a cause of postpartum hemorrhage. The balloon is filled with sterile saline according to manufacturer recommendations to provide

Table 4
Medications for postpartum hemorrhage

Medication	Dose	Potential Side Effects	Notes
Oxytocin (Pitocin)	IV: 10–40 U IM: 10 U	Rare Nausea, vomiting, hypotension with prolonged dosing	Recommended universally for active management of third stage of labor following birth of fetus or placenta Do not administer IV push
Misoprostol	600–1000 µg PO, SL, or PR	Nausea, vomiting, diarrhea, fever, chills	No contraindications
Methyl-ergonovine	IM: 0.2 mg every 2–4 h up to 5 doses	Hypertension, nausea, and vomiting	Contraindicated in hypertension, preeclampsia, coronary artery disease
15-methyl PGF$_2\alpha$	IM: 0.25 mg every 15–90 min up to 8 doses	Nausea, vomiting, diarrhea, flushing, fever, vasospasm, bronchospasm	Contraindicated if history of asthma; relative contraindication if active cardiac, pulmonary, or hepatic disease
TXA	IV: 1 g over 10 min; may repeat in 30 min; maximum dosage 2 g in 24 h	Rarely nausea, vomiting, hypotension, and dizziness	Administer within 3 h from onset of hemorrhage

Abbreviations: IM, intramuscular; IV, intravenous; PGF$_2\alpha$, prostaglandin F$_2\alpha$; PO, per mouth; PR, per rectum; SL, sublingual; U, units.

Data from ACOG Practice Bulletin #183. Postpartum hemorrhage. Obstetrics and Gynecology 2017;130(4): e168-e186. And Kennedy BB, Baird SM. Collaborative strategies for management of obstetric hemorrhage. In: O'Malley P., Foster J. (Eds). Critical Care Nurs Clin North Am 2017;29(3):315-330.

compression and to slow or stop bleeding within the first 5 minutes to 15 minutes after inflation. The balloon may be left in place for a maximum of 24 hours. Some devices also include a fluid collection bag to monitor hemostasis and measure any output. An indwelling urinary catheter is used in tandem if not already placed. After placement, the patient is carefully monitored for ongoing blood loss, including fundal height assessments, because concealed hemorrhage may occur superior to the device.[30,31] Data regarding effectiveness are limited; however, as many as 85.9% of patients do not require additional therapies.[29] The tamponade device may also act as a bridge to decrease bleeding while preparations are being made for aggressive interventions such as uterine artery embolization or hysterectomy.[30,31] A comparison of the 2 commercially available uterine balloon devices is outlined in **Table 5**.

An alternative to a uterine balloon placement is uterine packing with gauze. This procedure is more technically challenging, does not allow assessment of ongoing blood loss through a drainage port, and carries the risk of retained sponges, making the use of a tamponade device more practical, if available.

Table 5		
Uterine tamponade balloons		
Intrauterine Tamponade Device	**Maximum Device Volume**	**Details**
Bakri Postpartum Balloon	500 mL	• Rapid installation equipment available for use with IV bag • Allows monitoring of ongoing blood loss through drainage port • May require vaginal packing
Ebb Complete Tamponade System	Dual balloon system: 750-mL intrauterine balloon 300-mL vaginal balloon (optional inflation)	• Rapid fluid installation from IV bag or syringe • Vaginal balloon intended to decrease rates of expulsion • Dual balloon system requires 2 ports of installation • Allows monitoring of ongoing blood loss through drainage port
BT-Cath	500 mL	• Rapid fluid installation from IV bag or syringe • Allows monitoring of ongoing blood loss through drainage port • Intrauterine portion of drainage port does not extend beyond balloon

Data from Refs.[29–31]

Vacuum-induced uterine tamponade device

Recently, the US Food and Drug Administration (FDA) approved a new device for the treatment of postpartum hemorrhage. This device is introduced into the uterus through the cervix and exerts continuous low-level suction to evacuate clots and stimulate uterine contraction. In a recent prospective trial of 107 women, 94% were successfully managed with the device and had bleeding controlled in a median of 3 minutes (range, 2–5 minutes). Ninety eight percent of users reported that the device was easy to use.[32]

Surgical

The definitive management of obstetric hemorrhage remains surgical. If more conservative measures have failed to control bleeding, then a surgical approach to control of hemorrhage is indicated. Surgical options include uterine curettage, laceration repair, and laparotomy to perform uterine compression sutures, arterial ligation, or hysterectomy. The initial surgical option elected is targeted at the underlying cause of the bleeding. In patients with suspected retained placenta, uterine curettage may be considered, whereas, if the patient has a cervical or high vaginal laceration, then repair in an operating room may be necessary. For patients with uterine atony refractory to more conservative measures, laparotomy is indicated. The team should be prepared with necessary staff and instruments to perform hysterectomy if other surgical methods are not successful.

Before any surgical interventions, hemorrhagic shock is aggressively managed with blood products and crystalloids, with adequate venous access secured. If the patient is coagulopathic, this should be addressed with factor replacement (fresh frozen plasma [FFP], cryoprecipitate, or factor concentrates) before proceeding with general anesthesia and surgical intervention if possible. In these patients, use of a massive transfusion protocol is recommended to facilitate rapid distribution and administration of blood products.[9]

Arterial ligation

The intent of arterial ligation is to decrease pulse pressure and reduce volume of flow to the uterus. The techniques carry a high likelihood of success, estimated at 92%.[22] A common initial approach is to perform O'Leary sutures, ligating uterine arteries bilaterally at the cervicouterine isthmus. If this does not adequately control bleeding, then additional sutures may be placed to ligate the utero-ovarian vessels. Hypogastric (internal iliac) artery ligation has historically been used in attempts to manage uterine bleeding and avoid hysterectomy.[33,34] However, successful hypogastric artery ligation requires a surgeon skilled in dissection of the retroperitoneal space and can be further challenged by poor visualization and access from an enlarged postpartum uterus and active bleeding in the operative field. For these reasons, hypogastric artery ligation is rarely performed for this indication. However, arterial ligation does not seem to negatively affect fertility.[35]

Compression sutures

A variety of uterine compression suture techniques have been described to manage refractory uterine atony. The intent of the compression sutures is to provide constant compression of the myometrium using rapidly absorbable suture material such as chromic, and therefore control bleeding, similar to that achieved with manual compression. As the uterus involutes, the large loops of suture can create opportunities for bowel herniation and incarceration, hence the recommendation for rapidly absorbing suture material. The most widely known technique is the B-Lynch suture; however, different compression suture techniques have been described by others, including Cho and Hayman.[36,37] All of the techniques have similar reported success rates of 60% to 75%.[38–40] **Fig. 2** shows how to place a B-Lynch suture.

Hysterectomy

Hysterectomy is the definitive treatment of obstetric hemorrhage refractory to more conservative treatment approaches, regardless of the underlying cause.[9] In cases of placenta accreta spectrum disorder, hysterectomy is the recommended first-line treatment, whereas with other more common causes, such as uterine atony, hysterectomy may often be avoided if the patient responds to medications or other less aggressive therapies.

Any patient requiring laparotomy for management of obstetric hemorrhage should be considered a potential candidate for hysterectomy. If the patient is immediate post-cesarean, the Pfannenstiel incision may be reopened. However, if the patient is post–vaginal birth, a midline vertical incision should be considered to maximize exposure. The decision to perform a supracervical or total hysterectomy is left to the discretion of the surgeon, because data are inadequate to support 1 approach more than the other. In general, in this setting the technique that can be performed the most expeditiously and safest is recommended. Posthysterectomy surgical complications in the immediate peripartum period are common and most commonly involve bladder and ureteral injuries (in up to 40% of patients).[22]

Uterine artery embolization

Hemodynamically stable patients with slow, persistent bleeding who have failed other therapies may be candidates for uterine artery embolization (UAE). If the patient is a

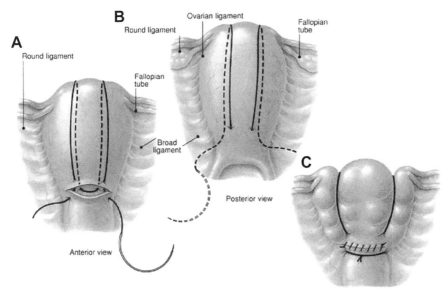

Fig. 2. B-Lynch suture. (*A*) Anterior view. (*B*) Posterior view. (*C*) Anterior view, post-completion. (*From* B-Lynch C, Coker A, Lawal AH, et al. The B-Lynch surgical technique for the control of massive postpartum haemorrhage: an alternative to hysterectomy? Five cases reported. BJOG Mar 1997. 104(3):372-5; Used with permission of Prof Christopher Balogun-Lynch.)

candidate and the procedure is successful, UAE offers the benefit of avoiding hysterectomy and its complications, and potentially maintaining fertility.

UAE requires placement of femoral arterial lines. Therefore, it is important that the patient be hemodynamically stable and not have DIC. The bleeding vessels are identified fluoroscopically and embolized with absorbable gelatin sponges, coils, or microparticles. UAE carries a high success rate (89%); however, approximately 15% of patients subsequently require hysterectomy.[22,41]

Potential post-UAE complications include venous thrombosis, uterine necrosis, and nerve damage, but occur uncommonly (<5% of patients).[22] Fertility and pregnancy complication rates do not seem to be significantly different postprocedure.[35]

Goal 3: Maintain Tissue Oxygenation and Perfusion

Volume replacement

In bleeding patients, maintaining adequate circulating volume is a primary focus of resuscitation and ensures adequate organ and tissue perfusion. Failure to adequately volume resuscitate the patient may lead to acidosis and multiorgan dysfunction. In obstetrics, volume resuscitation principles are often similar to trauma guidelines. At a minimum, the patient needs 2 large-bore peripheral intravenous catheters. If massive transfusion is necessary or if hemorrhagic shock develops, placement of a central line is warranted. Options for volume replacement include crystalloid solutions, colloids, and blood products. Adequacy of volume resuscitation may be assessed noninvasively by blood pressure, pulse, pulse pressure, oxygen saturation, capillary refill, and urine output.[42] In cases of anticipatory hemorrhage or shock, central line placement may be indicated.

Crystalloids

Isotonic crystalloids (lactated Ringer and normal saline) remain first-line solutions for intravascular volume expansion. Crystalloids have a low molecular weight with approximately 30% of infused volume remaining in the intravascular space, and the other two-thirds moving into the interstitial space. This redistribution can lead to tissue edema, pulmonary edema, and disruption in cellular metabolism.[43] In large volumes, crystalloids dilute red blood cells, decrease hematocrit levels and oncotic pressure, and increase mortality.[43,44] Therefore, newer resuscitation protocols prioritize early blood product replacement.

Colloids

Colloid solutions contain larger particles that do not pass through semipermeable membranes. Blood products are considered colloids but are addressed separately. The colloid works by increasing oncotic pressure intravascularly, which draws fluid in. Therefore, it is important that patients receiving colloid solutions be adequately prehydrated with crystalloids in order to provide a reservoir of fluid to be pulled intravascularly. In theory, colloid solutions produce more rapid and sustained increases in colloid oncotic pressure and plasma volume compared with crystalloid solutions. Data to support use of colloid solutions in resuscitation of hemorrhaging patients are limited; therefore, the use of colloid solutions in this setting should be limited. If a colloid solution is to be used, 25% albumin solution is preferred. An infusion of 25% albumin increases intravascular volume by roughly 300 to 500 mL over 60 minutes as a result of its oncotic activity.[45] However, studies have failed to show benefit of use. Further complicating hemorrhage, colloids, such as dextran and gelatins, have been associated with impaired platelet function, inhibition of fibrin polymerization, and increased fibrinolysis.[46] Hyperoncotic starch solutions are associated with an increased risk of kidney dysfunction and mortality and should not be used.[47]

Blood component therapy

For hemorrhaging patients, and particularly patients with hemorrhagic shock, aggressive replacement of packed red blood cells (PRBCs) and clotting factors is essential. Recommendations for blood replacement therapy are primarily derived from trauma literature and differ between patients requiring product replacement because of bleeding and those requiring massive transfusion. For those not requiring massive transfusion, recommended product ratios vary widely; however, 1 unit of FFP is typically given for every 2 to 3 units of PRBCs.[48,49] For massive transfusion, the recommended ratio of PRBC/FFP/platelets is typically 1:1:1 to mimic replacement of whole blood.[9]

Prevention of consumptive coagulopathy is an important component of blood product management in hemorrhaging patients and is accomplished primarily by administration of FFP and cryoprecipitate. A single unit of FFP or cryoprecipitate each increases the fibrinogen level the same amount :10 to 15 mg/dL/U. However, FFP contains all of the clotting factors and is a larger volume, hence its importance in the initial resuscitation. Cryoprecipitate contains fewer clotting factors and is a lower volume, but has the same effect on increasing fibrinogen.[50] Key management principles of massive transfusion are outlined in **Box 1**.

Cell salvage

The immediate recycling of blood lost during surgery or following trauma has become an accepted treatment modality, even in the obstetric realm. The use of autologous blood may eliminate or reduce the volume of allogeneic blood products transfused. Cell salvage systems can provide a 250-mL unit of blood with a hematocrit of 55%

Box 1
Massive transfusion management principles

Manage airway and breathing

Evaluate and address cause of hemorrhage

Establish 2 large-bore peripheral intravenous lines

Consider central line and arterial line placement

Administer 1 to 2 L of crystalloid initially

Initiate massive transfusion protocol

Administer FFP, PRBCs, and platelets 1:1:1

Maintain core temperature greater than 35°C

Monitor complete blood count, prothrombin time, partial thromboplastin time, fibrinogen every 30 min

Correct hypocalcemia

Correct hyperkalemia

Correct acidosis (pH = 7.4, normal base deficit, normal lactate level)

Continue product replacement until:
- Hemodynamically stable
- Platelet count greater than 50,000
- International Normalized Ratio less than 1.5

Data from Hall NR, Martin SR. Transfusion of Blood Components and Derivatives in the Intensive Care Patient. In: Foley MR, Strong TH, Garite TJ (eds). Obstetric Intensive Care Manual, 5th edition: The McGraw-Hill Companies. 2018.

---

in approximately 3 minutes.[51] Modern filtration techniques have essentially eliminated the concern for inducing amniotic fluid embolism by transfusing blood contaminated with amniotic fluid.[51–54] This safety record has prompted ACOG and others to recommend consideration of this technology for patients at risk for intraoperative hemorrhage when possible.[9,55] In situations such as a patient with known placenta accreta spectrum, advance planning can be done to ensure the availability of cell salvage intraoperatively. However, most obstetric hemorrhage scenarios are unanticipated, limiting the utility of cell salvage for many patients.

Goal 4: Monitor for Coagulopathy and Complications

Diagnosis of coagulopathies in the obstetric population can be a challenge because of normal hemostatic changes, such as increased fibrinogen levels and fibrinogen-fibrin degradation products.[11] There is no single laboratory test that diagnoses DIC alone. Therefore, multiple tests are obtained and trended. Obstetric hemorrhage is one of the most common conditions resulting in consumptive coagulopathy from the dilutional effect of massive transfusion without replacement of clotting factors, but it can also occur early in massive hemorrhage without another underlying cause.[56] Massive transfusion protocols are used to guide resuscitation efforts such that dilutional coagulopathy can be addressed and guide earlier transfusion of FFP. DIC scoring systems to assist in diagnosis have been introduced. Erez and colleagues[57] (2015) modified the International Society of Thrombosis and Hemostasis tool based on pregnancy-related hemostatic changes and showed a sensitivity of 88% and specificity of 96% for obstetric DIC. Because delay in diagnosis of DIC may lead to

Table 6
Hemorrhage preparation checklist

Bundle Component	Recommendation	Information
Recognition and prevention	Risk assessment	• Completed on admission, intrapartum, and postpartum
	Early warning signs and symptoms of compromise	• Implementation of a system surrounding recognition of early warning signs, timely communication, and provider presence at the bedside
	Active management of the third stage of labor	• Administer oxytocin after delivery of the shoulder or placenta • Uterine fundal massage after delivery of placenta
Readiness	Interprofessional team training and role delegation	• Each member of the hemorrhage response team trained to function with specific roles of resuscitation
	Interprofessional patient care conferences	• Preplanning for patients at risk of massive hemorrhage
	Simulation	• Interprofessional in situ simulation to practice team response, role delegation, processes, systems, and protocol effectiveness
	Hemorrhage protocol	• Evidence stage based and standardized
	MTP	• Collaboration with blood bank to determine simplified process for emergency release of blood products • Ratio for blood product administration • Determine simplified process for laboratory tests during MTP • Rapid infusion and warming of crystalloids and blood • Techniques to prevent hypothermia
	Hemorrhage cart	• Essential supplies, visual cognitive aids, and checklists for infrequently performed procedures readily available on all birthing units in the event of a hemorrhage
	Medication kit	• Immediate availability of all medications used in hemorrhage, including refrigerated medications

(continued on next page)

Table 6 (continued)		
Bundle Component	**Recommendation**	**Information**
Response	Checklist	• Align checklist with protocol • Start on recognition of hemorrhage. Antepartum/intrapartum checklist may differ from postpartum
	OR	• Anticipate and prepare for transport to OR • OR kits for hysterectomy readily available with staff trained to assist
	Support for patient, family, team members	• Team member role for real-time support of patient and/or family • Infrastructure for supporting mental health for clinicians and personnel following an event
Reporting	Huddles to plan patients at risk	• Interprofessional huddle to develop individualized plan of care before an event in a patient at high risk
	Debrief following hemorrhage event	• Immediate interprofessional, nonjudgmental debrief to review what went well and opportunities for improved response and/or outcome
	Interprofessional review	• Effective incident investigation and root cause analysis of sentinel events • Investigation of near-miss events or unsafe acts to improve safety
	Monitor outcomes and process metrics	• Use improvement science with data metrics to guide practice and implement interventions and measure results • Sustain gains in improvement

Abbreviations: MTP, massive transfusion protocol; OR, operating room.
Data from Refs.[9,20,59–61]

maternal morbidity and mortality, use of a scoring tool may assist in identifying the severity of the clinical situation in order to intervene and correct underlying coagulopathy.

Laboratory screening for coagulation status includes platelet count, prothrombin time (PT), activated partial thromboplastin time (aPTT), and International Normalized Ratio ; however, these values may remain within normal ranges until the hemorrhage progresses to a critical state. D-dimer values in normal pregnancy are increased and fluctuate dramatically; therefore, isolated values are not reliable for management. Decreasing plasma fibrinogen level reflects intravascular fibrin formation and is an early indicator of coagulopathy.[11]

Because length of time for obtaining laboratory results can contribute to delays in treatment, point-of-care testing during an acute hemorrhage is an effective method to determine management and decrease delays in laboratory evaluation and communication. In addition to DIC panels, electrolytes, complete blood count, and blood gases, point-of-care testing may also include thromboelastography (TEG; Haemoscope Inc, Niles, IL) and thromboelastometry (ROTEM, Tem International, Munich, Germany). TEG values provide a complete, rapid, closer-to-real-time assessment of the speed and quality of clot formation, which, in combination with clinical signs and symptoms, allows a pathophysiologic, logical guide to intervention to improve outcomes. TEG/ROTEM assays are tested on whole blood and provide information on coagulation factors, platelet function, fibrinogen level, and fibrinolysis in order to individualize and guide transfusion therapy.[58]

Trauma literature outlines 3 complications that increase morbidity and mortality related to hemorrhage and volume resuscitation: hypothermia, acidosis, and coagulopathy.[9,44] Inadequate tissue perfusion leading to lactate production and metabolic acidosis reduces clotting factor activation. Hypothermia following prolonged surgical procedure and/or massive volume replacement also inhibits clotting factor and platelet activity. Proactive warming of fluids, increasing ambient temperature in the operating room setting, following trends in blood gases in addition to clotting factors and blood chemistries, and correcting abnormalities are essential.

DISCUSSION

With continued high levels of maternal morbidity and mortality related to obstetric hemorrhage, there remain numerous opportunities for improvement. Readiness of obstetric and surgical teams to intervene at all times is essential. Interprofessional team training using simulation and use of protocols and checklists is part of a comprehensive strategy to safely and adequately address obstetric hemorrhage. Tools that guide providers and teams through evidence-based care in emergent situations optimize outcomes and have been recommended by state maternal morbidity and mortality review committees.[2] **Table 6** provides an example proactive preparation strategy for recognition, response, and reporting.

Clear and timely communication regarding hemorrhage is essential for improved outcomes.

All providers on a care team should be empowered and safe to speak up about abnormal assessment findings in order to facilitate appropriate treatment. Care culture that inhibits members of the team from communicating effectively adversely affect patient outcomes. Situational awareness is deliberate. Perception and understanding the meaning of care elements such as the environment, stage of hemorrhage, maternal assessment parameters, management plans, medications, and completed therapies require intention and are supported with ongoing, effective communication to the appropriate care providers and team members.

Regular interprofessional simulation is an essential method in preparation for obstetric emergencies. Data through simulation identify issues with communication, decrease time to intervention, and improve outcomes.[62–64]

One of the essential components of care for patients with hemorrhage is ensuring the appropriate level of care such that care can be specific to risk. Integrated systems that recognize the reality of limited resources and support coordinated transfer of care can enhance safety and reduce maternal risk of morbidity and mortality. In the event that a patient does not stabilize with routine protocol implementation, anticipation, communication, and collaboration for transfer to a higher level of care are necessary. This determination can be proactively regulated based on a clearly defined unit scope of service to mitigate risk and disparities.

Safe, effective, quality care in the event of an obstetric hemorrhage is also family centered. When an emergent response is required, adequate preparation of the family is challenging but remains a priority for effective communication. Information is provided as soon as possible, and the woman and family should be included in decision making. A team member or designee can remain with the family for sensitive support. Family presence in an intensive care unit setting is now widely accepted as beneficial. In obstetrics, family members are frequently, if not expected to be, present for other procedures, but rarely are discussions of family presence in the event of emergencies or resuscitation held in advance. The experience of witnessing a life-threatening emergency can be traumatic for partners and/or family members, with separation from their newborn or partner, and balancing anxiety with providing support, all noted as fears. In the event of a known complication that makes obstetric hemorrhage an anticipated event, efforts to prepare the family and determine preferences are essential. Postevent debriefings should include the patient and family to allow for questions. In all circumstances, communication is the hallmark of patient-centered care.

SUMMARY

Obstetric hemorrhage remains a leading cause of morbidity and mortality despite high rates of preventability. Improving the care of hemorrhaging patients requires a multidisciplinary, standardized approach to the recognition and management of these patients. This approach includes establishing maternal early warning signs that define when evaluation of the patient is warranted and which interventions should be considered, a process for ongoing objectification of blood loss, and a massive transfusion protocol. Quality-improvement processes should assess the effectiveness of these processes and guide practice evolution. Regular simulation is also a necessary component of team training and vetting of protocols designed to improve the care of hemorrhaging patients. Institutional and individual factors affect the preventability of maternal morbidity and mortality resulting from obstetric hemorrhage. Early recognition of clinical cues and readiness for rapid intervention to prevent severe hemorrhage are critical to optimizing maternal outcomes and reducing maternal morbidity and mortality. Common areas of concern in a collaborative care model include:

- Proactive preparation of all multidisciplinary team members with education, training, and simulated responses
- Adequate assessment and monitoring based on risk status
- Accurate measurement of blood loss
- Recognition of physiologic trends in maternal compromise
- Timely communication of assessment findings to all team members
- Underestimation of volume replacement and resuscitation needs for maternal hypovolemic shock
- Availability of blood products for massive transfusion protocols
- Delay of surgical intervention in the presence of ineffective manipulation and medication strategies
- Inconsistent integration and variability of adherence to stated processes, procedures/protocols, safety bundles, and checklists

Shared understanding of maternal risk, appropriate assessment skills, and preparation for a rapid, coordinated, team response is essential for multidisciplinary management of obstetric hemorrhage. Common errors and delay of treatment can be mitigated by use of key management principles and a sequenced progression of evidence-based strategies.[61]

CLINICS CARE POINTS

- Proactive preparation of all multidisciplinary team members with education, training, and simulated responses
- Adequate assessment and monitoring based on risk status
- Accurate measurement of blood loss
- Recognition of physiologic trends in maternal compromise
- Timely communication of assessment findings to all team members
- Underestimation of volume replacement and resuscitation needs for maternal hypovolemic shock
- Availability of blood products for massive transfusion protocols
- Delay of surgical intervention in the presence of ineffective manipulation and medication strategies
- Inconsistent integration and variability of adherence to stated processes, procedures/protocols, safety bundles, and checklists

DISCLOSURE

The authors have nothing to disclose.

REFERENCES

1. Petersen EE, Davis NL, Goodman D, et al. Vital signs: pregnancy-related deaths, United States, 2011–2015, and strategies for prevention, 13 states, 2013–2017. MMWR Morb Mortal Wkly Rep 2019;68:423–9.
2. Building U.S. Capacity to Review and Prevent Maternal Deaths. Report from nine maternal mortality review committees. 2018. Available at: https://www.cdcfoundation.org/sites/default/files/files/ReportfromNineMMRCs.pdf. Accessed September 4, 2020.
3. Creanga AA, Berg CJ, Syverson C, et al. Pregnancy-related mortality in the United States, 2006-2010. Obstet Gynecol 2015;125(1):5–12.
4. Say L, Chou D, Gemmill A, et al. Global causes of maternal death: a WHO systematic analysis. Lancet Glob Health 2014;2:e323.
5. Fingar, K.R., Hambrick, M.M., Heslin, K.C., Moore, J.E. Trends and disparities in delivery hospitalizations involving severe maternal morbidity, 2006-2015. 2018. Available at: https://hcup-us.ahrq.gov/reports/statbriefs/sb243-Severe-Maternal-Morbidity-Delivery-Trends-Disparities.jsp. Accessed September 4, 2020.
6. Guglielminotti J, Landau R, Wong CA, et al. Criticality of maternal complications during childbirths. J Patient Saf 2020;1–5. https://doi.org/10.1097/PTS.0000000000000511.
7. Nathan L. An overview of obstetric hemorrhage. Semin Perinatol 2019;43:2–4.
8. Gyamfi-Bannerman C, Srinivas SK, Wright JD, et al. Postpartum hemorrhage outcomes and race. Am J Obstet Gynecol 2018;219(2):185.e1–10.
9. ACOG Practice Bulletin #183. Postpartum hemorrhage. Obstet Gynecol 2017;130(4):e168–86.
10. Antony KM, Racusin DA, Aagaard K, et al. Maternal physiology. In: Landon MB, Galan H, Jauniaux E, et al, editors. Gabbe's obstetrics: normal and problem pregnancies. 8th edition. Amsterdam (the Netherlands): Elsevier; 2021.
11. Francois KE, Foley MR. (2021) Antepartum and postpartum hemorrhage. In: Landon MB, Galan H, Jauniaux E, et al, editors. Gabbe's obstetrics: normal and problem pregnancies. 8th edition. Amsterdam (the Netherlands): Elsevier; 2020. p. 343–74.

12. CMQCC OB Hemorrhage Task Force. OB hemorrhage emergency management plan: table chart. Available at: https://www.cmqcc.org/resource/ob-hem-emergency-management-plan-table-chart. Accessed August 30, 2020.

13. Carvajal JA, Ramos I, Kusanovic JP, et al. Damage-control resuscitation in obstetrics. J Matern Fetal Neonatal Med 2020. https://doi.org/10.1080/14767058.2020.1730800.

14. Quantitative blood loss in obstetric hemorrhage. ACOG Committee Opinion No. 794. American College of Obstetricians and Gynecologists. Obstet Gynecol 2019;134:e150–6.

15. Rubenstein AF, Zamudio S, Al-Khan A, et al. Clinical experience with the implementation of accurate measurement of blood loss during cesarean delivery: influences on hemorrhage recognition and allogeneic transfusion. Am J Perinatol 2018;35:655–9.

16. Lertbunnaphong T, Lapthanapat N, Leetheeragul J, et al. Postpartum blood loss: visual estimation versus objective quantification with a novel birthing drape. Singapore Med J 2016;57(6):325–8.

17. Al Kadri HM, Al Anazi BK, Tamim HM. Visual estimation versus gravimetric measurement of postpartum blood loss: a prospective cohort study. Arch Gynecol Obstet 2011;283:1207–13.

18. AWHONN Practice Brief. Quantification of blood loss: AWHONN practice brief number 1. J Obstet Gynecol Neonatal Nurs 2015;44:158–60.

19. Diaz V, Abalos E, Carroli G. Methods for blood loss estimation after vaginal birth. Cochrane Database Syst Rev 2018;9:CD010980.

20. Main EK, Cape V, Abredo A, et al. Reduction of severe maternal morbidity from hemorrhage using a state perinatal quality collaborative. Am J Obstet Gynecol 2017;216(3):289.e1–11.

21. Association of Women's Health, obstetric and neonatal nurses. Oxytocin administration for management of third stage of labor. Practice brief number 2. Available at: http://www.pphproject.org/downloads/awhonn_oxytocin.pdf. Accessed September 14, 2020.

22. Likis FE, Sathe NA, Morgans AK, et al. Management of postpartum hemorrhage. Comparative effectiveness review No. 151. (Prepared by the vanderbilt evidence-based practice center under Contract No. 290-2012-00009-I.) AHRQ Publication No. 15-EHC013-EF. Rockville (MD): Agency for Healthcare Research and Quality; 2015. Available at: www.effectivehealthcare.ahrq.gov/reports/final.cfm.

23. WOMAN Trial Collaborators. Effect of early tranexamic acid administration on mortality, hysterectomy, and other morbidities in women with post-partum haemorrhage (WOMAN): an international, randomised, double-blind, placebo-controlled trial [published correction appears in Lancet. 2017 May 27;389(10084):2104]. Lancet 2017;389(10084):2105–16.

24. Ahonen J, Jokela R, Korttila K. An open non-randomized study of recombinant activated factor VII in major postpartum haemorrhage. Acta Anaesthesiol Scand 2007;51:929–36.

25. Bhuskute N, Kritzinger S, Dakin M. Recombinant factor VIIa in massive obstetric haemorrhage [letter]. Eur J Anaesthesiol 2008;25:250–1.

26. Alfirevic Z, Elbourne D, Pavord S, et al. Use of recombinant activated factor VII in primary postpartum hemorrhage: the Northern European registry 2000-2004. Obstet Gynecol 2007;110:1270–8.

27. Franchini M, Lippi G, Franchi M. The use of recombinant activated factor VII in obstetric and gynaecological haemorrhage. BJOG 2007;114(1):8.

28. Rossaint R, Bouillon B, Cerny V, et al. Management of bleeding following major trauma: an updated European guideline. Task force for advanced bleeding care in Trauma. Crit Care 2010;14(2):R52.

29. Suarez S, Conde-Agudelo A, Borovac-Pinheiro A, et al. Uterine balloon tamponade for the treatment of postpartum hemorrhage: a systematic review and meta-analysis. Am J Obstet Gynecol 2020;222:293.e1-52.

30. Georgiou C. Balloon tamponade in the management of postpartum haemorrhage: a review. BJOG 2009;116(6):748.

31. Dildy GA, Belfort MA, Adair CD, et al, ebb Surveillance Study Team. Initial experience with a dual-balloon catheter for the management of postpartum hemorrhage. Am J Obstet Gynecol 2014;210(2):136.e1.

32. D'Alton ME, Rood KM, Smid MC, et al. Intrauterine vacuum-induced hemorrhage control device for rapid treatment of postpartum hemorrhage. Obstet Gynecol 2020;136(5):882–91.

33. Evans S, McShane P. The efficacy of internal iliac artery ligation in obstetric hemorrhage. Surg Gynecol Obstet 1985;160(3):250.

34. Clark SL, Phelan JP, Yeh SY, et al. Hypogastric artery ligation for obstetric hemorrhage. Obstet Gynecol 1985;66:353–6.

35. Doumouchtsis SK, Nikolopoulos K, Talaulikar V, et al. Menstrual and fertility outcomes following the surgical management of postpartum haemorrhage: a systematic review. BJOG 2014;121(4):382.

36. Cho JH, Jun HS, Lee CN. Hemostatic suturing technique for uterine bleeding during cesarean delivery. Obstet Gynecol 2000;96:129–31.

37. Hayman RG, Arulkumaran S, Steer PJ. Uterine com- pression sutures: surgical management of postpartum hemorrhage. Obstet Gynecol 2002;99:502–6.

38. B-Lynch C, Coker A, Lawal AH, et al. The B-Lynch surgical technique for the control of massive postpartum haemorrhage: an alternative to hysterectomy? Five cases reported. Br J Obstet Gynaecol 1997;104:372–5.

39. Kayem G, Kurinczuk JJ, Alfirevic Z, et al. Specific second-line therapies for postpartum haemorrhage: a national cohort study. BJOG 2011;118:856–64.

40. Kayem G, Kurinczuk JJ, Alfirevic Z, et al. Uterine compression sutures for the management of severe postpartum hemorrhage. U.K. Obstetric Surveillance System (UKOSS). Obstet Gynecol 2011;117:14–20.

41. Zwart JJ, Dijk PD, van Roosmalen J. Peripartum hysterectomy and arterial embolization for major obstetric hemorrhage: a 2-year nationwide cohort study in the Netherlands. Am J Obstet Gynecol 2010;202:150.e1-7.

42. Dell'Anna AM, Torrini F, Antonelli M. Shock: definition and recognition. In: Pinsky M, Teboul JL, Vincent JL, editors. Hemodynamic monitoring. Lessons from the ICU (under the Auspices of the European society of intensive care medicine). Cham (Switzerland): Springer; 2019.

43. Feinman M, Cotton BA, Haut ER. Optimal fluid resuscitation in trauma: type, timing, and total. Curr Opin Crit Care 2014;20(4):366–72.

44. ATLS Subcommittee; American College of Surgeons' Committee on Trauma; International ATLS working group. Advanced trauma life support 10th edition. 2018. Available at: https://viaaerearcp.files.wordpress.com/2018/02/atls-2018.pdf. Accessed September 15, 2020.

45. Hasselgren E, Zdolsek M, Zdolsek JH, et al. Hahn RG long intravascular persistence of 20% albumin in postoperative patients. Anesth Analg 2019;129(5):1232.

46. Bolliger D, Gorlinger K, Tanaka KA. Pathophysiology and treatment of coagulopathy in massive hemorrhage and hemodilution. Anesthesiology 2010;113:1205–19.

47. Perel P, Roberts I, Ker K. Colloids versus crystalloid for fluid resuscitation in critically ill patients. Cochrane Database Syst Rev 2013;(Issue 2):CD000567.
48. Roback JD, Caldwell S, Carson J, et al. Evidence-based practice guidelines for plasma transfusion. American association for the study of liver, American academy of pediatrics, United States Army, American Society of Anesthesiology, American Society of Hematology. Transfusion 2010;50(6):1227.
49. Spahn DR, Bouillon B, Cerny V, et al. Management of bleeding and coagulopathy following major trauma: an updated European guideline. Crit Care 2013; 17(2):R76.
50. Hall NR, Martin SR. Transfusion of blood components and derivatives in the intensive care patient. In: Foley MR, Strong TH, Garite TJ, editors. For obstetric intensive care manual. 5th edition. New York: The McGraw-Hill Companies; 2018.
51. Waters JH, Biscotti C, Potter PS, et al. Amniotic fluid removal during cell salvage in the cesarean section patient. Anesthesiology 2000;92:1531–6.
52. Goucher H, Wong CA, Patel SK, et al. Cell salvage in obstetrics. Anesth Analg 2015;121:465–8.
53. Liumbruno GM, Liumbruno C, Rafanelli D. Intraoperative cell salvage in obstetrics: is it a real therapeutic option? Transfusion 2011;51:2244–56.
54. Waters JH. Intraoperative blood recovery. ASAIO J 2013;59(1):11–7.
55. Placenta accreta spectrum. Obstetric Care Consensus No. 7. Amer- ican College of Obstetricians and Gynecologists. Obstet Gynecol 2018;132:e259–75.
56. Cunningham G, Nelson D. Disseminated intravascular coagulation syndromes in obstetrics. Obstet Gynecol 2015;126(5):999–1011.
57. Erez O, Novack L, Beer-Weisel R, et al. DIC score in pregnant women–a population based modification of the international society on thrombosis and hemostasis score. PLoS One 2014;9(4):e93240.
58. Othman M, Elbatarny HK, Abdul-Kadir RA. (2019) The use of viscoelastic hemostatic tests in pregnancy and the puerperium: review of the current evidence-communication from the Women's Health SSC of the ISTH. J Thromb Haemost 2019;17:1184–9.
59. Seacrist M, Vanotterloo L, Morton C, et al. Quality improvement opportunities identified through case review of pregnancy related death from obstetric hemorrhage. J Obstet Gynecol Neonatal Nurs 2019;48(3):P288–99.
60. Main EK, Goffman D, Scavone BM, et al. National partnership for maternal safety: consensus bundle on obstetric hemorrhage. Anesth Analg 2019;129(6):e206.
61. Main EK, Goffman D, Scavone BM, et al. National partnership for maternal safety: consensus bundle on obstetric hemorrhage. Obstet Gynecol 2015;126(5):1111.
62. Theilen U, Frasera L, Jones P, et al. Regular in-situ simulation training of paediatric Medical Emergency Team leads to sustained improvements in hospital response to deteriorating patients, improved outcomes in intensive care and financial savings. Resuscitation 2017;115:61–7.
63. Draycott T, Sibanda T, Owen L, et al. Does training in obstetric emergencies improve neonatal outcome? BJOG 2006;113:177–82.
64. Park C, Grant J, Dumas RP, et al. Does simulation work? Monthly trauma simulation and procedural training are associated with decreased time to intervention. J Trauma Acute Care Surg 2020;2(88):242–6.

Role of Lipid Management in Women's Health Preventive Care

Pardis Hosseinzadeh, MD, Robert Wild, MD, MPH, PhD*

KEYWORDS

- Women's health • Lipids • Dyslipidemia • Hypertriglyceridemia

KEY POINTS

- Understanding opportunities to diagnose and manage dyslipidemia across a woman's life span has major implications for cardiovascular disease risk prevention for the entire population.
- Obstetricians/gynecologists are uniquely positioned to raise awareness on the early diagnose and management of dyslipidemias and thus impact the overall health of the women they care for throughout different stages in life.
- Contraceptives can impact one's lipid profile and care should be taken when counseling for different options regarding baseline comorbidities, including the dyslipidemias.

INTRODUCTION

Dyslipidemia and its sequelae such as atherosclerosis can affect a woman throughout her life and lead to long-term comorbidities for both the mother and the child.[1] Many women rely only on their obstetrician/gynecologists (OB/GYN) for primary care during their reproductive ages. Acknowledging the principle that lipid awareness is critical throughout the life of the individual is therefore paramount for OB/GYNs. This article aims to discuss some unique women's health issues that are important in lipid management because of the epidemic of the metabolic syndrome and obesity in our society. Practitioners caring for women of reproductive age are ideally placed to help decrease atherosclerosis development for the entire population by screening for and managing abnormal lipid levels during gestation.[1]

Atherosclerotic cardiovascular disease (ASCVD), which increases with age, is caused by multiple interrelating factors such as hypertension, diabetes mellitus, dyslipidemia, and obesity. Some of these factors relate to one's lifestyle and are

Section of Reproductive Endocrinology and Infertility, Department of Obstetrics and Gynecology, University of Oklahoma Health and Sciences Center, 800 Stanton L. Young Boulevard, Suite 2000, Oklahoma City, OK 73104, USA
* Corresponding author.
E-mail address: robert-wild@ouhsc.edu

Obstet Gynecol Clin N Am 48 (2021) 173–191
https://doi.org/10.1016/j.ogc.2020.11.003
0889-8545/21/© 2020 Elsevier Inc. All rights reserved.

obgyn.theclinics.com

considered modifiable; others are nonmodifiable. We now know that 90% of women have at least 1 risk factor for developing heart disease, although ASCVD is recognized an average of 10 years later than for their same age male counterparts. This factor has led to an inadvertent decreased emphasis on atherosclerosis prevention for women. Given that dyslipidemia imparts the highest population-adjusted cardiovascular risk for women at 47%, a working knowledge of issues important for managing dyslipidemia is essential for OB/GYNs who serve as the primary care provider for majority of women of childbearing age.[2] Recognition of high-risk areas and how lipids are affected by major reproductive events affecting women's health should be areas of high priority.

Understanding the opportunities to decrease dyslipidemia before, during, and after pregnancy has major implication for ASCVD risk prevention for the entire population. Understanding how contraceptive and hormone choices affect clinical lipid management for women is essential.

PREGNANCY
Alterations of Lipid Values in Pregnancy

As pregnancy progresses, lipids levels steadily increase during the pregnancy with a noticeable increase in the third trimester.[3] This lipid metabolism throughout pregnancy allows for proper nutrients for the fetus. The natural increase reflects the increasing insulin resistance for the mother as pregnancy progresses through term. Total cholesterol (TC), low-density lipoprotein cholesterol (LDL-C), high-density lipoprotein cholesterol (HDL-C), and triglycerides (TG) average values have been measured in normal women followed before, during, and after pregnancy in a large cohort of women proceeding through normal pregnancy and delivery (**Fig. 1**).[4] Most of the women are of young reproductive age and as such their values before pregnancy are in the normal range for nonpregnant women.

Understanding lipids alteration pattern throughout pregnancy and postpartum is essential. As depicted in **Fig. 1**, there may be a decrease in levels in the first 8 weeks of gestation and then a noticeable increase discerned by the end of the first trimester. There begins a steady increase throughout pregnancy in the major lipoprotein lipids. By the third trimester, levels peak to maximize near term.[4] It is important to note that

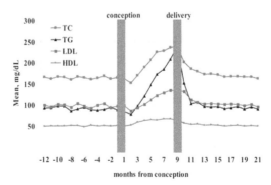

Fig. 1. TC, triglycerides (TG), high-density lipoprotein (HDL) cholesterol, and low-density lipoprotein (LDL) cholesterol 1 year before, during, and after pregnancy. (*From* Wiznitzer A, Mayer A, Novack V, et al. Association of lipid levels during gestation with preeclampsia and gestational diabetes mellitus: a population-based study. Am J Obstet Gynecol 2009;201(5):482.e1–8; with permission.)

the values in this population do not exceed 250 mg/dL at any time during pregnancy. TC seems to return to prepregnancy levels within 1 year,[5] and in some populations these peak values are lower (Chinese). Levels of HDL-C decrease postpartum and remains lower than prepregnancy for multiple years. With less consistent evidence TG can remain elevated.[5] TG levels decrease rapidly in the postpartum period, whereas LDL levels remain elevated for at least 6 to 7 weeks.[6] Postpartum factors can also influence this return. Lactation is associated with an earlier or more complete return.[7]

The sequential average fasting lipid and lipoproteins measured in the different population is shown in **Fig. 2**. **Fig. 2** illustrates mean lipid levels also; however, these measurements also include persons with pregnancy complications. Likewise, TG and TC increase to term; however, values exceed 300 mg/dL[6]. There is also a significant increase in TG content in all circulating lipoprotein fractions during pregnancy.[3]

Fig. 3 shows the first trimester maternal TG in relationship to pregnancy complications. TG levels exceeding 250 mg/dL are associated with pregnancy-induced hypertension, preeclampsia, gestational diabetes, and large for gestational age babies.[8]

Screening for Dyslipidemia in Pregnancy

The prevalence of dyslipidemia during pregnancy varies significantly depending on which criteria are used; however, it is higher with comorbidities.[9] Many women have out of normal range undiscovered dyslipidemia before pregnancy. The early identification of any woman at risk for severe gestational hypertriglyceridemia is essential. Ideally, this process happens at the preconception counseling visit or soon after pregnancy diagnosis.

Women with a history of pancreatitis or abdominal pain associated with prior estrogen use and those with a family history of hypertriglyceridemia are at risk during pregnancy. Individuals with known hypertriglyceridemia should have their TG levels monitored during pregnancy. Signs suggestive of hypertriglyceridemia include eruptive xanthomata skin lesions, lipemia retinalis, and hepatosplenomegaly. Not all patients with severe hypertriglyceridemia have these signs, however. The dyslipidemia is often associated with other health conditions, making that woman at risk for obstetric and fetal complications. These include uncontrolled diabetes mellitus, polycystic ovarian syndrome (PCOS), and genetic lipid disorders. These put the mother at risk for problems, they put her offspring at risk, and possibly put future generations at

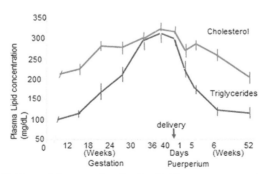

Fig. 2. Pregnancy, lipids, and lipoproteins. Fasting lipids were measured serially throughout pregnancy, at delivery, and in the puerperium and at 12 months. Results are standard error of the mean and include normal and complicated pregnancies. (*Adapted from* Potter JM, Nestel PJ. The hyperlipidemia of pregnancy in normal and complicated pregnancies. Am J Obstet Gynecol 1979;133(2):165–70; with permission.)

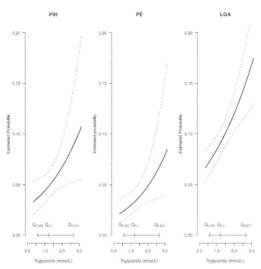

Fig. 3. First trimester maternal TG relationships. The estimated probability of PIH, pre-eclampsia, and LGA. TG levels in the first trimester of pregnancy are a significant, but modest, contributor in the expression of PIH, PE, induced preterm birth, and children to be born large for gestational age. With this observation, inclusion of a lipid profile may be considered in early pregnancy and in the preconception screening. 1 mmol/L of TG = 135 mg/dL; 2 mmol/L of TG = 176 mg/dL. Q0.025, Q0.5, and Q0.875 represent the 2.5th, 50th, and 97.5th percentiles of the studied population. PIH, pregnancy induced hypertension; PE, preeclampsia; LGA, large for gestational age. (*Adapted from* Vrijkotte TG, Krukziener N, Hutten BA, et al. Maternal lipid profile during early pregnancy and pregnancy complications and outcomes: the ABCD study. J Clin Endocrinol Metab 2012;97(11):3917–25; with permission.)

risk. High levels of maternal TC and/or TG are associated with preterm birth,[10] pregnancy-induced hypertension,[11] and large for gestational age.[12] Conversely, decreased levels of TC during pregnancy are associated with preterm birth,[13] with a greater risk for a small for gestational age fetus.[10] Familial hyperlipidemia (FH) is more common than any of the genetic diseases routinely screened for in pregnancy,[14] yet there are currently no obstetrician recommendations in place to screen for FH. Severe hypertriglyceridemia is sometimes encountered because of screening for other genetic or acquired conditions. Ultimately, pregnancy is as a cardiometabolic stress test where those at risk can manifest severe disease. It follows that maternal and fetal complications are better prevented and managed by proper screening with a detailed metabolic and pregnancy history, as well as a lipid profile sampling. A careful cardiometabolic history can provide insight as to the future cardiometabolic risk of mother and child. It also can be a starting point for cascade family screening initiated by the OB/GYN.

Screening should be repeated routinely after the pregnancy is concluded, usually at the 6-week routine postpartum visit. This time is critical because of transitioning in provider health care and competing pressures of new mothers, who can be lost to follow-up. Women who experience complications of pregnancy or who gain excessive weight before or during pregnancy likely have abnormal cardiometabolic profiles.[15] In patients whose primary provider changes, continuity plans with attention to a long-term assessment of hyperlipidemia during the extended puerperal period and beyond is prudent. Attention to and avoiding this gap can go a long way in preventing disease.

Hypertriglyceridemia in Pregnancy

The differential diagnosis of hypertriglyceridemia in pregnancy is the same as in a nonpregnant woman, with the exception that OB/GYNs need to be aware of obstetric complications associated with hypertriglyceridemia. The evaluation of hypertriglyceridemia is as in nonpregnant women, with the realization that there is an expected 2- to 3-fold TG level increase by the third trimester. Women diagnosed with gestational diabetes and/or preeclampsia often have abnormal TG levels greater and additive to their persistent hypertriglyceridemia before the pregnancy. In the United States, the average values in persons with these disorders can exceed 300 mg/dL and levels escalate as pregnancy progresses. Hypertriglyceridemia at the end of gestation is associated with the development of dyslipidemia in the postpartum period, and there is a greater risk of the child being large for gestational age[16] and at risk of greater atherosclerosis burden going in to in adult life.[17] The most common etiology for hypertriglyceridemia is poorly controlled or undiscovered diabetes mellitus. Other etiologies include medications that aggravate TG metabolism, psychiatric and/or human immunodeficiency virus medications, illicit drugs, and/or alcohol. Undiagnosed hypothyroidism and/or genetic dyslipidemias lead to hyperlipidemia in pregnancy.

In summary, women with hypertriglyceridemia need a careful analysis of family history for hypertriglyceridemia, pancreatitis, diabetes, hypertension, smoking status, cardiometabolic disease, illicit drugs, or dietary carbohydrate and alcohol intake, as well as the use of prescription medicines and/or supplements. Glycemic, thyroid, hepatic, and renal evaluations are also indicated.

Management of Dyslipidemia Associated with Pregnancy

For women with a diagnosis of dyslipidemia before pregnancy, any lipid level-lowering medications aside from bile acid sequestrates or omega-3 fatty acids should be stopped. Recommendations for the best time to stop statins range from 3 months to 1 month before conception. When an unplanned pregnancy occurs, statins should be stopped immediately when the pregnancy is discovered. These recommendations are based on expert opinion alone, without definitive evidence. Statins have been used in animal models of preeclampsia to revert the angiogenic imbalance, a hallmark of preeclampsia, and restore endothelial dysfunction. This biological plausibility and data from preclinical animal studies support a role for statins in preeclampsia prevention.[18] A recent randomized controlled trial, provides preliminary safety and pharmacokinetic data regarding the use of pravastatin for preventing preeclampsia in high-risk pregnant women. They reported no identifiable safety risks associated with pravastatin use in this cohort.[19]

Table 1	
Historical FDA classification of lipid level-lowering agents and pregnancy classification	
Lipid Level-Lowering Agent	**Pregnancy Class**
Statins	X
Fibrates	C
Ezetimibe	C
Niacin	C
Cholestyramine	C
Colesevelam	B

Despite this finding, and because of animal data that found that very high doses of lipophilic statins caused birth defects, the US Food and Drug Administration (FDA) historically categorized stains as pregnancy category X. **Table 1** provides the pregnancy classification of widely used lipid level-lowering agents. This classification is no longer advised by the FDA, conceding that the potential risk of harm and possible benefits should always be considered. Most cardiologists advise against their use because of unknowns and potential liability.

Unfortunately, despite the known benefits of many antihyperlipidemic therapies on atherogenic lipid profiles and clinical outcomes, there is a paucity of studies that have been performed in pregnancy. In fact, pregnant women are routinely excluded from clinical trials. As a result, recommendations on the treatment of significant dyslipidemia in pregnant women are limited.

Dyslipidemia discovered during pregnancy should be treated with a diet and exercise intervention, as well as glycemic control when associated with diabetes types 1 and 2. Common agents used are glyburide and metformin as well as insulin to control blood glucose. Omega-3 fatty acids are frequently used and are thought to be safe in pregnancy as monotherapy to decrease maternal TG levels. Hypercholesterolemia can be treated with bile acid sequestrates; notably, colesevelam is in pregnancy category B.

Severe hypertriglyceridemia (including at levels associated with pancreatitis) can be treated with omega-3 fatty acids, parenteral nutrition, plasmapheresis, or historically with gemfibrozil in the mid to late trimesters (pregnancy class C medication).[20] It is recommended that lipids be monitored every trimester or within 6 weeks of an intervention to evaluate for compliance, response, and dose adjustment if needed. Close postpartum follow-up of mothers and children with FH or dysmetabolic issues of pregnancy is required. States of severe hypertriglyceridemia, hypertension of pregnancy, preeclampsia, gestational diabetes, and/or albuminuria need to be evaluated for residual cardiometabolic risk.

Familial Hyperlipidemia and Pregnancy

Cholesterol levels increase in pregnancy, with a similar percentage increase in normal women and those with heterozygous FH. Women with FH do not seem to have a higher risk of preterm delivery or to have low birth weight infants or infants with congenital malformation (undetected bias cannot be ruled out).[21] An experienced lipid specialist should be consulted for women with homozygous FH whose care is beyond the OB/GYN scope of practice. Because TG levels increase progressively with each trimester, women with TG levels of 500 mg/dL or greater at the onset of pregnancy may develop severe hypertriglyceridemia during the third trimester, leading to pancreatitis.[22]

A complete lipid profile assessment during each trimester of pregnancy is recommended. For women with FH, following brain natriuretic peptide, or B-type natriuretic peptide, as a useful monitor for potential coronary ischemia has been suggested.[23] FH can be treated with lifestyle interventions, bile acid sequestrants, and monitoring of potential TG level increases in response. If adequate control is not obtained with these regimens, Colesevelam (pregnancy class B medication), and/or LDL apheresis may be necessary.[24] Given the complex nature of treatment in such cases, patients with FH are best followed in tertiary care centers in a multidisciplinary approach setting with experienced OB/GYNs, endocrinologists, and a cardiologists involved.

Dyslipidemia and Breastfeeding

Lactation may attenuate unfavorable metabolic risk factor changes that occur with pregnancy, with effects of masking apparent after weaning. As a modifiable behavior, lactation may affect women's future risk of cardiovascular and metabolic diseases.[25] For disorders with high TG levels, it is advisable to avoid estrogenic oral contraception, even with late breastfeeding. However, breastfeeding does not guarantee lactational anovulation and thereby contraception. Approximately 1 in 3 women ovulate during prolonged breast feeding, highlighting the need to advise patients regarding the best contraceptives despite breastfeeding. Diet, nutritional consultation, and regular exercise should be considered for patients affected with dyslipidemia during and after the pregnancy.

Long-Term Implications of Complications in Pregnancy

Several conditions specific to women (eg, hypertensive disorders during pregnancy, preeclampsia, gestational diabetes mellitus, delivering a preterm or low birth weight infant)[26,27] have been shown to increase ASCVD risk. Contributions of dyslipidemia, obesity, the presence of the metabolic syndrome, or insulin resistance states before pregnancy[28,29] also host important future ASCVD risk scenarios. The accumulated weight gain during successive pregnancies and the inability to effect adequate weight loss during middle age are well-known risk factors for ASCVD.[30] The increase in lipid components during pregnancy, notably TG and their metabolically dangerous atherogenic particle metabolites, may not be corrected postpartum. Thus, after pregnancy and throughout the life course of every woman, a thorough pregnancy history should be obtained, and risk factors and risk-enhancing factors should be identified. Interventions should include aggressive lifestyle counseling to decrease ASCVD risk and, when appropriate, statin therapy, if ASCVD risk estimation indicates that the potential for benefit from statin therapy outweighs the potential for adverse effects.

POLYCYSTIC OVARIAN SYNDROME

PCOS is the most common endocrine disorder among women of reproductive age. Depending on the population and diagnostic criteria used, PCOS affects between 4% and 19% of reproductive-aged women.[31] Women with PCOS are at an increased risk for the metabolic syndrome, diabetes mellitus, complications of pregnancy, and endometrial cancer.[29] Most individuals with PCOS show insulin resistance, which is intensified by obesity and often the pregnant state, potentially leading to attendant complications. In addition, women with PCOS are at greater risk for obstetric complications irrespective of whether they have developed overt metabolic syndrome. Lipid abnormalities are found in women affected by PCOS. A recent study showed that mild hypercholesterolemia is frequently encountered in women with PCOS.[32] Different lipid patterns have been shown to be present in PCOS, including low levels of HDL; high TG, TC, and LDL-C; and significantly higher lipoprotein concentrations.[33] Concomitantly, the HDL-C level is often decreased, TG production increases, and circulating atherogenic small LDL particles increase, all of which are further aggravated if women with PCOS are obese.

Women with PCOS frequently develop dyslipidemia and/or the metabolic syndrome at any age, including at the onset of menses and continuing throughout the adolescent years. The standard medication used to control menses, to decrease endometrial and ovarian cancer risk, and to decrease hirsutism is the combined oral contraceptive (COC).

Depending on which COC is chosen for which clinical manifestation of PCOS, TG levels may increase, HDL-C levels may increase, and LDL-C levels may decrease when COCs are given to women with PCOS who have associated dyslipidemia.

Rarely, a genetic lipid disorder is uncovered when screening for dyslipidemia in women with PCOS. Very high TG levels (ie, >500 mg/dL) are rarely caused by PCOS alone. Using an oral contraceptive can further aggravate hypertriglyceridemia of this magnitude and can precipitate pancreatitis.

Screening for Associated Dyslipidemia in Polycystic Ovarian Syndrome

We recommend that all patients with PCOS, regardless of age, undergo lipid and diabetes screening given the increased prevalence of dyslipidemia and insulin resistance in this population.[18,34] We also recommend an increased frequency of monitoring for such clinical changes compared with the general population, even if the initial values are normal, because the risk of developing these conditions increases with age. Some experts have suggested 2-year screening intervals. Given that normalizing dyslipidemia and glucose intolerance can decrease atherogenesis, OB/GYNs need to be familiar with the principles of management for such conditions throughout the reproductive period. We recommend similar, if not tighter, lipid level goals in dyslipidemia as those used in the metabolic syndrome. The Androgen Excess Society consensus document recommends the target values. These values have been updated according to the American Association of Clinical Endocrinologists and the American College of Endocrinology **Table 2**. Lipid management of women with PCOS (ref#59).

Treatment of Dyslipidemia in Polycystic Ovarian Syndrome

Diet and exercise are the foundations of intervention. The available evidence suggests that lifestyle interventions (diet, exercise, and behavioral interventions) are more effective than minimal treatment for weight loss and for improving insulin resistance and dyslipidemia.[35] The use of medication to control lipids has special considerations

Table 2 PCOS risk categories and lipid target values			
	Risk	LDL Target Values, mg/dL (mmol/L)[a]	Non-HDL Target Values, mg/dL (mmol/L)[a]
PCOS	At optimal	≤100 (2.59)	≤130 (3.37)
PCOS (obesity, hypertension, dyslipidemia, cigarette smoking, IGT, subvascular disease)	At risk	≤100 (2.59)	≤100 (2.59)
PCOS with MetS	High risk	≤100 (2.59)	≤130 (3.37)
PCOS[b] with MetS and T2DM, overt renal disease, or other vascular disease	—	≤70 (1.81)	≤100 (2.59)

Values are based on a 12-hour fast. For secondary prevention post events LDL targets are less than 55 mg/dL.

Abbreviations: IGT, impaired glucose tolerance; MetS, metabolic syndrome; T2DM, type 2 diabetes mellitus.

[a] To convert mg/dL to mmol/L, divide by 39.

[b] Odds for CVD increase with number of MetS components and with other risk factors, smoking, poor diet, inactivity, obesity, family history of premature CVD (men <55 years old or women <65 years old), and subclinical vascular disease.

Adapted from Wild RA, Carmina E, Diamanti-Kandarakis E, et al. Assessment of cardiovascular risk and prevention of cardiovascular disease in women with the polycystic ovary syndrome: a consensus statement by the Androgen Excess and Polycystic Ovary Syndrome (AE-PCOS) Society. J Clin Endocrinol Metab 2010;95(5);2038–49; with permission.

for women with PCOS. Therapy should be focused on reversing all components of the metabolic syndrome through diet, exercise, and medication only if needed.[36]

In general, metformin is widely used because of its low cost, long-term safety data, and low side effect profile. However, treatment of type 2 diabetes mellitus is the only approved indication for metformin. Nevertheless, it has been used off-label to treat or prevent several clinical problems associated with PCOS, including oligomenorrhea, hirsutism, anovulatory infertility, prevention of pregnancy complications, and obesity.[37] However, available data do not support the use of metformin for the treatment of hirsutism or as a first-line treatment for ovulation induction, oligomenorrhea, and many other features of PCOS, except insulin resistance. Data regarding the effect of metformin on dyslipidemia are controversial and it has been suggested to improve the lipid profile through an increase in LDL-C and decreased weight, waist circumference, and blood pressure in patients with PCOS.[38] Metformin is not considered as a first-line therapy for dyslipidemia in women with PCOS. Numerous medications have been used for PCOS, including weight loss medications (as of this writing, 8 have been FDA approved). Glucagon-like peptide 1 receptor agonists, sodium glucose cotransporter inhibitors, which have a glucosuria effect that results in a decreased hemoglobin A1C, weight, and systolic blood pressure have been used in women with PCOS with significant comorbidities. Dipeptidyl peptidase 4 inhibitors exert anti hyperglycemic effects by inhibiting dipeptidyl peptidase 4 to enhance glucagon-like peptide 1 and other incretin hormones. They are weight neutral, have modest hemoglobin A1C–lowering effects, and are available in combinations with metformin, a sodium glucose cotransporter inhibitor, and thiazolidinediones. Pioglitazone has been used in PCOS; however, weight gain, bone fracture risk in postmenopausal women, and an increased risk of chronic edema and heart failure have limited the use of all thiazolidinediones. Of the numerous diet interventions available, Heart Healthy, Mediterranean, and the Dietary Approaches to Stop Hypertension diets have shown short-term improved lipid and other biomarker effects for women with PCOS.[39] High carbohydrate diets tend to aggravate insulin resistance and severely restricting low carbohydrate diets acutely offer weight loss; however, this is not sustainable with long-term lipid reduction and normalization. Weight loss should be targeted in all overweight women with PCOS by decreasing caloric intake in the setting of adequate nutritional intake and healthy food choices, irrespective of diet composition.[40] There is no perfect diet for all patients and national nutritional guidelines should be followed to encourage diets that work for a given individual.

Statins are an ideal choice to treat elevated LDL-C and are the most important primary and secondary prevention medications for cardiovascular diseases (CVD). Statins are used in women with PCOS to treat their metabolic syndrome as well as to decrease testosterone and androstenedione levels. Statins decrease LDL-C and non–HDL-C levels. In 1 clinical trial, atorvastatin therapy improved chronic inflammation and the lipid profile and also decreased the testosterone level in women with PCOS.[41] However, statins impair insulin sensitivity.[42] Because women with PCOS are at an increased risk of developing type 2 diabetes mellitus, statin therapy should be initiated from the generally accepted American Health association or American college of Cardiology or National Lipid Association guidelines, criteria after individual risk assessment of ASCVD risk, and not solely in the setting of a diagnosis of PCOS.[43]

Among the statins, atorvastatin, simvastatin, and lovastatin are the most commonly used statins and can inhibit DNA synthesis and growth of follicular mesenchymal cells. Other statins have a lower risk of minor side effects and are commonly substituted. Simvastatin has been shown to improve menstrual cyclicity and to decrease hirsutism, acne, and ovarian volume. The decrease in ovarian volume likely occurs in parallel with a decrease reduction in the number of theca cells, resulting in decreased androgen production.[44] Given the current categorization of statins use in pregnancy owing to concern for teratogenic risk, women who are at risk of becoming pregnant must be counseled extensively[45] as to the need for a reliable form of contraception. Stains can be useful in treating fatty liver, which is common in women with PCOS who have the metabolic syndrome.[46]

Other lipid level-lowering medications used successfully in women with PCOS include. Nicotinic acid, also known as vitamin B_3, is involved in lipid metabolism through the conversion to nicotinamide. Nicotinic acid inhibits hydrolysis, reduces the release of nonesterified fatty acids into the liver, and subsequently decrease the hepatic synthesis and release of very low-density lipoprotein TGs by binding to nicotinic receptors in adipose tissue. Moreover, nicotinic acid can improve the lipid profile by lowering LDL particles and increasing HDL in the serum of PCOS patients as TG are lowered.[47]

CONTRACEPTION

Family planning optimizes pregnancy and maternal outcomes. OB/GYNs must have insight into the effects of contraceptive type on lipid metabolism and the effects of lipid management because of contraceptive choice, keeping in mind the risks associated with being pregnant if contraception is not used.

Most surveys show that approximately 50% of pregnancies are unexpected in the United States.[48] No contraceptive method fits everyone. The risk of complications associated with pregnancy, contraceptive efficacy in preventing pregnancy (which most often carries greater risk to the mother if the contraceptive is not used or fails), as well as the cardiometabolic impact of the method chosen are important considerations.

Screening for lipid levels should be kept up to date, commensurate with childhood, adolescent, and adult guidelines for population screening (see the National Lipid Association guidelines). Special thought must be used to identify persons with FH, hypertriglyceridemia, or rare genetic forms of hyperlipidemia on routine screening and/or family history. A detailed metabolic and pregnancy history provides insight as to the cardiometabolic future risk of the mother and her children.

Lipid Changes with Different Forms of Contraception

Combined oral contraceptives

COCs have multiple tissue effects, including estrogenic, progestational, androgenic, antiestrogenic, and antiandrogenic effects. All forms decrease the risk for endometrial and ovarian cancers. The major risk associated with all COCs is thromboembolic disease. Women with various medical comorbidities including obesity, older age, and tobacco use are at an increased risk for these cardiovascular events. There are 2 types of estrogen (ethinyl-estradiol and mestranol) used in the United States. Various doses of estrogen within COCs are available. Higher estrogen doses carry a greater risk of thromboembolic events. Few 50-mg estrogen-containing pills are available on the market today for this reason. At present, most COCs contain 35 mg of ethinyl-estradiol or less and there are multiple types of progestins used in the COCs currently marketed.

In healthy women, COC use decreases insulin sensitivity, but in general, this decrease is not clinically significant.[49] Evidence for the effects of COCs on insulin sensitivity in women with PCOS is conflicting. Studies have reported improvement,[50] worsening,[51] or no change[52] in insulin sensitivity. Nevertheless, there is no evidence that COC use influences the risk of developing diabetes or affects glycemic control.[53]

COCs can negatively impact lipid and carbohydrate metabolism, but usually not with a clinically meaningful effect size. For certain subgroups, such as those with PCOS, these changes can be significant.[54] The estrogenic effect of COCs increases levels of TGs and HDL-C and decreases levels of LDL-C. Androgenic progestins (such as norgestrel and levonorgestrel) can increase LDL-C levels and decrease HDL-C levels. The progestational effect is lipid neutral. For example, desogestrel, a third-generation COC that uses low-dose norethindrone, decrease LDL-C levels and increases HDL-C levels. In addition, the more overall estrogenic a COC is, the more it seems to increase TG and HDL levels. This effect carries a greater risk of precipitating pancreatitis in scenarios in which baseline TG levels are increased and increase further with estrogenic COC use. Transdermal or vaginal combination contraceptives (estrogenic plus progestin) do not decrease the risk of a thrombotic event compared with COCs. Transdermal estrogenic do not aggravate TG levels.

Intrauterine devices

Persons with known severe hyperlipidemia can be given a progestin-impregnated intrauterine device (level 2 recommendation). Less overall bleeding is noted with this method, but irregular and unpredictable bleeding is common. A nonhormonal option is the copper intrauterine device, which can be used for up to 10 years per device and is a lipid-neutral option. In regards to progestin-only intrauterine devices, randomized comparative studies have shown that this method is safe regarding effects on lipid metabolism, blood pressure, and liver function tests.[55,56]

Progestin only

Oral, implantable, or injectable progestins are widely used, especially for persons at risk of noncompliance. In general, progestin-only methods are lipid neutral. There is some evidence that injectable depo-medroxyprogesterone is associated with weight gain. Weight gain is associated with creating or aggravating a current metabolic syndrome with the associated risks of diabetes and mixed dyslipidemia. Despite this finding, implantable and injectable progestin forms of contraception are extremely efficacious for preventing pregnancy. Newer and older progestin-only oral contraceptives are available and are often used when estrogenic preparations are contraindicated or when the risk/benefit ratio is a concern with a COC. However, progestin-only formulations are associated with increased breakthrough bleeding and decreased contraceptive efficacy.

Permanent Sterilization

Male and female permanent sterilization procedures are widely used and highly effective forms of contraception. Although nonhormonal and thus lipid neutral, permanent sterilization can unfortunately lead to loss of general-care follow-up as patients are no longer seeking medical care for pregnancy. As primary care providers offering such contraceptive options, it is prudent to recognize the importance of continuing screening for ASCVD risk factors.

MENOPAUSE TRANSITION
Lipid Changes During Menopause

With the onset of waning of ovarian function, lipid changes are noticeable on both a population and an individual basis. The changes tend to occur primarily during the later phases of menopause transition. The magnitude of change toward dyslipidemia is like and additive to the changes that occur with aging. The relative odds of having an

LDL-C level of 130 mg/dL before to after menopause has been reported to be 2.1 (95% confidence interval, 1.5–2.9).[57]

An increase in serum cholesterol in postmenopausal women is generally considered as result of a decrease in serum estradiol and a decrease in the number of LDL-C receptors. Changes in body fat distribution are also observed during this transitional time.[58]

Fig. 4 shows the natural changes of the major lipid and apolipoprotein lipid levels using cross-sectional panel design analysis as these women transitioned through the menopause years, studied in the multiethnic Study of Women's Health Across the Nation (SWAN) dataset. Note that the levels are assessed and measured as annual mean data comparing years before and after the final menstrual period. Menopause is defined in retrospect as 1 year with no menses during this transition. Day 0 in the graphs is labeled and standardized as the final menstrual period. Importantly, apolipoprotein B levels increase noticeably.

The absolute risk for CVD increases substantially in midlife for women. Rates associated with an adverse effect on lipid metabolism increase at the time of menopause. Those persons with significant risk factors before menopause are additionally affected. A high LDL-C level is a strong predictor of CVD risk in women younger than 65 years and a low HDL-C level is a stronger predictor of CHD mortality in women than in men and particularly so in women 65 years of age and older.[59] In the Framingham Heart Study, the 8-year risk of heart disease was 7% for women with a total/HDL-C ratio of less than 5%, 12% for those with ratios of 5% to 7%, and 20% for those with ratios of greater than 7.[60] It is important for OB/GYNs to identify these individuals early to plan for the best control of these same risk factors during the menopause transition.[57,61]

In addition, there is a link to an increased prevalence of the metabolic syndrome.[62] With expert treatment, it has been shown that carotid atherosclerosis is observed more frequently beginning in the menopause transition, and a significant number of women also possess coronary calcium deposition before this time.[63]

Annual rates of change in carotid intima media thickness and adventitial diameter have been reported, as noted in **Fig. 5**. The rate of change at the late perimenopausal stage significantly differs from that at the premenopausal stage. The rate of change at the late perimenopausal stage significantly differs from that at the early perimenopausal stage. The rate of change at the postmenopausal stage significantly differs from that at the premenopausal stage ($P<.05$).

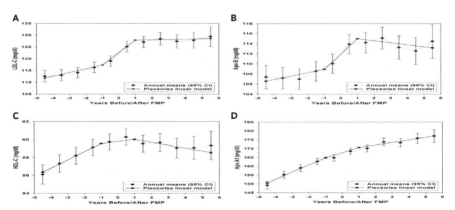

Fig. 4. Lipids annual and estimated means pattern of LDL-C (*A*), apolipoprotein (Apo) B (*B*), HDL-C (*C*), and Apo A-I (*D*) across the SWAN study follow-up period.

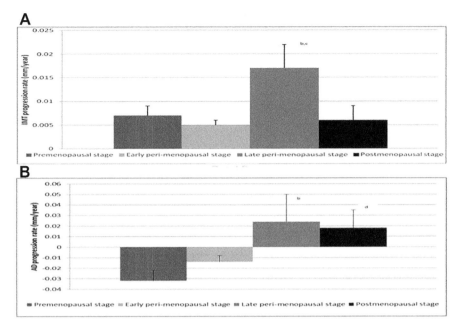

Fig. 5. Annual rates of change in (*A*) carotid intima media thickness (IMT) and (*B*) adventitial diameter (AD). (*From* El Khoudary SR, Wildman RP, Matthews K, et al. Progression rates of carotid intima-media thickness and adventitial diameter during the menopausal transition. Menopause 2013;20(1):8–14; with permission.)

Considerations for Hormone Replacement Therapy

The hormonal changes of menopause are associated with an increasingly atherogenic lipid profile. This factor provides both an opportunity and a challenge for the aggressive management of dyslipidemia. Menopausal hormone replacement therapy is primarily indicated to control menopause-related quality-of-life issues. Replacement therapy should not be prescribed to reduce cardiovascular events (ie, for prevention or treatment of vascular diseases). Identifying appropriate candidates for menopausal hormone therapy is challenging given the complex profile of risks and benefits associated with treatment.[64,65] Most professional societies agree that hormone therapy should not be used for chronic disease prevention. Note the results from an analysis of the Women's Health Initiative (WHI), in which oral estrogen plus progestin and estrogen alone were used in the randomized clinical trial (**Table 3**). Accordingly, there is a black box warning by the FDA for women with known coronary artery disease, thromboembolic disorders, or who have had a cerebrovascular accident because these preparations carry thrombotic risk and critical events in persons with these disorders involving thrombotic pathophysiology.

The WHI, a 15-year longitudinal study of morbidity and mortality in more than 160,000 healthy, postmenopausal women (average age 63 years at baseline), found a lack of a cardioprotective effect associated with hormone replacement therapy.[66] Although estrogen replacement did decrease LDL-C and increase HDL-C, it also increased TG and small, dense LDL particles, 2 of the 3 components that characterize atherogenic dyslipidemia.[67] Based on this, WHI findings are consistent with previous trials in which hormone replacement therapy was not shown to protect against ASCVD

Table 3
CHD risk in the Women's Health Initiative hormone therapy trials (estrogen and progestin and estrogen alone) according to baseline levels of biomarkers

Biomarker P Value for Interaction	Odds Ratio (95% CL) for Hormone Therapy Treatment Effect	P for Interaction
LDL-C (mg/dL)		
<130	0.66 (0.34−1.27)	.03
≥130		
LDL-C/HDL-C ratio		
<2.5	0.66 (0.34−1.27)	.002
≥2.5	1.73 (1.18−2.53)	
Hs-CRP (mg/dL)		
<2.0	1.01 (0.63−1.62)	.16
≥2.0	1.58 (1.05−2.39)	
MetS	2.26 (1.26−4.07)	.03
No MetS	0.97 (0.58−1.61)	—

Abbreviations: CL, confidence limit; hs-CRP, high-sensitivity C-reactive protein.
Adapted from Wild RA, Manson JE. Insights from the Women's Health Initiative: individualizing risk assessment for hormone therapy decisions. Semin Reprod Med 2014;32(6):433–37; with permission.

or cerebrovascular accident. This analysis suggests that persons at higher risk for CVD events (increased dyslipidemia or the presence of the metabolic syndrome or with a family history of thrombotic disease) are more likely to have this risk aggravated by the administration of oral hormone replacement therapy. Findings from the WHI and other randomized trials suggest that a woman's age, proximity to menopause, underlying cardiovascular risk factor status, and various biological characteristics may modify health outcomes with hormone therapy.

The message is clear: assessing CVD risk before hormone therapy is given for menopausal symptoms is prudent to identify persons who may be at increased adverse event risk with oral hormone therapy.

An emerging body of evidence suggests that it may be possible to assess an individual's risk and, therefore, better predict who is likely to have favorable outcomes versus adverse effects when taking hormone therapy. There are also several biomarkers under study to determine whether they provide incremental risk prediction for CVD in women taking hormone therapy. However, thus far none have been shown to provide added risk prediction and currently they are not recommended for clinical use. Several risk estimators are available to estimate risk, including the Framingham Risk Assessment tool (https://www.framinghamstudy.org/risk-functions/coronary-heart-disease/hard-10-year-risk.php), the Reynold Risk Score, which includes C-reactive protein (https://www.reynold'srisksscore.org), and the Multi-Ethnic Study Atherosclerosis 10-year risk score (https://mesa-nhlbi.org/MESACHDRiks/MesaRiskScore/RiskScore.aspx), which are increasingly validated for women 40 years and older. Many of these estimators are embedded within the electronic medical records systems. Thus, once a woman is identified as a potential candidate for hormone therapy because of moderate to severe menopausal symptoms or other indications, risk stratification may be an important tool for minimizing patient CVD risk factors and for assessing suitability for hormone therapy.[64,65,68]

This individualized approach holds great promise for improving the safety of hormone therapy. A treatment decision to provide symptom relief should be made with a patient's full understanding of the potential risks and benefits, and considering her personal preferences. To better integrate patient values, practical considerations, and emerging clinical experience, recent research from observational studies and randomized clinical trials on hormone therapy should be considered.

Systemic estrogens induce a dose-dependent decrease in TC and LDL-C, as well as an increase in HDL-C concentrations; these effects are more prominent with oral administration. Micronized progesterone or dydrogesterone are the preferred progestogens owing to their neutral effect on the lipid profile. Using the lowest effective dose of hormone therapy is recommended, regardless of the clinical scenario. In general, doses of less than 0.3 mg of oral conjugated estrogen daily do not control hot flashes for most women. However, this dose is protective against bone loss from estrogen deficiency osteopenia.[64] Transdermal rather than oral estrogens should be used in women with hypertriglyceridemia. Delivering the medication transdermally may be associated with fewer adverse events than when given by the oral route.[69] Tissue effects may differ depending on whether there is a first-pass hepatic effect, as is the case with oral estrogen. Ospemifene, an oral selective estrogen receptor modulator, and vaginal dehydroepiandrosterone are both recently FDA approved for the treatment of moderate to severe symptomatic vulvovaginal atrophy in postmenopausal women who are not candidates for vaginal estrogen therapy. Ospemifene exerts a favorable effect on the lipid profile, but data are scant regarding dehydroepiandrosterone.[70]

With vaginal and transdermal preparations, there is less of an effect on clotting factors, lipid metabolism, inflammatory biomarkers, and sex hormone–binding globulin synthesis. Differences in the dose, route, and formulations, in conjunction with genetic metabolic differences, may lead to different outcomes. Observational studies, although limited in number, suggest that transdermal delivery may be associated with a lower risk of venous thromboembolism and stroke than with oral estrogen administration; however, these studies do not prove a cause–effect relationship.[71] Randomized clinical trial evidence is needed to answer this question more definitively.

SUMMARY

Advances in research, technology, and pharmacology increase the options available for women, but this rapidly changing knowledge-based presents a challenge for clinicians. Moreover, the delivery of care for women has been historically fragmented. To overcome this barriers, multidisciplinary curriculums in women's health education have been created. Care for women is optimized by education on a range of medical concerns provided by experts from a wide variety of medical specialties. Given the complexity of care, interdisciplinary approaches are becoming an increasingly important aspect of care by health care providers, with needs that cross many areas of medical expertise.

DISCLOSURE

The authors have nothing to disclose.

REFERENCES

1. de Oliveira Y, Cavalcante RGS, Cavalcanti Neto MP, et al. Oral administration of Lactobacillus fermentum post-weaning improves the lipid profile and autonomic

dysfunction in rat offspring exposed to maternal dyslipidemia. Food Funct 2020; 11(6):5581–94.

2. Eckel RH, Jakicic JM, Ard JD, et al. 2013 AHA/ACC guideline on lifestyle management to reduce cardiovascular risk: a report of the American College of Cardiology/American Heart Association Task Force on Practice Guidelines. Circulation 2014;129(25 Suppl 2):S76–99.

3. Piechota W, Staszewski A. Reference ranges of lipids and apolipoproteins in pregnancy. Eur J Obstet Gynecol Reprod Biol 1992;45(1):27–35.

4. Wiznitzer A, Mayer A, Novack V, et al. Association of lipid levels during gestation with preeclampsia and gestational diabetes mellitus: a population-based study. Am J Obstet Gynecol 2009;201(5):482.e1-8.

5. Mankuta D, Elami-Suzin M, Elhayani A, et al. Lipid profile in consecutive pregnancies. Lipids Health Dis 2010;9:58.

6. Potter JM, Nestel PJ. The hyperlipidemia of pregnancy in normal and complicated pregnancies. Am J Obstet Gynecol 1979;133(2):165–70.

7. Stuebe AM, Rich-Edwards JW. The reset hypothesis: lactation and maternal metabolism. Am J Perinatol 2009;26(1):81–8.

8. Vrijkotte TG, Krukziener N, Hutten BA, et al. Maternal lipid profile during early pregnancy and pregnancy complications and outcomes: the ABCD study. J Clin Endocrinol Metab 2012;97(11):3917–25.

9. Feitosa ACR, Barreto LT, Silva IMD, et al. Impact of the use of different diagnostic criteria in the prevalence of dyslipidemia in pregnant women. Arq Bras Cardiol 2017;109(1):30–8.

10. Catov JM, Ness RB, Wellons MF, et al. Prepregnancy lipids related to preterm birth risk: the coronary artery risk development in young adults study. J Clin Endocrinol Metab 2010;95(8):3711–8.

11. Jan MR, Nazli R, Shah J, et al. A study of lipoproteins in normal and pregnancy induced hypertensive women in tertiary care hospitals of the north west frontier province-Pakistan. Hypertens Pregnancy 2012;31(2):292–9.

12. Kushtagi P, Arvapally S. Maternal mid-pregnancy serum triglyceride levels and neonatal birth weight. Int J Gynaecol Obstet 2009;106(3):258–9.

13. Edison RJ, Berg K, Remaley A, et al. Adverse birth outcome among mothers with low serum cholesterol. Pediatrics 2007;120(4):723–33.

14. Nordestgaard BG, Chapman MJ, Humphries SE, et al. Familial hypercholesterolaemia is underdiagnosed and undertreated in the general population: guidance for clinicians to prevent coronary heart disease: consensus statement of the European Atherosclerosis Society. Eur Heart J 2013;34(45):3478–3490a.

15. Smith GN, Walker MC, Liu A, et al. A history of preeclampsia identifies women who have underlying cardiovascular risk factors. Am J Obstet Gynecol 2009; 200(1):58.e1-8.

16. Son GH, Kwon JY, Kim YH, et al. Maternal serum triglycerides as predictive factors for large-for-gestational age newborns in women with gestational diabetes mellitus. Acta Obstet Gynecol Scand 2010;89(5):700–4.

17. Brown HL, Warner JJ, Gianos E, et al. Promoting risk identification and reduction of cardiovascular disease in women through collaboration with obstetricians and gynecologists: a presidential advisory from the American Heart Association and the American College of Obstetricians and Gynecologists. Circulation 2018; 137(24):e843–52.

18. Costantine MM, Cleary K, Eunice Kennedy Shriver National Institute of Child Health and Human Development Obstetric–Fetal Pharmacology Research Units

Network. Pravastatin for the prevention of preeclampsia in high-risk pregnant women. Obstet Gynecol 2013;121(2 Pt 1):349–53.

19. Costantine MM, Cleary K, Hebert MF, et al. Safety and pharmacokinetics of pravastatin used for the prevention of preeclampsia in high-risk pregnant women: a pilot randomized controlled trial. Am J Obstet Gynecol 2016;214(6):720.e1-7.

20. Goldberg AS, Hegele RA. Severe hypertriglyceridemia in pregnancy. J Clin Endocrinol Metab 2012;97(8):2589–96.

21. Toleikyte I, Retterstol K, Leren TP, et al. Pregnancy outcomes in familial hypercholesterolemia: a registry-based study. Circulation 2011;124(15):1606–14.

22. Jeon HR, Kim SY, Cho YJ, et al. Hypertriglyceridemia-induced acute pancreatitis in pregnancy causing maternal death. Obstet Gynecol Sci 2016;59(2):148–51.

23. Tanous D, Siu SC, Mason J, et al. B-type natriuretic peptide in pregnant women with heart disease. J Am Coll Cardiol 2010;56(15):1247–53.

24. Kusters DM, Homsma SJ, Hutten BA, et al. Dilemmas in treatment of women with familial hypercholesterolaemia during pregnancy. Neth J Med 2010;68(1):299–303.

25. Zarrati M, Shidfar F, Moradof M, et al. Relationship between breast feeding and obesity in children with low birth weight. Iran Red Crescent Med J 2013;15(8):676–82.

26. Grandi SM, Vallee-Pouliot K, Reynier P, et al. Hypertensive disorders in pregnancy and the risk of subsequent cardiovascular disease. Paediatr Perinat Epidemiol 2017;31(5):412–21.

27. Shostrom DCV, Sun Y, Oleson JJ, et al. History of gestational diabetes mellitus in relation to cardiovascular disease and cardiovascular risk factors in US women. Front Endocrinol 2017;8:144.

28. Charlton F, Tooher J, Rye KA, et al. Cardiovascular risk, lipids and pregnancy: preeclampsia and the risk of later life cardiovascular disease. Heart Lung Circ 2014;23(3):203–12.

29. Kjerulff LE, Sanchez-Ramos L, Duffy D. Pregnancy outcomes in women with polycystic ovary syndrome: a metaanalysis. Am J Obstet Gynecol 2011;204(6): 558.e1-6.

30. Gunderson EP. Childbearing and obesity in women: weight before, during, and after pregnancy. Obstet Gynecol Clin North Am 2009;36(2):317–32, ix.

31. Yildiz BO, Bozdag G, Yapici Z, et al. Prevalence, phenotype and cardiometabolic risk of polycystic ovary syndrome under different diagnostic criteria. Hum Reprod 2012;27(10):3067–73.

32. Pergialiotis V, Trakakis E, Chrelias C, et al. The impact of mild hypercholesterolemia on glycemic and hormonal profiles, menstrual characteristics and the ovarian morphology of women with polycystic ovarian syndrome. Horm Mol Biol Clin Invest 2018;34(3):20180002.

33. Ghaffarzad A, Amani R, Mehrzad Sadaghiani M, et al. Correlation of serum lipoprotein ratios with insulin resistance in infertile women with polycystic ovarian syndrome: a case control study. Int J Fertil Steril 2016;10(1):29–35.

34. Moran LJ, Misso ML, Wild RA, et al. Impaired glucose tolerance, type 2 diabetes and metabolic syndrome in polycystic ovary syndrome: a systematic review and meta-analysis. Hum Reprod Update 2010;16(4):347–63.

35. Moran LJ, Hutchison SK, Norman RJ, et al. Lifestyle changes in women with polycystic ovary syndrome. Cochrane Database Syst Rev 2011;(2):CD007506.

36. Diabetes Prevention Program Research G, Knowler WC, Fowler SE, et al. 10-year follow-up of diabetes incidence and weight loss in the diabetes prevention program outcomes study. Lancet 2009;374(9702):1677–86.

37. Nestler JE. Metformin for the treatment of the polycystic ovary syndrome. N Engl J Med 2008;358(1):47–54.

38. Kumar DRN, Seshadri KG, Pandurangi M. Effect of metformin-sustained release therapy on low-density lipoprotein size and adiponectin in the south Indian women with polycystic ovary syndrome. Indian J Endocrinol Metab 2017;21(5): 679–83.
39. Asemi Z, Esmaillzadeh A. DASH diet, insulin resistance, and serum hs-CRP in polycystic ovary syndrome: a randomized controlled clinical trial. Horm Metab Res 2015;47(3):232–8.
40. Moran LJ, Ko H, Misso M, et al. Dietary composition in the treatment of polycystic ovary syndrome: a systematic review to inform evidence-based guidelines. J Acad Nutr Diet 2013;113(4):520–45.
41. Duleba AJ, Banaszewska B, Spaczynski RZ, et al. Simvastatin improves biochemical parameters in women with polycystic ovary syndrome: results of a prospective, randomized trial. Fertil Steril 2006;85(4):996–1001.
42. Hyun MH, Jang JW, Choi BG, et al. Risk of insulin resistance with statin therapy in individuals without dyslipidemia: a propensity-matched analysis in a registry population. Clin Exp Pharmacol Physiol 2020;47(6):947–54.
43. Puurunen J, Piltonen T, Puukka K, et al. Statin therapy worsens insulin sensitivity in women with polycystic ovary syndrome (PCOS): a prospective, randomized, double-blind, placebo-controlled study. J Clin Endocrinol Metab 2013;98(12): 4798–807.
44. Banaszewska B, Pawelczyk L, Spaczynski RZ, et al. Effects of simvastatin and metformin on polycystic ovary syndrome after six months of treatment. J Clin Endocrinol Metab 2011;96(11):3493–501.
45. Zarek J, Koren G. The fetal safety of statins: a systematic review and meta-analysis. J Obstet Gynaecol Can 2014;36(6):506–9.
46. Setji TL, Brown AJ. Polycystic ovary syndrome: update on diagnosis and treatment. Am J Med 2014;127(10):912–9.
47. Aye MM, Kilpatrick ES, Afolabi P, et al. Postprandial effects of long-term niacin/ laropiprant use on glucose and lipid metabolism and on cardiovascular risk in patients with polycystic ovary syndrome. Diabetes Obes Metab 2014;16(6):545–52.
48. Sanga K, Mola G, Wattimena J, et al. Unintended pregnancy amongst women attending antenatal clinics at the Port Moresby General Hospital. Aust N Z J Obstet Gynaecol 2014;54(4):360–5.
49. Wang A, Mo T, Li Q, et al. The effectiveness of metformin, oral contraceptives, and lifestyle modification in improving the metabolism of overweight women with polycystic ovary syndrome: a network meta-analysis. Endocrine 2019; 64(2):220–32.
50. Pasquali R, Gambineri A, Anconetani B, et al. The natural history of the metabolic syndrome in young women with the polycystic ovary syndrome and the effect of long-term oestrogen-progestagen treatment. Clin Endocrinol 1999;50(4):517–27.
51. Korytkowski MT, Mokan M, Horwitz MJ, et al. Metabolic effects of oral contraceptives in women with polycystic ovary syndrome. J Clin Endocrinol Metab 1995; 80(11):3327–34.
52. Cibula D, Sindelka G, Hill M, et al. Insulin sensitivity in non-obese women with polycystic ovary syndrome during treatment with oral contraceptives containing low-androgenic progestin. Hum Reprod 2002;17(1):76–82.
53. Gourdy P. Diabetes and oral contraception. Best Pract Res Clin Endocrinol Metab 2013;27(1):67–76.
54. Bargiota A, Diamanti-Kandarakis E. The effects of old, new and emerging medicines on metabolic aberrations in PCOS. Ther Adv Endocrinol Metab 2012; 3(1):27–47.

55. Ng YW, Liang S, Singh K. Effects of Mirena (levonorgestrel-releasing intrauterine system) and Ortho Gynae T380 intrauterine copper device on lipid metabolism–a randomized comparative study. Contraception 2009;79(1):24–8.
56. Kayikcioglu F, Gunes M, Ozdegirmenci O, et al. Effects of levonorgestrel-releasing intrauterine system on glucose and lipid metabolism: a 1-year follow-up study. Contraception 2006;73(5):528–31.
57. Derby CA, Crawford SL, Pasternak RC, et al. Lipid changes during the menopause transition in relation to age and weight: the Study of Women's Health Across the Nation. Am J Epidemiol 2009;169(11):1352–61.
58. Park JK, Lim YH, Kim KS, et al. Changes in body fat distribution through menopause increase blood pressure independently of total body fat in middle-aged women: the Korean National Health and Nutrition Examination Survey 2007-2010. Hypertens Res 2013;36(5):444–9.
59. Garber AJ, Abrahamson MJ, Barzilay JI, et al. Consensus Statement by the American Association of Clinical Endocrinologists and American College of Endocrinology on the comprehensive type 2 diabetes management algorithm - 2018 executive summary. Endocr Pract 2018;24(1):91–120.
60. Trinder M, Uddin MM, Finneran P, et al. Clinical utility of lipoprotein(a) and LPA genetic risk score in risk prediction of incident atherosclerotic cardiovascular disease. JAMA Cardiol 2020;e205398 [Epub ahead of print].
61. Matthews KA, Gibson CJ, El Khoudary SR, et al. Changes in cardiovascular risk factors by hysterectomy status with and without oophorectomy: Study of Women's Health Across the Nation. J Am Coll Cardiol 2013;62(3):191–200.
62. Mendes KG, Theodoro H, Rodrigues AD, et al. Prevalence of metabolic syndrome and its components in the menopausal transition: a systematic review. Cad Saude Publica 2012;28(8):1423–37 [in Portuguese].
63. El Khoudary SR, Wildman RP, Matthews K, et al. Progression rates of carotid intima-media thickness and adventitial diameter during the menopausal transition. Menopause 2013;20(1):8–14.
64. Mizunuma H, Shiraki M, Shintani M, et al. Randomized trial comparing low-dose hormone replacement therapy and HRT plus 1alpha-OH-vitamin D3 (alfacalcidol) for treatment of postmenopausal bone loss. J Bone Miner Metab 2006;24(1):11–5.
65. Wild RA, Manson JE. Insights from the Women's Health Initiative: individualizing risk assessment for hormone therapy decisions. Semin Reprod Med 2014;32(6):433–7.
66. Rossouw JE, Anderson GL, Prentice RL, et al. Risks and benefits of estrogen plus progestin in healthy postmenopausal women: principal results From the Women's Health Initiative randomized controlled trial. JAMA 2002;288(3):321–33.
67. Blum CB, Adult Treatment Panel IIIoTNCEP. Perspectives: some thoughts on the adult treatment panel III report. Prev Cardiol 2002;5(2):87–9, 93.
68. Mosca L, Appel LJ, Benjamin EJ, et al. Evidence-based guidelines for cardiovascular disease prevention in women. Circulation 2004;109(5):672–93.
69. North American Menopause S. The 2012 hormone therapy position statement of: the North American Menopause Society. Menopause 2012;19(3):257–71.
70. Anagnostis P, Bitzer J, Cano A, et al. Menopause symptom management in women with dyslipidemias: an EMAS clinical guide. Maturitas 2020;135:82–8.
71. Canonico M, Oger E, Plu-Bureau G, et al. Hormone therapy and venous thromboembolism among postmenopausal women: impact of the route of estrogen administration and progestogens: the ESTHER study. Circulation 2007;115(7):840–5.

Benign Uterine Disease
The Added Role of Imaging

Stephanie Nougaret, MD, PhD[a,b,]*, Teresa Margarida Cunha, MD[c],
Nadia Benadla, MD[b], Mathias Neron, MD[d], Jessica B. Robbins, MD[e]

KEYWORDS

- Leiomyoma • Polyp • Adenomyosis • MRI • Uterus

KEY POINTS

- Benign uterine disease is mainly composed of adenomyosis, leiomyomas, and endometrial polyps.
- MRI is used for the detection, localization, and characterization of benign uterine disease and their differential diagnosis.
- MRI is the imaging modality for pretreatment evaluation, assessing potential procedural risk, predicting treatment response, and monitoring patient outcomes.

INTRODUCTION

Benign uterine diseases are very frequent gynecologic conditions affecting women of all ages,[1–6] but mostly during the reproductive range. All of them may cause similar symptoms such as pelvic pain, abnormal vaginal bleeding, and reproductive dysfunction.[1–6] Although ultrasound examination is the first-line imaging technique for the examination of the uterus, MRI has become more and more important, not only to establish the diagnosis, but also to guide patient management.[7–13] Additional benefits of MRI include absence of ionizing radiation and iodinated contrast material. As such, MRI has been incorporated into the clinical workflow for the assessment and management of gynecologic conditions. MRI is particularly helpful in evaluating the atypical features that can mimic malignancy.[10,14–16] MRI also helps to triage symptomatic patients into the most accurate treatment modality, including surgical management

[a] Montpellier Cancer Research Institute, Montpellier, France; [b] Department of Radiology, Montpellier Cancer Institute, INSERM, U1194, University of Montpellier, 208 Avenue des Apothicaires, Montpellier 34295, France; [c] Department of Radiology, Instituto Português de Oncologia de Lisboa Francisco Gentil, R. Prof. Lima Basto, Lisboa Codex 1099-023, Portugal; [d] Department of Surgery, Montpellier Cancer Institute, 208 Avenue des Apothicaires, Montpellier 34295, France; [e] University of Wisconsin School of Medicine and Public Health, Madison, WI, USA
* Corresponding author. Department of Radiology, Institut du Cancer de Montpellier, 208 Rue des Apothicaires, Montpellier 34 295, France.
E-mail address: stephanienougaret@free.fr

Obstet Gynecol Clin N Am 48 (2021) 193–214
https://doi.org/10.1016/j.ogc.2020.12.002
0889-8545/21/© 2021 Elsevier Inc. All rights reserved.

(hysterectomy, myomectomy), interventional procedures (uterine artery embolization [UAE]), and medical therapy, according to the extent, location, and morphologic characteristics of the disease.[17–19] Hysterectomy is curative, but uterus-sparing therapies may offer a valid alternative for eligible women of reproductive age.

In this article, we highlight the usefulness of MRI in the diagnosis of the most common benign uterine diseases, such as leiomyomas and adenomyosis; discuss their typical and atypical MRI findings; and describe the therapeutic options and the role of MRI in the treatment planning.

MRI PROTOCOL

Recommendations for diagnostic and management of patients with uterine lesions are extensive.[1,20,21] Recently, guidelines for MRI were proposed by the European Society of Urogenital Radiology.[13]

Patient Preparation

The majority of pelvic MRI examinations require intravenous injection of contrast media. To decrease motion artifacts, an antiperistaltic agent is recommended before the examination. Patients with a tumor involving the vagina or cervix should be informed that vaginal gel may be needed. **Box 1** summarizes the information that can be given to the patient before MRI.

Imaging Protocol

High-resolution thin-section images acquired at 1.5 T or 3.0 T are recommended. The optimal protocol, according to recent European Society of Urogenital Radiology guidelines,[13] includes the following.

- High-resolution T2 sequences in the axial, oblique, sagittal, and coronal planes. The axial oblique T2-weighted sequence perpendicular to the corpus of the uterus is particularly useful to evaluate the location of the lesion relative to the endometrial cavity.

Box 1
Information that can be given to the patient prior to their MRI exam

- MRI is a noninvasive test that uses a magnetic field and pulses of radio wave energy to make pictures of the organs and structures inside the body.

- Before the test:
  - You will remove all metal objects, such as hearing aids, dentures, jewelry, watches, and hairpins.
  - You may be asked to change into a gown.
  - You may have contrast material (dye) put into your arm through a tube called an IV. Contrast material helps doctors see specific organs, blood vessels, and most tumors.
  - An antiperistaltic (Buscopan/Glucagon) may be given as well to decrease the images artifacts related to bowel movement.
  - Some examinations require putting a small amount of gel lubricant into your vagina. This lubricant helps the doctor to define your anatomy.

- During the test:
  - You will lie on your back on a table that is part of the MRI scanner.
  - Inside the scanner you will hear a fan and feel air moving. You may hear tapping, thumping, or snapping noises. You may be given earplugs or headphones to reduce the noise.
  - You will be asked to hold still during the scan. You may be asked to hold your breath for short periods.

- An axial T1-weighted sequence of the pelvis with and without fat suppression. Axial T1-weighted sequence is useful to evaluate the presence of fat or blood contents in an adnexal lesion and can be used to detect the presence of lymph nodes and bone marrow abnormalities.
- Large field of view T1-weighted or T2-weighted sequences of the upper abdomen allow visualization of the secondary signs of pelvic mass effect such as hydronephrosis and malignant disease such as lymph nodes or peritoneal carcinomatosis.
- Contrast-enhanced axial T1-weighted images of the pelvis with fat saturation allows further lesion characterization, vascularization, and its differentiation from an adnexal mass.
- Dynamic contrast injection/MR angiography is recommended if UAE may be a possibility to evaluate uterine artery anatomy and collateral gonadal arterial supply in case of a leiomyoma.
- Diffusion-weighted imaging has shown added value for lesion characterization and distinction between leiomyoma and leiomyosarcoma (as discussed elsewhere in this article). Diffusion-weighted imaging is particularly helpful in the case of endometrial thickening to differentiate between endometrial hypertrophy or polyp and endometrial cancer.

LEIOMYOMAS
Epidemiology and Pathophysiology

Leiomyomas (also referred to as myomas or fibroids) are the most common benign uterine tumor that affect up to 20% to 30% of women during their reproductive age[11] and may be solitary or multiple.[22] Their cause is unknown. Leiomyomas frequently grow during pregnancy and with oral contraceptive use, and tend to regress after menopause.[22] They are symptomatic in 20% to 50% of women. Symptoms can be menorrhagia, dysmenorrhea, urinary frequency, pelvic pressure and back pain, and dyspareunia.[5] Leiomyomas usually involve the myometrium and are classified by their location as submucosal, intramural, or subserosal (PALM-COEIN) (**Fig. 1**).[23] Very briefly, submucosal leiomyomas can be pedunculated (type 0) or intracavitary with more than 50% (type 1) or less than 50% (type 2) of the leiomyoma within the endometrial cavity. A type 3 leiomyoma contacts the endometrium but does not extend into the endometrium. The type 4 leiomyoma is purely intramural without contacting the endometrium or the uterine serosa. A type 5 leiomyoma contacts the serosa and has more than 50 of its content intramural, whereas type 6 is subserosal with less than 50% intramural. A pedunculated subserosal leiomyoma is type 7 and all others are type 8 (eg, cervical or broad ligament).

MRI Features

MRI is useful for distinguishing leiomyomas from other myometrial pathology, especially in patients with nondiagnostic or equivocal ultrasound findings.[24] MRI is particularly useful for the detection of aggressive features indicating leiomyosarcomas, which, although rare, are of pivotal importance if the tumor is considered for laparoscopic removal.[20] Failure to detect leiomyosarcoma before intervention, especially in the era of minimally invasive surgery including morcellation, can pose a great threat of intraperitoneal dissemination and inappropriate treatment, as well as a delay in the initiation of appropriate therapy.[25–27] As such, MRI has become the recommended imaging modality for uterine mass characterization.[28–30]

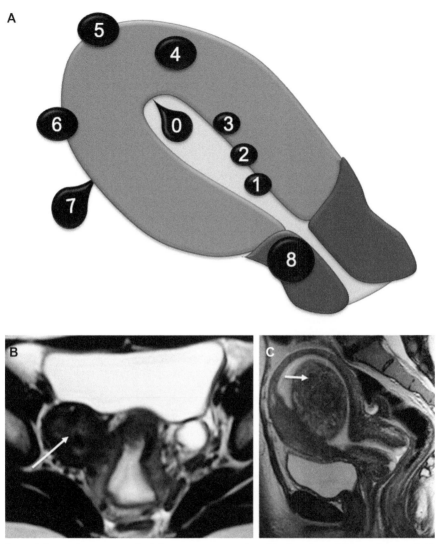

Fig. 1. (*A*) Drawing reports the leiomyoma International Federation of Gynecology and Obstetrics (FIGO) classification as FIGO 0, pedunculated intracavitary; FIGO 1, submucosal less than 50% intramural; FIGO 2, submucosal 50% or greater intramural; FIGO 3, contacts endometrium, 100% intramural; FIGO 4, intramural; FIGO 5, subserosal 50% or greater intramural; FIGO 6, subserosal less than 50% intramural; FIGO 7, subserosal pedunculated; and FIGO 8, other (specify eg, cervical, parasitic). (*B*) Axial T2-weighted image showing a subserosal leiomyoma (*white arrow* FIGO 6). (*C*) sagittal T2-weighted image showing a submucosal leiomyoma (*white arrow* FIGO 1).

On MRI, most leiomyomas without degeneration present as well-delineated round or ovoid lesions homogeneously hypointense on T2-weighted imaging and isointense on T1-weighted imaging, with heterogeneous and variable enhancement after contrast injection. The presence of a T2-hyperintense rim indicates a pseudocapsule of edema owing to dilated lymphatic vessels and veins[31] (**Fig. 2**). Typical leiomyomas

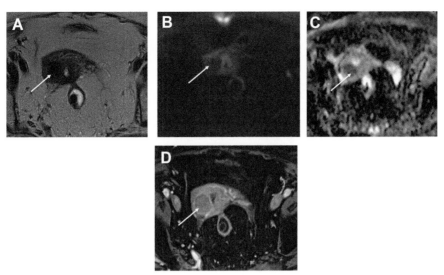

Fig. 2. Typical leiomyoma. (*A*) Axial T2-weighted images, (*B*) axial diffusion-weighted image with (*C*) the corresponding apparent diffusion coefficient (ADC) map, and (*D*) gadolinium-enhanced axial T1-weighted fat-saturated image show a myometrial lesion in keeping with a leiomyoma (*arrow*). Nondegenerated leiomyoma appears as a well-defined lesion with hypointense signal intensity on T2-weighted images related to the outer myometrium (*A*) and homogeneous contrast enhancement after gadolinium injection (*D*). No signs of restricted diffusion: low signal intensity on diffusion-weighted image (*B*) and on corresponding ADC map (*C*), as a "blackout phenomenon."

do not have restricted diffusion, showing low signal both on diffusion weighted images and on the corresponding apparent diffusion coefficient (ADC) map, called the "blackout phenomenon"[10] (see **Fig. 2**). This feature is highly suggestive of a benign myometrial lesion, in contrast with leiomyosarcomas.

When leiomyomas enlarge and outgrow their blood supply ($\geq$5 cm in size), they may degenerate.[22,24] The types of degeneration are hyaline, myxoid, cystic, calcific, hemorrhagic, and hydropic. **Table 1** highlights the different types of leiomyomas degeneration (**Figs. 3–6**).

Besides Degeneration, Two Subtypes Have to Be Mentioned

Cellular leiomyoma is a histologic subtype with more compact smooth muscle cells and less collagen. On MRI, cellular leiomyoma demonstrates hyperintense signal on T2-weighted imaging and avid enhancement after injection of contrast material[11] (**Fig. 7**), features that can make it difficult to differentiate them from leiomyosarcoma[32] (**Fig. 8**).

Lipoleiomyoma is a rare histologic subtype generally affecting postmenopausal women. Lipoleiomyomas are composed of smooth muscle, as well as adipose and fibrous tissue. Owing to their fat content, on MRI they demonstrates hyperintense signal on T1-weighted imaging and T2-weighted imaging and loss of SI on fat-saturated sequences.[10]

Differential diagnosis on MRI

Focal myometrial contractions. Contractions may appear as hypointense T2 myometrial masses and may mimic uterine leiomyomas. However, because they are transient

Table 1
MRI features of leiomyomas and leiomyosarcomas

	T2-Weighted Imaging Signal	T2-Weighted Imaging Border	T1-Weighted Images	Contrast-enhanced T1-Weighted Images	Diffusion-Weighted Imaging/ADC
Type of leiomyoma					
Nondegenerated	Hypointense	Well-defined	Isointense	Variable	Hypointense
Cellular subtype	Hyperintense	Well-defined	Isointense	Vivid enhancement	Hyperintense
Lipoleiomyoma subtype	Variable -Fat component	Well-defined	Variable fat component (hyperintense)	Variable	Hypointense
Degeneration type					
Hyaline	Most common type (60%)	Well-defined	Isointense	Avid enhancement	Hypointense
Cystic (see **Fig. 3**)	Presence of cystic areas cobblestone appearance	Well-defined	Hypointense	No enhancement	Hypointense
Myxoid (**Fig. 4**)	Rare Presence of gelatinous intralesional foci Very hyperintense	Well-defined	Hypointense	Delayed enhancement	Hypointense
Hemorrhagic (red degeneration) (**Fig. 5**)	Owing to hemorrhagic infarction Associated with pregnancy and oral contraceptives May also occur after uterine artery embolization Variable	Well-defined	Hyperintense	Variable	Hypointense
Calcific	Associated with end-stage hyaline degeneration and after uterine artery embolization treatment changes Hypointense	Well-defined	Hypointense	No enhancement	Hypointense

Hydroptic (**Fig. 6**)	Very rare. Watery oedema combined with hyalinization, resulting in a cord-like pattern growth of the tumoral cells. The accumulation of watery oedema can sometimes be misinterpreted as a myxoid matrix and, therefore, these types of leiomyomas may be misdiagnosed as myxoid leiomyomas	Hyperintense and hypointense cord like element	Variable	Hypointense	Enhancing cord-like solid components	Variable
Specific entity						
STUMP	Rare heterogeneous tumor that cannot be definitively classified histologically as leiomyoma or leiomyosarcoma. No specific features	Variable	Variable	Variable	Variable	
Leiomyosarcoma (see **Fig. 8**)	T2 Dark areas	Nodular border	Presence of high T1 SI related to blood	Enhancement with central necrosis	High diffusion-weighted images/low ADC	

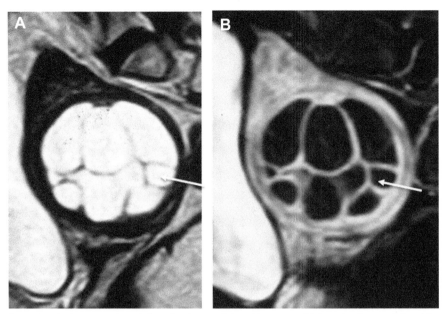

Fig. 3. Cystic degeneration. (*A*) Sagittal T2-weighted image and (*B*) sagittal T1-weighted fat-saturated postcontrast image show a large well-defined multicystic lesion (*arrow*) consistent with leiomyoma with cystic degeneration.

and do not persist on all sequences, they can be easily differentiated from leiomyomas (**Fig. 9**).

Endometrial polyp. Submucosal leiomyoma may be mistaken for an endometrial polyp. Polyps usually demonstrate hyperintense signal on T2-weighted imaging. In

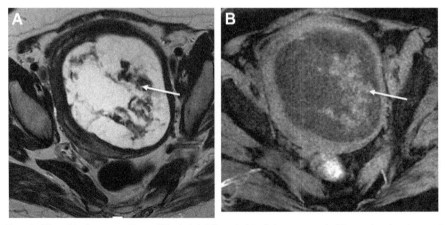

Fig. 4. Myxoid degeneration. (*A*) Axial T2-weighted image and (*B*) contrast-enhanced sagittal T1-weighted fat-saturated image show a leiomyoma (*arrow*) presenting areas with high signal intensity on T2-weighted imaging and enhancement after gadolinium injection, except for gelatinous intratumoral lakes that do not enhance, suggesting a myxoid leiomyoma.

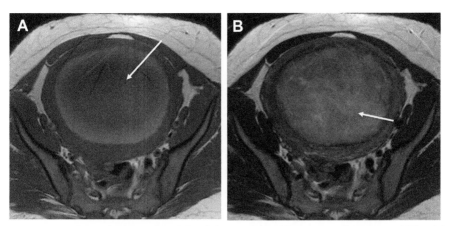

Fig. 5. Hemorrhagic degeneration. (*A*) Axial T1-weighted fat-saturated image and (*B*) axial T2-weighted image show a large uterine lesion (*white arrow*) with a component of very high signal intensity on T1-weighted imaging and heterogeneous signal intensity on T2-weighted imaging, suggesting intralesional hemorrhage.

contrast, pedunculated submucosal leiomyomas are hypointense on T2-weighted imaging and have a stalk that arises from the myometrium.

Adenomyomas. See the Adenomyosis section, elsewhere in this article.

Ovarian mass. In some situations, the distinction between an ovarian lesion and an uterine mass is not easy. Several signs have been described to distinguish ovarian from uterine mass location.

- A sharp angle between the ovary and the lesion is known as the "beak sign," indicating an ovarian origin.
- The claw sign (uterine tissue seen draped around the mass) or the bridging vessels sign (enlarged and tortuous vessels that extend from the uterus to supply the lesion) suggest the diagnosis of a uterine mass.

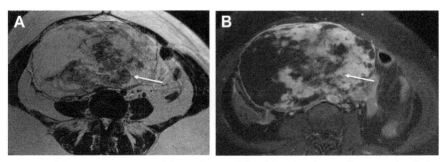

Fig. 6. Hydroptic degeneration. (*A*) Axial T2-weighted images show a large uterine lesion with high signal intensity on T2-weighted imaging associated with a dark cord-like signal on T2-weighted imaging (*arrow*). (*B*) Contrast-enhanced axial oblique T1-weighted fat-saturated image shows cord-like enhancing foci (*arrow*) among large nonenhancing areas.

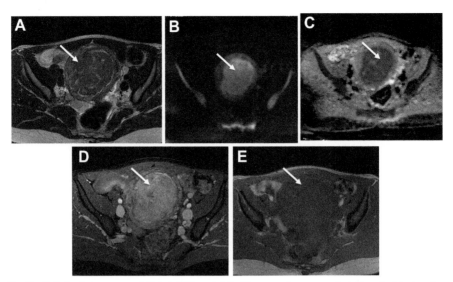

Fig. 7. Cellular leiomyoma. (*A*) Axial T2-weighted images show a well-delineated lesion (*arrow*) of intermediate to high signal intensity without T2 dark areas. (*B*) Axial oblique diffusion-weighted image (b = 1000) show high signal intensity (*arrow*) with restriction on a (*C*) corresponding ADC map (*arrow*). (*D*) Contrast-enhanced axial oblique T1-weighted fat-saturated image shows avid and heterogeneous enhancement (*arrow*). The absence of hemorrhage on T1 precontrast image (*E*), T2 dark area (*A*), the presence of well-defined border and an ADC value of greater than 1 (*C*) were favoring a cellular leiomyoma to a leiomyosarcoma; this diagnosis was confirmed histologically.

Leiomyosarcomas. Leiomyosarcomas arise de novo and have no biologic link to leiomyomas.[33,34] They require prompt surgical management.[35] Leiomyosarcomas may present with similar symptoms and imaging features as leiomyomas, which makes the diagnosis difficult. Large size and rapid growth are unreliable signs of malignancy.[33] The growth of a uterine mass after menopause and elevated lactose dehydrogenase, particularly lactose dehydrogenase isozyme type 3, should be viewed as suspicious for leiomyosarcoma.[33] Endometrial sampling may aid in the diagnosis of uterine sarcoma, but its sensitivity is limited owing to the myometrial origin of leiomyosarcomas.[33,35] No single MRI feature can reliably distinguish leiomyosarcomas from atypical leiomyomas,[36,37] although a combination of MRI features may suggest the correct diagnosis. In a study from Lakhman and colleagues,[14] the combination of 3 or more out of 4 discriminative features including nodular borders, hemorrhage (high SI on T1-weighted imaging), T2-weighted dark areas, and central unenhanced areas were associated with an improved sensitivity and specificity for the diagnosis of leiomyosarcoma. Diffusion restriction alone is insufficient for the diagnosis, because there is considerable overlap in ADC values between leiomyomas and leiomyosarcoma, and leiomyomas may demonstrate restricted diffusion, especially cellular leiomyomas[39] (see **Figs. 7** and **8**). One point worth discussing is that the presence of restricted diffusion and a T2 blackout effect is highly specific of a leiomyoma[15] (see **Fig. 2**). Thomassin-Naggara and colleagues[40] reported that using a recursive model combining T2 SI, b=1000 images and ADC map with a cut off value 1.23, MRI achieved a 92.4% accuracy in distinguishing benign and uncertain or malignant myometrial tumors. The authors concluded that diffusion-weighted images may be of interest to distinguish uterine sarcomas from benign leiomyomas.[40] More recently,

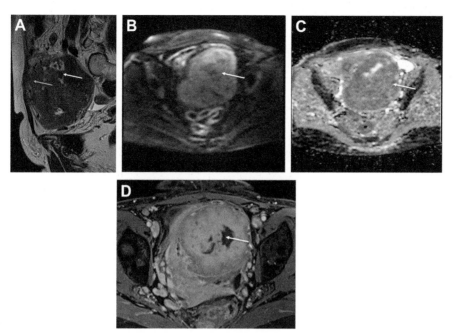

Fig. 8. Leiomyosarcoma. (*A*) Sagittal T2-weighted images, (*B*) axial diffusion-weighted image with ADC map (*C*) and (*D*) gadolinium-enhanced axial T1-weighted fat-saturated image. Axial T2-weighted image shows dark T2 area (*arrows, A*) and ill-defined borders (*orange arrow*). (*B*) Axial oblique diffusion-weighted image (b = 1000) show high signal intensity (*arrow*) with low signal on corresponding ADC map (*C*). (*D*) Contrast-enhanced axial oblique T1-weighted fat-saturated image shows heterogeneous enhancement with central necrosis (*arrow*). Those combined features are suggestive of leiomyosarcoma, which was confirmed histologically.

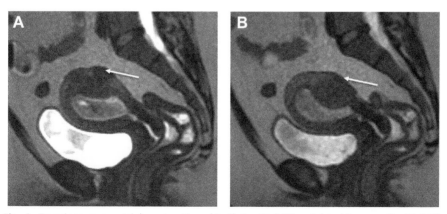

Fig. 9. Transient myometrial contraction. (*A, B*) Sagittal T2-weighted images. Sagittal T2-weighted image shows hypointense lesions in the posterior myometrium (*arrows, A*). This finding is absent on the subsequent sagittal T2-weighted image that shows a normal uterus with a thin and distinct junctional zone (*arrow, B*), confirming the diagnosis of transient myometrial contraction.

Wahab and colleagues found that uterine masses were classified as certainly benign if they showed a global or focal area of a low T2 signal and/or a low or an intermediate diffusion-weighted images signal (lower than that in the endometrium or lymph nodes).[41] If they did not meet these criteria (ie, intermediate T2 signal and high diffusion-weighted images signal [higher than in the endometrium or lymph nodes]), they were classified as probably benign (ADC of >0.905) or highly suspicious (ADC of <0.905) in the most restricted portion. The resulting algorithm achieved a sensitivity and specificity of 98% and 96%, respectively, in the training set, and was validated in 2 independent sets. **Fig. 10** shows a possible algorithm to help distinguish between leiomyoma and leiomyosarcoma.

How to Help the Gynecologist

Several surgical or minimally invasive therapeutic modalities are now available for treating uterine leiomyomas, including hysterectomy, laparoscopic surgery, high-intensity focused ultrasound (HIFU), and UAE. MRI is particularly helpful in treatment planning and monitoring these therapies.

Diagnosis

As discussed elsewhere in this article, MRI is particularly helpful for differentiation between leiomyomas and leiomyosarcomas, thereby avoiding the risk of morcellation of a malignant lesion.[10,14,38]

International Federation of Gynecology and Obstetrics classification

MRI excels in leiomyoma mapping and gives an accurate International Federation of Gynecology and Obstetrics classification. Indeed, management approaches according to International Federation of Gynecology and Obstetrics classification has been widely proposed.[17,19]

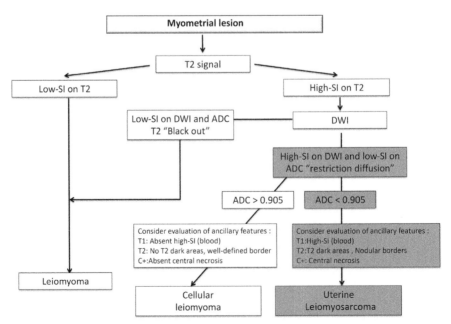

Fig. 10. Potential role for MRI in differentiating leiomyoma and uterine leiomyosarcoma. DWI, diffusion-weighted imaging; SI, signal intensity.

Types 0 and 1 myomas can be resected by hysteroscopy.[42–44] MRI helps in the visualization of the stalk of the leiomyoma and its location within the endometrial cavity.

Location
Leiomyomas can be classified according to their position: anterior wall, fundus, posterior wall, or cervix. Again, MRI is highly accurate for anatomic mapping.[45] The location of the leiomyoma is particularly important if HIFU is being considered.[46] In that case, tumors on the anterior wall or fundus can benefit from the heat accumulation during ablation in contrast to posterior location.[46] Distance between posterior wall leiomyomas and the skin surface is larger than that between anterior leiomyoma and skin surface; this has been negatively correlated to the ablation efficacy.[47]

Number
Uterine leiomyomas can be divided into single leiomyoma and multiple leiomyomas. It is crucial to avoid laparoscopic myomectomies in patients who have more than 5 leiomyomas. Furthermore, patients with 5 or more leiomyomas have an increased risk of technical failure of HIFU treatment. Again, MRI excels in lesion mapping.

Size
The size of the leiomyoma often impacts management decisions. Leiomyoma size is accurately evaluated on MRI.

Signal on T2-weighted imaging
MRI T2 signal has shown interesting results in predicting response to therapy. T2 SI classification has been used for determining patient suitability to HIFU. Type I T2 SI is defined as SI lower than or equal to that of skeletal muscles, type II is when the T2 SI is lower than that of the myometrium but higher than that of skeletal muscles, and type III is when the T2 SI higher than that of the myometrium.[48] The authors found that type I leiomyomas were suitable for HIFU treatment because of greater improvements in clinical symptoms and volume reduction after treatment.[48] In contrast, type III fibroids were unsuitable for HIFU treatment because of worse outcomes.[48] High T2 SI leiomyomas have been shown to be associated with larger volume reduction after UAE compared with low T2 SI leiomyomas.[49]

Contrast enhancement
Hypervascularity on contrast-enhanced studies has been correlated with a good response to UAE.[50] Leiomyomas with high pretreatment T1 signal related to blood product are less likely to benefit from UAE because they have already undergone hemorrhagic degeneration.[50]

ADENOMYOSIS
Epidemiology, Clinical Symptoms, and Pathophysiology
Adenomyosis is a benign condition occurring in around 20% to 30% of women and defined as "the ectopic presence of endometrial glands and stroma in the myometrium more than 2.5 mm from the endometrium–myometrium interface."[5,51] Furthermore, adenomyosis and leiomyomas occur concomitantly in 20% to 75% of cases.[52–54] The symptoms of adenomyosis are common but nonspecific, including dysmenorrhea, menorrhagia, and abnormal vaginal bleeding. The etiology of adenomyosis remains unclear.[4,55] Exposure to estrogen, prior uterine surgery, and parity are known risk factors. The theories with the greatest consensus propose that adenomyosis

results from invagination of the endometrial basalis layer into the myometrium or from embryologically misplaced pluripotent Müllerian remnants.[6]

MRI Features

MRI is highly accurate for the diagnosis of adenomyosis. In a prospective cohort, Stamatopoulos and colleagues[56] described a sensitivity of 46.1%, a specificity of 99.2%, and a positive predictive value of 92.3% of MRI in the diagnosis of adenomyosis. An MRI classification of adenomyosis was recently proposed by Bazot and Darai,[57] and another one by Kobayashi and Matsubara.[58] This classification describes the different forms of adenomyosis.

Classic MRI appearance of adenomyosis

- *Subendometrial cysts* are a direct sign of adenomyosis and represent the presence of endometrial glands within the myometrium. They correspond with foci of fluid embedded within the myometrium, varying in size from 2 to 9 mm. These microcysts typically have a T1 hypointense signal and a T2 hyperintense signal. Hemorrhagic content may accumulate within the cysts resulting in hyperintense T1 signal.[4] They are mainly located in the superficial myometrium and are highly specific (98%). However, they are only detected in 50% of cases[25–28,59] (**Fig. 11**).
- *Thickening of the junctional zone* (JZ) is an indirect sign related to myometrial hypertrophy, secondary to the presence of ectopic endometrial glands within the myometrium. A JZ thickness of greater than 12 mm has a diagnostic accuracy of 85%, specificity of 96%, and sensitivity of 63% to predict adenomyosis,[25] although recently debated by Tellum and colleagues.[29] The JZ differential sign was described by Dueholm and associates[30] as the difference between the

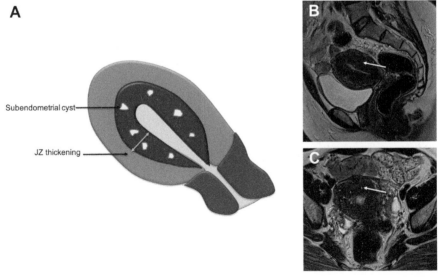

Fig. 11. Adenomyosis. (*A*) Classic features of adenomyosis: subendometrial cysts and diffuse thickening (*orange arrow*) of the junctional zone (JZ). (*B*) Sagittal T2-weighted image shows an enlarged uterus with the classic MRI appearance of adenomyosis, as thickening of the JZ. (*C*) Axial T2-weighted image show a high T2 focus (*arrow, C*) in keeping with subendometrial cyst.

maximal and minimal thicknesses in the anterior and posterior uterine JZ; a differential of greater than 5 mm may be a more reliable marker than a JZ thickness of greater than 12 mm (see **Fig. 11**).

Subtypes of adenomyosis
MRI differential diagnosis

- *Nonmeasurable JZ:* The JZ may not be measurable in postmenopausal patients and in patients using contraceptive drugs (**Table 2**) (**Figs. 12** and **13**).[2,9,60–65]
- *Physiologic changes of the uterus during the menstrual cycle (pseudo-thickening of the JZ)*: The thickness of the JZ is a hormone-dependent feature and changes according to the menstrual cycle. The JZ may appear diffusely thickened during menstruation, mimicking adenomyosis. Preferably, MRI should be not performed during menstruation to avoid this pitfall.[66,67]
- *Myometrial contractions*: Transient uterine contractions appear as T2 hypointense T2-weighted imaging bands perpendicular to the JZ or focal thickening of the JZ and can mimic focal adenomyosis[68] (see **Fig. 9**).
- *Endometrial cancer:* Adenomyosis can be seen in 20% of patients with endometrial cancer.[3] The evaluation of myometrial invasion may be difficult with the coexistence of adenomyosis as pseudo widening of the endometrium and be confused with myometrial invasion may be present and must not be mistaken with myometrial invasion.[3,69–71] Diffusion-weighted imaging may help to define the depth of myometrial invasion in case of coexisting adenomyosis; adenomyosis does not restrict diffusion, in contrast with endometrial cancer, which does restrict diffusion.[72]

Table 2
Different subtypes of adenomyosis

Types	Features
Adenoma (see **Fig. 12**)	Mass-like confluence of ectopic endometrial glands within the myometrium, distinct from the JZ. May bulge into the endometrium. Ill-defined low signal T2-weighted mass, which may contain punctate foci of high T2 signal.
Hemorrhagic cystic adenomyosis (adenomyotic cyst; see **Fig. 13**)	Rare subtype. Frequently symptomatic with dysmenorrhea and menorrhagia. Develops after spontaneous hemorrhage of ectopic endometrial glands. The hemorrhage is contained by a partial or complete rim of myometrial tissue, resulting in a cyst-like appearance with high signal on T1-weighted images and a low signal rim on T2-weighted imaging. The cyst may be submucosal, intramural, or subserosal.
External adenomyosis	Arises in the outer part of the uterus, most likely in the posterior myometrium disrupting the serosa but not affecting the JZ. Usually associated with deep endometriosis. On MRI, it appears as an ill-defined subserosal posterior T2 hypointense mass/pseudomass and may contain T2 hyperintense small cystic areas.
Adenomyomatous polyp or polypoid adenomyoma	Presents as a polypoid mass in the lower uterine endometrium or endocervix, and account for about 2% of all endometrial polyps. On MRI, the lesion presents as a hypointense polypoid mass associated with hyperintense foci on T2-weighted imaging.

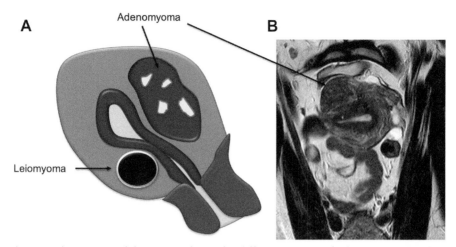

A

Adenomyoma

B

Leiomyoma

Fig. 12. Adenomyoma. (*A*) Drawing shows the different aspects of adenomyoma and leiomyoma. Note that adenomyoma is a dark lesion with bright foci inside owing to endometrial glands, whereas a typical leiomyoma is a homogeneous dark lesion with bright peripheral rim owing to perilesional edema that generally causes an adjacent mass effect more than adenomyoma. (*B*) Axial T2-weighted images show an ill-defined, low signal intensity mass with embedded hyperintense foci in the myometrium (*arrow, B*), suggesting an adenomyoma.

- *Leiomyoma:* Adenomyoma present as a T2-weighted imaging hypointense mass with ill-defined borders, minimal mass effect and with multiple bright foci. In contrast, leiomyoma, presents with well defined borders, adjacent mass effect, and large vessels surrounding the lesion.[73]

How to Help the Gynecologist

Symptomatic adenomyosis has traditionally been treated with hysterectomy.[74] The absence of a surgical plane separating adenomyotic tissue from normal myometrium makes adenomyomectomy difficult, leaving hysterectomy as the only viable surgical

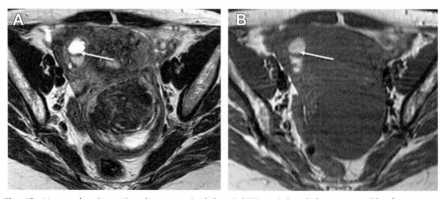

Fig. 13. Hemorrhagic cystic adenomyosis. (*A*) Axial T2-weighted show a cyst-like focus myometrial mass (*arrow*) with high signal focus on a T1-weighted sequence (*B*) (*arrow*), confirming hemorrhagic content.

option if hormone therapy fails. However, uterine-sparing techniques, including either complete or partial adenomyomectomy via open or laparoscopic approaches, can be considered. MRI can help by giving a description of the lesion and its delineation, and in triaging the appropriate surgical management. For example, MRI is able to differentiate superficial from deep adenomyosis, which is particularly important when rollerball ablation is considered.[75,76]

ENDOMETRIAL BENIGN PATHOLOGY

Endometrial polyps are common gynecologic lesions with an incidence of 10% to 24%, usually seen in premenopausal patients with postmenopausal bleeding. Polyps can be sessile or pedunculated masses of variable size that distend the endometrial cavity. Their diagnosis is usually confirmed with endometrial cytology, biopsy, or curettage. Because these procedures are usually performed in a blind manner, it is not always possible to make a definitive diagnosis. Moreover, it can be difficult or impossible in some cases with vaginal or cervical stenosis. MRI has shown to be particularly accurate in the diagnosis of endometrial polyp and distinction from endometrial cancer. On T2-weighted imaging, a fibrous core (T2 hypointense) and intratumoral cysts (T2 hyperintense foci) are highly representative of an endometrial polyp. In contrast with endometrial carcinoma, there is no myometrial invasion and necrosis with endometrial polyps. After gadolinium administration, intense enhancement of the fibrous core may be seen. With diffusion-weighted images, Fujii and colleagues[77] and Tamai and colleagues[78] showed that there was no overlap between ADC values of endometrial cancers and those of benign pathologies such as polyp dePolypsmonstrate a higher ADC value compared with endometrial cancer with a proposed diagnostic cut off of approximately 1.

BENIGN PATHOLOGY OF THE CERVIX AND VAGINA

MRI is particularly helpful in the diagnosis of cervical and vaginal cysts.

Nabothian Cysts

Nabothian cysts are very frequent and related to the distension of the endocervical glands. Cysts may be multiple, measuring up to 4 cm in size. On MRI, cysts typically have high a T2 SI. Cysts may demonstrate a bright signal on DWI owing to the mucinous content but lack restriction on ADC maps (also known as "T2 shine through").[79] Only the thin wall of the cyst enhances after gadolinium injection. Differential diagnosis includes the rare entity of adenocarcinoma, HPV independent, gastric type previously termed as adenoma malignum, a cervical carcinoma that seems to be cystic and mucin rich, but that also has enhancing components and restricted diffusion.[80–82]

Bartholin's Cysts, Gartner Cysts, and Skene Gland Cysts

Bartholin's cysts are caused by retained secretions within the vulvovaginal glands and are located in the posterolateral aspect of the lower vagina and vulva. In contrast, Gartner cysts are typically located in the anterolateral wall of the vagina above the inferior margin of the symphysis pubis. They correspond with an incomplete involution of the vaginal portion of the mesonephric duct. Skene gland cysts are located near the external urethral meatus.[83,84] The usually demonstrates high T2 signal with variable T1 signal owing to their mucinous/proteinaceous content; on DWI, skene gland cysts may have bright signal but lack restriction on the ADC map owing to the mucinous content.[79] Only the thin wall of the cyst enhances after gadolinium injection.[83,84]

SUMMARY

Benign uterine diseases are common conditions affecting women of all ages. Ultrasound examination is often the initial imaging study obtained in these patients. However, MRI is the preferred modality for additional lesion characterization and provides critical information to assist in selecting the appropriate therapies for symptomatic patients.

REFERENCES

1. American Association of Gynecologic Laparoscopists. Advancing Minimally Invasive Gynecology W: AAGL practice report: practice guidelines for the diagnosis and management of submucous leiomyomas. J Minim Invasive Gynecol 2012;19: 152–71.
2. Brosens JJ, de Souza NM, Barker FG. Uterine junctional zone: function and disease. Lancet 1995;346:558–60.
3. Habiba M, Pluchino N, Petignat P, et al. Adenomyosis and endometrial cancer: literature review. Gynecol Obstet Invest 2018;83:313–28.
4. Krentel H, Cezar C, Becker S, et al. From clinical symptoms to MR imaging: diagnostic steps in adenomyosis. Biomed Res Int 2017;1514029:2017.
5. Munro MG. Uterine polyps, adenomyosis, leiomyomas, and endometrial receptivity. Fertil Steril 2019;111:629–40.
6. Vannuccini S, Petraglia F. Recent advances in understanding and managing adenomyosis. F1000Res 2019;8. https://doi.org/10.12688/f1000research.17242.1.
7. Agostinho L, Cruz R, Osorio F, et al. MRI for adenomyosis: a pictorial review. Insights Imaging 2017;8:549–56.
8. Bolan C, Caserta MP. MR imaging of atypical fibroids. Abdom Radiol (N Y) 2016; 41:2332–49.
9. Brown HK, Stoll BS, Nicosia SV, et al. Uterine junctional zone: correlation between histologic findings and MR imaging. Radiology 1991;179:409–13.
10. DeMulder D, Ascher SM. Uterine leiomyosarcoma: can MRI differentiate leiomyosarcoma from benign leiomyoma before treatment? AJR Am J Roentgenol 2018; 211:1405–15.
11. Deshmukh SP, Gonsalves CF, Guglielmo FF, et al. Role of MR imaging of uterine leiomyomas before and after embolization. Radiographics 2012;32:E251–81.
12. Dudiak CM, Turner DA, Patel SK, et al. Uterine leiomyomas in the infertile patient: preoperative localization with MR imaging versus US and hysterosalpingography. Radiology 1988;167:627–30.
13. Kubik-Huch RA, Weston M, Nougaret S, et al. European Society of Urogenital Radiology (ESUR) Guidelines: MR imaging of leiomyomas. Eur Radiol 2018;28: 3125–37.
14. Lakhman Y, Veeraraghavan H, Chaim J, et al. Differentiation of uterine leiomyosarcoma from atypical leiomyoma: diagnostic accuracy of qualitative MR imaging features and feasibility of texture analysis. Eur Radiol 2017;27:2903–15.
15. Sato K, Yuasa N, Fujita M, et al. Clinical application of diffusion-weighted imaging for preoperative differentiation between uterine leiomyoma and leiomyosarcoma. Am J Obstet Gynecol 2014;210:368.e1-e8.
16. Wang L, Li S, Zhang Z, et al. Prevalence and occult rates of uterine leiomyosarcoma. Medicine (Baltimore) 2020;99:e21766.

17. Dubuisson J. The current place of mini-invasive surgery in uterine leiomyoma management. J Gynecol Obstet Hum Reprod 2019;48:77–81.

18. Lewis TD, Malik M, Britten J, et al. A comprehensive review of the pharmacologic management of uterine leiomyoma. Biomed Res Int 2018;2018:2414609.

19. Owen C, Armstrong AY. Clinical management of leiomyoma. Obstet Gynecol Clin North Am 2015;42:67–85.

20. Stokes LS, Wallace MJ, Godwin RB, et al. Quality improvement guidelines for uterine artery embolization for symptomatic leiomyomas. J Vasc Interv Radiol 2010;21:1153–63.

21. Burke CT, Funaki BS, Ray CE Jr, et al. ACR Appropriateness Criteria(R) on treatment of uterine leiomyomas. J Am Coll Radiol 2011;8:228–34.

22. Murase E, Siegelman ES, Outwater EK, et al. Uterine leiomyomas: histopathologic features, MR imaging findings, differential diagnosis, and treatment. Radiographics 1999;19:1179–97.

23. Munro MG, Critchley HO, Broder MS, et al. FIGO classification system (PALM-COEIN) for causes of abnormal uterine bleeding in nongravid women of reproductive age. Int J Gynaecol Obstet 2011;113:3–13.

24. Hricak H, Tscholakoff D, Heinrichs L, et al. Uterine leiomyomas: correlation of MR, histopathologic findings, and symptoms. Radiology 1986;158:385–91.

25. Reinhold C, McCarthy S, Bret PM, et al. Diffuse adenomyosis: comparison of endovaginal US and MR imaging with histopathologic correlation. Radiology 1996; 199:151–8.

26. Reinhold C, Tafazoli F, Mehio A, et al. Uterine adenomyosis: endovaginal US and MR imaging features with histopathologic correlation. Radiographics 1999;(19 Spec No):S147–60.

27. Reinhold C, Tafazoli F, Wang L. Imaging features of adenomyosis. Hum Reprod Update 1998;4:337–49.

28. Tafazoli F, Reinhold C. Uterine adenomyosis: current concepts in imaging. Semin Ultrasound CT MR 1999;20:267–77.

29. Tellum T, Matic GV, Dormagen JB, et al. Diagnosing adenomyosis with MRI: a prospective study revisiting the junctional zone thickness cutoff of 12 mm as a diagnostic marker. Eur Radiol 2019;29:6971–81.

30. Dueholm M, Lundorf E, Hansen ES, et al. Magnetic resonance imaging and transvaginal ultrasonography for the diagnosis of adenomyosis. Fertil Steril 2001;76: 588–94.

31. Mittl RL Jr, Yeh IT, Kressel HY. High-signal-intensity rim surrounding uterine leiomyomas on MR images: pathologic correlation. Radiology 1991;180:81–3.

32. Nougaret S, Horta M, Sala E, et al. Endometrial cancer MRI staging: updated guidelines of the European Society of Urogenital Radiology. Eur Radiol 2019; 29:792–805.

33. Ricci S, Stone RL, Fader AN. Uterine leiomyosarcoma: epidemiology, contemporary treatment strategies and the impact of uterine morcellation. Gynecol Oncol 2017;145:208–16.

34. Astolfi A, Nannini M, Indio V, et al. Genomic database analysis of uterine leiomyosarcoma mutational profile. Cancers (Basel) 2020;12:2126.

35. Rieber A, Aschoff A, Nussle K, et al. MRI in the diagnosis of small bowel disease: use of positive and negative oral contrast media in combination with enteroclysis. Eur Radiol 2000;10:1377–82.

36. Bi Q, Wu K, Lv F, et al. The value of clinical parameters combined with magnetic resonance imaging (MRI) features for preoperatively distinguishing different

subtypes of uterine sarcomas: an observational study (STROBE compliant). Medicine (Baltimore) 2020;99:e19787.

37. Shushkevich A, Thaker PH, Littell RD, et al. State of the science: uterine sarcomas: from pathology to practice. Gynecol Oncol 2020;159(1):3–7.

38. Rio G, Lima M, Gil R, et al. T2 hyperintense myometrial tumors: can MRI features differentiate leiomyomas from leiomyosarcomas? Abdom Radiol (N Y) 2019;44: 3388–97.

39. Namimoto T, Yamashita Y, Awai K, et al. Combined use of T2-weighted and diffusion-weighted 3-T MR imaging for differentiating uterine sarcomas from benign leiomyomas. Eur Radiol 2009;19:2756–64.

40. Thomassin-Naggara I, Dechoux S, Bonneau C, et al. How to differentiate benign from malignant myometrial tumours using MR imaging. Eur Radiol 2013;23: 2306–14.

41. Wahab CA, Jannot A, Bonaffini PA, et al. Diagnostic algorithm to differentiate benign atypical leiomyomas from malignant uterine sarcomas with diffusion-weighted MRI. Radiology 2020;297(2):361–71.

42. Lagana AS, Alonso Pacheco L, Tinelli A, et al. Management of asymptomatic submucous myomas in women of reproductive age: a consensus statement from the global congress on hysteroscopy scientific committee. J Minim Invasive Gynecol 2019;26:381–3.

43. Takeda A, Manabe S, Hosono S, et al. Preoperative evaluation of submucosal myoma by virtual hysteroscopy. J Am Assoc Gynecol Laparosc 2004;11:404–9.

44. Zhang RC, Wu W, Zou Q, et al. Comparison of clinical outcomes and postoperative quality of life after surgical treatment of type II submucous myoma via laparoscopy or hysteroscopy. J Int Med Res 2019;47:4126–33.

45. Yabuta M, Kishi Y, Koike N, et al. The importance of the accurate diagnostic preoperational magnetic resonance imaging (MRI) examinations: review of 1059 cases that undergoing laparoscopic surgery for diagnosed benign uterine myoma. J Minim Invasive Gynecol 2015;22:S196.

46. Kim YS, Kim JH, Rhim H, et al. Volumetric MR-guided high-intensity focused ultrasound ablation with a one-layer strategy to treat large uterine fibroids: initial clinical outcomes. Radiology 2012;263:600–9.

47. Froling V, Kroncke TJ, Schreiter NF, et al. Technical eligibility for treatment of magnetic resonance-guided focused ultrasound surgery. Cardiovasc Intervent Radiol 2014;37:445–50.

48. Funaki K, Fukunishi H, Funaki T, et al. Magnetic resonance-guided focused ultrasound surgery for uterine fibroids: relationship between the therapeutic effects and signal intensity of preexisting T2-weighted magnetic resonance images. Am J Obstet Gynecol 2007;196:184 e1-6.

49. Chang S, Kim MD, Lee M, et al. Uterine artery embolization for symptomatic fibroids with high signal intensity on T2-weighted MR imaging. Korean J Radiol 2012;13:618–24.

50. deSouza NM, Williams AD. Uterine arterial embolization for leiomyomas: perfusion and volume changes at MR imaging and relation to clinical outcome. Radiology 2002;222:367–74.

51. Tetikkurt S, Celik E, Tas H, et al. Coexistence of adenomyosis, adenocarcinoma, endometrial and myometrial lesions in resected uterine specimens. Mol Clin Oncol 2018;9:231–7.

52. Vercellini P, Parazzini F, Oldani S, et al. Adenomyosis at hysterectomy: a study on frequency distribution and patient characteristics. Hum Reprod 1995;10:1160–2.

53. Vavilis D, Agorastos T, Tzafetas J, et al. Adenomyosis at hysterectomy: prevalence and relationship to operative findings and reproductive and menstrual factors. Clin Exp Obstet Gynecol 1997;24:36–8.

54. Weiss G, Maseelall P, Schott LL, et al. Adenomyosis a variant, not a disease? Evidence from hysterectomized menopausal women in the Study of Women's Health Across the Nation (SWAN). Fertil Steril 2009;91:201–6.

55. Maruyama S, Imanaka S, Nagayasu M, et al. Relationship between adenomyosis and endometriosis; Different phenotypes of a single disease? Eur J Obstet Gynecol Reprod Biol 2020;253:191–7.

56. Stamatopoulos CP, Mikos T, Grimbizis GF, et al. Value of magnetic resonance imaging in diagnosis of adenomyosis and myomas of the uterus. J Minim Invasive Gynecol 2012;19:620–6.

57. Bazot M, Darai E. Role of transvaginal sonography and magnetic resonance imaging in the diagnosis of uterine adenomyosis. Fertil Steril 2018;109:389–97.

58. Kobayashi H, Matsubara S. A classification proposal for adenomyosis based on magnetic resonance imaging. Gynecol Obstet Invest 2020;85:118–26.

59. Reinhold C, Atri M, Mehio A, et al. Diffuse uterine adenomyosis: morphologic criteria and diagnostic accuracy of endovaginal sonography. Radiology 1995; 197:609–14.

60. McCarthy S, Scott G, Majumdar S, et al. Uterine junctional zone: MR study of water content and relaxation properties. Radiology 1989;171:241–3.

61. Scoutt LM, Flynn SD, Luthringer DJ, et al. Junctional zone of the uterus: correlation of MR imaging and histologic examination of hysterectomy specimens. Radiology 1991;179:403–7.

62. Masui T, Katayama M, Kobayashi S, et al. Changes in myometrial and junctional zone thickness and signal intensity: demonstration with kinematic T2-weighted MR imaging. Radiology 2001;221:75–85.

63. Lesny P, Killick SR. The junctional zone of the uterus and its contractions. BJOG 2004;111:1182–9.

64. Fusi L, Cloke B, Brosens JJ. The uterine junctional zone. Best Pract Res Clin Obstet Gynaecol 2006;20:479–91.

65. Kiguchi K, Kido A, Kataoka M, et al. Uterine peristalsis and junctional zone: correlation with age and postmenopausal status. Acta Radiol 2017;58:224–31.

66. Takeuchi M, Matsuzaki K. Adenomyosis: usual and unusual imaging manifestations, pitfalls, and problem-solving MR imaging techniques. Radiographics 2011;31:99–115.

67. Tamai K, Togashi K, Ito T, et al. MR imaging findings of adenomyosis: correlation with histopathologic features and diagnostic pitfalls. Radiographics 2005;25: 21–40.

68. Ozsarlak O, Schepens E, de Schepper AM, et al. Transient uterine contraction mimicking adenomyosis on MRI. Eur Radiol 1998;8:54–6.

69. Hertlein L, Rath J, Zeder-Goss C, et al. Coexistence of adenomyosis uteri and endometrial cancer is associated with an improved prognosis compared with endometrial cancer only. Oncol Lett 2017;14:3302–8.

70. Aydin HA, Toptas T, Bozkurt S, et al. Impact of coexistent adenomyosis on outcomes of patients with endometrioid endometrial cancer: a propensity score-matched analysis. Tumori 2018;104:60–5.

71. Erkilinc S, Taylan E, Gulseren V, et al. The effect of adenomyosis in myometrial invasion and overall survival in endometrial cancer. Int J Gynecol Cancer 2018; 28:145–51.

72. Jha RC, Zanello PA, Ascher SM, et al. Diffusion-weighted imaging (DWI) of adenomyosis and fibroids of the uterus. Abdom Imaging 2014;39:562–9.
73. Mark AS, Hricak H, Heinrichs LW, et al. Adenomyosis and leiomyoma: differential diagnosis with MR imaging. Radiology 1987;163:527–9.
74. Garcia L, Isaacson K. Adenomyosis: review of the literature. J Minim Invasive Gynecol 2011;18:428–37.
75. Li Z, Zhang J, Song Y, et al. Utilization of radiomics to predict long-term outcome of magnetic resonance-guided focused ultrasound ablation therapy in adenomyosis. Eur Radiol 2020. https://doi.org/10.1007/s00330-020-07076-1.
76. McCausland AM, McCausland VM. Depth of endometrial penetration in adenomyosis helps determine outcome of rollerball ablation. Am J Obstet Gynecol 1996;174:1786–93, 1793-4.
77. Fujii S, Matsusue E, Kigawa J, et al. Diagnostic accuracy of the apparent diffusion coefficient in differentiating benign from malignant uterine endometrial cavity lesions: initial results. Eur Radiol 2008;18:384–9.
78. Tamai K, Koyama T, Saga T, et al. The utility of diffusion-weighted MR imaging for differentiating uterine sarcomas from benign leiomyomas. Eur Radiol 2008;18: 723–30.
79. Oguri H, Maeda N, Izumiya C, et al. MRI of endocervical glandular disorders: three cases of a deep Nabothian cyst and three cases of a minimal-deviation adenocarcinoma. Magn Reson Imaging 2004;22:1333–7.
80. Doi T, Yamashita Y, Yasunaga T, et al. Adenoma malignum: MR imaging and pathologic study. Radiology 1997;204:39–42.
81. Sugiyama K, Takehara Y. MR findings of pseudoneoplastic lesions in the uterine cervix mimicking adenoma malignum. Br J Radiol 2007;80:878–83.
82. Yamashita Y, Takahashi M, Katabuchi H, et al. Adenoma malignum: MR appearances mimicking Nabothian cysts. AJR Am J Roentgenol 1994;162:649–50.
83. Siegelman ES, Outwater EK, Banner MP, et al. High-resolution MR imaging of the vagina. Radiographics 1997;17:1183–203.
84. Walker DK, Salibian RA, Salibian AD, et al. Overlooked diseases of the vagina: a directed anatomic-pathologic approach for imaging assessment. Radiographics 2011;31:1583–98.

The Midlife Transition, Depression, and Its Clinical Management

Claudio N. Soares, MD, PhD, FRCPC, MBA[a],*,
Alison K. Shea, MD, PhD, FRCPC[b]

KEYWORDS

- Depression • Menopause • Midlife transition • Anxiety • Sleep • Estrogen therapy
- Cognition • Nonhormonal interventions

KEY POINTS

- Depression is a highly prevalent and quite disabling condition, which often leads to significant personal, societal, and economic costs.
- Some women experience windows of vulnerability for the development of depression across the life span, in part because of greater sensitivity to hormonal changes.
- Management of depression during midlife years should be tailored to address symptomatic and functional improvement across various domains.
- Estrogen has neuromodulatory effects and may contribute to both the occurrence and the alleviation of depressive symptoms in midlife women.
- Antidepressants and behavioral therapies remain the treatments of choice for depression across the life cycle, but treatments should be tailored to improve multiple domains.

INTRODUCTION

Depression is a highly prevalent and quite disabling condition. The World Health Organization estimates that more than 260 million people are affected by it (one in every 5 adults in North America), with significant costs for individuals, their families, and the society at large.[1] Women seem to be disproportionately more affected by depression than men, as they experience a 2-fold increased risk (on average) across their life span.[2] The cause of this increased risk has long been the subject of debate, ranging from cultural aspects, hormonal influences, and gender-related determinants of health. Over the past few decades, however, a paradigm shift has been witnessed

a Department of Psychiatry, Queen's University School of Medicine, Providence Care Hospital, 752 King Street West, Kingston, Ontario K7L 4X3, Canada; b Department of Obstetrics and Gynecology, Faculty of Health Sciences, McMaster University, 1280 Main Street West, Hamilton, Ontario L8S 4L8, Canada
* Corresponding author.
E-mail address: c.soares@queensu.ca

Obstet Gynecol Clin N Am 48 (2021) 215–229
https://doi.org/10.1016/j.ogc.2020.11.009
0889-8545/21/© 2020 Elsevier Inc. All rights reserved.

obgyn.theclinics.com

in the understanding of mood disorders and how they affect women across their life cycle. It is now clear that some women may experience a particularly increased vulnerability for depression at certain reproductive stages (or *windows*) across their life span.[3] In other words, the occurrence of depression (new onset, recurrence), for some women, could be linked at least in part to the existence of *windows of vulnerability*, during which an increased sensitivity to hormonal changes could contribute to the emergence of mood symptoms and/or influence its clinical presentation, that would be the case, for example, of women experiencing increased dysphoria or irritability during luteal phases of their menstrual cycles, or depressive symptoms during puerperium or the menopausal transition.[4,5]

The female midlife period, which spans the decades between ages of 45 and 64 years and encompasses the menopause transition, may pose significant challenges to a woman's overall health. For some women, the combination of age and a heightened prevalence of metabolic syndrome, hypertension, diabetes, osteoporosis, and osteoarthritis could result in a progressive decline in the quality of life (QOL) and functioning.[6] The presence of significant, bothersome vasomotor symptoms (VMS) and sleep problems, in isolation or concomitant to other health-related issues, can certainly have a compounded, deleterious effect on a woman's overall health and QOL.[7]

Depression and Menopause: What Is the Evidence?

The heightened burden associated with a major depressive disorder (MDD) is undeniable at any given point in the life cycle, both for men and for women. As one takes a closer look into the occurrence of mood symptoms during midlife years, however, it would be helpful to make a distinction between depressive symptoms (those not fully meeting criteria for depression) and MDD (new-onset or recurrent episodes). Depressive symptoms, usually characterized by low mood, decreased motivation, reduced enjoyment from usual activities, and disrupted sleep, do occur more often than MDD. Depressive symptoms seem to be increased during the menopause transition and have been associated with psychosocial impairment and poorer QOL.[8–10] Major depressive episodes (new onset or recurrent), on the other hand, although less common than depressive symptoms, still occur more often during midlife years. In fact, existing data suggest a 2- to 4-fold increased risk for MDD during the menopause transition compared with the premenopausal or postmenopausal years.[11] Therefore, it is paramount that clinicians caring for women, including gynecologists and primary care providers, not only become familiarized with clinical presentations of MDD but also periodically assess the occurrence of bothersome depressive symptoms and their treatment options, including pharmacologic agents and behavioral or lifestyle interventions.

The putative associations between menopause staging and the occurrence of depression (MDD or depressive symptoms) have now been exhaustively investigated and well documented in cross-sectional and prospective studies. Data from cross-sectional studies indicate that depressive symptoms might be endorsed by a significant percentage of women during perimenopause compared with those in premenopausal years.[12,13] Longitudinal studies, perhaps constituting a better way to assess this potential association, have indicated an increased risk (1.5- to 3.0-fold) for the occurrence of depressive symptoms during the menopause transition, even among those with no history of depression.[14,15] Finally, cohort studies have documented an increased risk for clinical depression (MDD, 2- to 4-fold increased risk) throughout the menopause transition and early postmenopausal years, particularly among those with prior history of MDD.[14]

Risk factors for depression (MDD or depressive symptoms) during midlife years can be categorized into 2 groups: (1) continuum-related risk factors and (2) window-related risk factors.

Continuum-related risk factors
Continuum-related risk factors are likely to be pervasive throughout the life span and act as moderating factors. Those include demographic or socioeconomic factors (eg, unemployment, low education, being black or Hispanic); health-related factors (eg, greater body mass index, being a smoker, having poorer overall health, or reporting impaired functioning owing to chronic medical conditions); and psychosocial factors (eg, poor social support, history of stressful life events). It is important to highlight that the strongest predictor for MDD during midlife years is a previous depressive episode. On the other hand, history of hormone-related mood symptoms (premenstrual syndrome, premenstrual dysphoric disorder, or postpartum depression) seems to be moderately linked to depressive symptoms during the menopause transition.

Window-related risk factors
Window-related risk factors are timing- or context-related factors and likely act as mediating or precipitating factors for the occurrence of menopause-related depression. They include hormone variations during the transition (for example, wider fluctuations in follicle-stimulating hormone [FSH] and estradiol levels that might be precursors of mood changes); menopause-related symptoms (sleep problems, VMS); chronic medical conditions with particular worsening during midlife years; early life adversity; recent stressful life events, particularly when occurring close to the menopause transition.[16,17]

Proper recognition of and better understanding of the relative contribution of moderating (continuum-related) and mediating (window-related) factors may be critical for clinicians in their efforts to prevent, early detect, or promptly intervene against midlife depression.

Course of illness
Recent prospective data have examined mediators for distinct trajectories of depressive symptoms throughout the menopause transition and beyond. The Study of Women's Health Across the Nation (SWAN), a prospective study that followed women as they transitioned through the midlife years, determined that about 30% of women who developed depression at some point during the study ultimately experienced a persistent or recurrent condition, even for new-onset cases. Sleep problems and recent upsetting life events were among contributing factors to more persistent and/or recurrent depressive outcomes.[18,19] The Australian Longitudinal Study on Women's Health identified 4 distinct patterns for the evolution of depressive symptoms over a 15-year follow-up, based on standardized scores: the majority (80.0%) were stable and low, followed by increasing scores (9.0%), decreasing scores (8.5%), and stable high (2.5%). Individuals exhibiting stable high or increasing depressive symptoms over time (around 10%) were likely to experience a continuum of risk factors, such as previous diagnosis or treatment of depression and socioeconomic challenges. There were also context-related risk factors, such as the exposure to a prolonged perimenopause, and hence, a longer duration of bothersome VMS, or a surgically induced menopause.[20]

Anxiety, cognition, and sleep
Anxiety, cognitive issues, and sleep problems are often identified as concurrent issues that might contribute to poorer QOL among midlife women. SWAN investigators

explored different components or symptoms of anxiety (eg, irritability, nervousness or tension, fearfulness, and heart racing) and categorized their occurrence as high or low anxiety based on their scoring on the General Anxiety Disorder-7 scale.[21] Overall, women with greater symptoms of anxiety at study entry maintained significant rates of anxiety throughout the 10-year follow-up period. However, high anxiety declined significantly as women entered the postmenopausal period, which provides an important psychoeducational point when discussing the natural course of symptoms with women during this time. Moreover, those who reported high anxiety at baseline experienced a peak in symptoms during the late perimenopausal years (13.5%), suggesting that, for some women, midlife years could also represent a window of vulnerability for increased anxiety. Freeman and Sammel[22] examined the association between anxiety and hot flashes over a 14-year follow-up interval (Penn Ovarian Aging Cohort). Somatic anxiety, including symptoms such as abdominal pain, chest pain, fatigue, dizziness, insomnia, and headache, was strongly associated with hot flashes in the menopause transition, even after adjusting for important factors, such as age, menopausal staging, reproductive hormone levels, history of depression, and others. Importantly, somatic anxiety often *preceded* the development of moderate to severe hot flashes. Others have found that both perimenopausal and postmenopausal years may be associated with greater risk for anxiety, regardless of the presence of VMS.[23]

Many women present with changes in their cognitive function during midlife years, with most reporting "forgetfulness" or a worsening of verbal memory (which is tested in real life through their ability to remember names or recall other information that was told verbally). Commonly, women describe suffering from a "brain fog," which may worsen during the first year after the final menstrual period.[24] Challenges include difficulty concentrating or organizing tasks; there have been some discussions on whether these changes would often emerge in the context of concomitant stressors or symptoms of depression/anxiety, rather than signaling a primary problem or even a heightened risk for the development of dementia. There are some transient changes that are more prevalent during the menopause transition, suggesting a possible association with fluctuations in sex hormones.[25,26]

One should keep in mind that some decline in cognitive functions is expected to occur in women during midlife years, usually around the age of 50 years. An important, and frequently asked, question is whether changes observed during this period would signal a greater risk for developing more significant cognitive impairment later in life. While addressing this question, clinicians should reassure their patients that most common changes in cognitive functions observed during midlife years, particularly during the menopause transition, are transient by nature, and even if some symptoms persist beyond this transition, most women will show significant adaptation and normal (age-compatible) performance over time. A distinction should be made, however, with respect to the occurrence of mild cognitive impairment (MCI). MCI is rare among individuals younger than 50 years but may be considered as women mature. Those diagnosed with MCI have an increased risk of developing dementia, such as Alzheimer disease (AD), later in life, with conversion rates around 10% to 20% per year.[27] Some clinical guidelines for the distinction between MCI and dementia can be found in **Table 1**.

The SWAN study followed more than 200 women prospectively over a mean follow-up of 6.5 years and reported on cognitive changes over time. As women matured, there was a progressive decline in cognitive speed and episodic memory, which was accentuated by time since the final menstrual period. These findings remained significant even when adjusted for age, race/ethnicity, education, language, use of hormone therapy, VMS, sleep problems, and other conditions, such as depression

Table 1
Distinctions between mild cognitive impairment and dementia

	MCI	Dementia
Daily functioning	Cognitive issues do not affect daily performance; patients completed daily activities without difficulties Might experience mild difficulties in completing complex tasks	Cognitive issues do interfere with the individual's performance and affects daily activities at work, home, social activities, and relationships with others Cannot complete complex tasks
Language, thought processing	Normal speech, reasoning, vocabulary. Occasional difficulty in finding a word, but can usually hold a conversation	Impairment in reasoning ability, impaired language
Visuospatial ability, orientation	Generally intact, may pause for directions but can reorient easily	Impaired, lost or disoriented frequently
Memory	Slightly affected in standardized tests, others may notice	Significantly affected in standardized tests

or anxiety, VMS, sleep disturbance, and the effects of practice/learning the tasks.[28] Others have demonstrated the compounding adverse effects of VMS and depression on cognitive performance (eg, memory tasks).[29,30]

In addition to changes in cognitive function, women commonly report poor sleep disturbance during and following the menopause transition. Cross-sectional and longitudinal studies suggest that about 30% of midlife women suffer from poor or disrupted sleep.[31] In the SWAN cohort, the actigraphy data from women who experienced VMS showed more sleep-related movement and sleep fragmentation as well as reduced sleep efficiency. Although sleep disruption may be associated with an underlying problem (eg, presence of VMS or depression), it can often persist after the bothersome symptom has been addressed.[32,33]

Subjectively, women experiencing depression and VMS report poorer perceived sleep quality, despite the lack of objective measures of sleep disruption, such as increased number of awakenings, night sweats, or changes in wakefulness after sleep onset (WASO) time.[34,35] The contribution of hot flashes and sleep disturbances to the occurrence of depressive symptoms was investigated by Joffe and colleagues[36] in an interesting study involving 39 asymptomatic premenopausal women. Study participants were exposed to gonadal hormone suppression with the use of leuprolide for 4 weeks; after 4 weeks of estrogen suppression, most women (n = 20 or 69%) developed hot flashes, whereas only 1 subject developed clinical depression. Only nocturnal hot flashes were significantly associated with an increase in depressive symptoms. Depressive symptoms, on the other hand, were more common and seemed to be associated with objective and subjective sleep changes. Others have examined the effects of aging and hormone changes on the sleep architecture across the midlife years,[37] revealing that both aging and increased FSH concentration could affect sleep patterns. Aging was associated with shorter total sleep time, lower sleep efficiency, and greater sleep fragmentation, whereas increased FSH levels were associated with higher proportion of slow-wave sleep and increased WASO time. In addition, a greater body mass index and waist-to-hip ratio have also been associated with poor sleep efficiency, suggesting that poor sleep may be multifactorial.[33]

The neuromodulatory effects of estrogen

Estrogen impacts brain function through its mediating effects on monoaminergic systems and brain regions that are thought to be involved in mood, sleep, and cognitive regulation; more specifically, it regulates serotonin (5-hydroxytryptamine [5-HT]) and noradrenaline (NE) neurotransmission and interacts with estrogen receptors that are widely distributed in key areas, such as the prefrontal cortex and hippocampus.[38,39] Overall, the effects of E on 5-HT and NE could be considered beneficial to mood.[40] E2 may favor serotonin synthesis by limiting the activity of monoamine oxidases (MAOs) A and B, which are enzymes involved in 5-HT degradation and by increasing tryptophan hydroxylase, an enzyme that is necessary for serotonin synthesis. Thus, E2 administration could potentially result in an overall net increase in 5-HT synthesis. Estrogen also increases serotonin availability by downregulating 5-HT_{1a} autoreceptors and upregulating 5-HT_{2a} receptors in the synaptic cleft, resulting in an increase in serotonin found in the synapse and consequently more serotonin available for postsynaptic transmission.[41,42] Given that there is an intimate relationship between E2 and 5-HT, it is not surprising that women note change in mood, sleep, and cognition when levels are dramatically fluctuating during the perimenopause and depleted following the final menstrual period.

Other monoaminergic systems are also impacted by estrogen. Estrogen promotes greater NE synthesis through similar mechanisms to those described for serotonin, that is, decrease in the expression of MAOs and increase in the activity of tyrosine hydroxylase, the rate-limiting enzyme in the synthesis of catecholamine.[43] Moreover, acute E2 administration catalyzes the hydroxylation of dopamine to produce more NE. Last, estrogen may also have neuroprotective properties because of its stimulating effect on brain-derived neurotrophic factor.[44]

Estrogen-based therapy for depression: a closer look

The overall acceptability of estrogen therapy (ET) as part of the therapeutic armamentarium for depression among perimenopausal and postmenopausal women remains limited. A 2015 systematic review[40] on the efficacy of estrogen-based interventions for depression in this age group revealed a very limited number (5) of randomized controlled trials (RCTs) that examined the benefits of ET on clinically depressed women. From these 5 studies, it was suggested that there is some evidence to support the antidepressant efficacy of estradiol treatment of perimenopausal, but not postmenopausal women.

Positive results from 2 RCTs[45,46] on the use of transdermal estradiol for the treatment of MDD led to the inclusion of E2 therapy into the 2016 Clinical Guidelines of the Canadian Network for Mood and Anxiety Treatments, as a second-line treatment (level 2) for the management of MDD during perimenopause.[47] The 2 RCTs (Soares and Schmidt) had similar designs and were considered of high quality because of the utilization of standardized tools to confirm the diagnosis of depression and the characterization of menopausal staging using FSH levels and history of menstrual irregularity. In addition, treatment compliance was monitored by serum E2 measurements in both studies. Antidepressant effects were well documented, and significant mood improvement was observed among those suffering from new-onset or recurrent MDD in the presence or absence of concomitant VMS. Moreover, the antidepressant effects of E2 persisted after a 4-week washout period, even when women experienced reemergence of hot flashes and night sweats.[46] The same hormone intervention (transdermal E2), however, had failed to show efficacy for MDD in late *postmenopausal* women,[48] suggesting that the menopause transition not only might be a critical window of risk for depression but also may be a *window of opportunity* for the antidepressant benefits of estrogen during midlife years.[49]

A recent RCT examined the efficacy of estrogen in *preventing* the onset of depressive symptoms in midlife women.[50] Participants received either transdermal estradiol (0.1 mg/d) plus intermittent oral micronized progesterone (200 mg/d for 12 days every 3 months) or placebo (patches and pills) for 12 months. Those receiving active hormone therapy were less likely to develop depressive symptoms compared with women receiving placebo (32.3% vs 17.3%; odds ratio, 2.5; 95%confidence interval, 1.1–5.7; P = .03). Interestingly, the group of women who benefited the most from this preventive strategy was composed of those in early perimenopause and those who had experienced stressful life events in the preceding 6 months of the study; prior history of depression or presence/severity of VMS did not modify the preventive effects of E2. The prophylactic use of HT against depression, although promising, still warrants further investigation to confirm its efficacy and safety.

Clinicians should consider all existing options in order to best tailor treatments for symptomatic midlife women. Given the accumulated clinical experience over the past decade with estrogen-based therapies, it is reasonable to consider a brief trial (4–6 weeks) of transdermal estradiol for women in the menopause transition who present with bothersome VMS and concurrent depressive symptoms.[49] Estradiol therapy could also be an option for women with depression who are unable or unwilling to initiate treatment with antidepressants. After an initial trial of estrogen, the need for antidepressants (either as monotherapy or in combination with estrogen) or other therapies could be reassessed.

Last, data on the use of various progestogens (progestins vs progesterone) on mood symptoms in midlife depression are quite limited; most trials used intermittent progesterone with good tolerability, but appropriate endometrial protection needs to be considered as well in women with an intact uterus.

There are a couple of newly available HT formulations that may also provide promise: tibolone (a precursor molecule to estradiol, progesterone, and testosterone) and the combination product of conjugated equine estrogens/bazedoxefine. Although the latter has not yet been formally studied for efficacy of treating mood symptoms, the lack of need for the progesterone component owing to the bazedoxefine component for endometrial protection presents an exciting option. The effect of tibolone on depressive symptoms has been studied in a 2017 RCT.[51] After 12 weeks of treatment with tibolone, perimenopausal women with MDD showed a significant improvement, as scored using the Montgomery Asberg depression scale.

Table 2 summarizes existing data on estrogen-based therapies for depressed perimenopausal and postmenopausal women.

Estrogen-based therapies for cognition and sleep

The relationship between estrogen and cognitive function has proven to be complicated because of multiple variables, including use of different formulations/combinations, age, and menopause staging at the time of initiating hormone therapy, just to name a few.[52] Some early observational studies had suggested a decreased risk for AD in women receiving hormone therapy.[53] Data from the SWAN cohort[54] showed better cognitive performance among hormone therapy users during the menopause transition and early postmenopausal years. Prospective studies and randomized controlled interventions, however, have revealed a different scenario. Almeida and colleagues[55] examined the benefits of ET (oral E2, 2 mg/d) for cognition, mood, and QOL in *older, postmenopausal* women (n = 115, average age 73 years) in a 20-week randomized double-blind placebo-controlled trial. Outcome measures included

Table 2
Randomized trials on estrogen therapies for symptomatic or depressed perimenopausal and postmenopausal women

Authors	Population Studied (Type, n)	Design	Intervention	Outcome Measures	Key Findings
Schmidt et al,[45] 2001	Perimenopause-related depression (n = 31)	DB, PL Parallel study followed by crossover, PL-controlled	ET (transdermal E2), followed by MPA	HDRS, CES-D scores	ET led to significant improvements in depressive symptoms (HDRS and CES-D scores)
Soares et al,[46] 2001	Perimenopause-related depression (n = 45)	DB, PL Parallel study	ET (transdermal E2)	MADRS scores	ET led to significant improvements in depressive symptoms (MADRS scores)
Rudolph et al,[73] 2004; Santoro,[74] 2005	Postmenopausal women with mild or moderate depressive symptoms (n = 129)	DB, PL Parallel study	EPT (oral E2 valerate + progestin [dienogest])	HDRS scores	EPT led to improvements in HDRS scores; high attrition rates in both groups
Morrison etal,[48] 2004	Postmenopausal women with depressive disorders (n = 57)	DB, PL Parallel study	ET (transdermal E2) followed by MPA	HDRS, CES-D scores	No differences with active treatment (both groups showed improvement)
Joffe et al,[75] 2011	Mixed perimenopausal and postmenopausal women with depressive symptoms, VMS, and insomnia (n = 72)	DB, PL Parallel study	ET (transdermal E2), Zolpidem	MADRS, BDI, PSQI scores	No significant differences with respect to mood changes between treatment and PL groups

Abbreviations: DB, double-blind; PL, placebo; PSQI, Pittsburgh Sleep Quality Index.
Data from Refs.[45,46,48,73–75]

changes in the depressive scores and cognitive function assessed through a battery of tests, including CAMCOG, Block Design, Memory for Faces, California Verbal Learning Test, and verbal fluency. After 20 weeks of treatment, unopposed estrogen administered orally was not associated with significant changes in cognitive function, mood, or QOL. However, starting HT more than 10 years after the menopause transition is not currently recommended by the North American Menopause Society. There is a certain window of opportunity to start HT, and beyond this time, initiation may come with risks.[56]

Disappointingly, both the Kronos Early Estrogen Prevention Study (KEEPS) cognitive study and the Women's Health Initiative (young cohort) did not reveal significant improvements in cognitive assessments following several years of hormone therapy in early postmenopausal women.[57,58]

It is important to note that other factors could be contributing to cognitive function in midlife women, such as life stressors, depression, sleep disorders, anxiety, substance use and abuse, as well as the use of antidepressants and/or sleeping medications. If VMS, sleep disturbance, or psychiatric symptoms are present, these should be treated first.

Lifestyle changes could be targeted for optimal cognitive health, including healthy diet, reduction in cigarette smoking, and regular, intense exercise.[59] Unfortunately, vitamins and supplements, including omega-3, green tea extract, and vitamin E, have not proven to prevent cognitive decline in women.[60–63] However, a diet rich in vegetables and fish may be helpful for healthy brain function.[64,65]

In terms of sleep, data from the KEEPS indicated that both oral and transdermal HT improved sleep quality and satisfaction in early menopausal women, with transdermal HT reducing the WASO time as well.[66] In another study,[67] the use of daily transdermal estradiol (0.1 mg/d) with 200-mg progesterone used cyclically for 12 days every 3 months led to reductions in time to fall asleep and the number of awakenings among perimenopausal and early postmenopausal women, even after controlling for VMS. Low-dose estradiol (0.5 mg/d) and venlafaxine (37.5 mg/d) were superior to placebo in reducing insomnia and in improving subjective sleep quality among perimenopausal and postmenopausal women following 8 weeks of treatment.[68]

Last, progesterone alone, 300 mg/d, has been studied in postmenopausal women, leading to greater reduction in WASO time and greater increase in duration and intensity of deep sleep compared with placebo.[69]

The role of nonhormonal interventions

Antidepressants and behavioral interventions remain the first-line treatment of depression across the life span, including midlife years. Pharmacologic interventions should be first considered particularly for those who experienced multiple depressive episodes in the past (ie, not exclusively hormone related), those reporting severe symptoms or significant functional impairment, or those expressing suicidal ideation. For recurrent episodes, a previous response to a specific antidepressant (agent, class) should guide the primary decision as to what to try first. For those experiencing depression for the first time, those who are treatment-naive, or those presenting with history of partial or no response to antidepressants in the past, existing data support the efficacy and tolerability of various selective serotonin reuptake inhibitors (SSRIs) and serotonin-norepinephrine reuptake inhibitors at usual doses. There is evidence for fluoxetine, sertraline, venlafaxine, citalopram, escitalopram, duloxetine, desvenlafaxine, and vortioxetine on depression scores in menopausal women.[70–78]

Existing data do not support superior efficacy of a particular antidepressant agent or class over the others for the management of midlife depression. Some key points, however, should be taken into consideration. Information on tolerability could guide the discussion, particularly when sexual dysfunction and changes in weight are of concern. Existing data on the efficacy of some agents for menopause-related symptoms (VMS, pain, disrupted sleep) and QOL improvement could guide clinicians. Furthermore, information regarding drug-drug interactions should be considered, as multiple medications are often prescribed to women during midlife years. For example, some SSRIs, such as paroxetine, duloxetine, and sertraline, are cytochrome CYP450 2D6 enzyme substrates. Caution is advised when taking other medications that require this enzyme for metabolism, such as tamoxifen. Use of both these medications together may decrease the efficacy of tamoxifen.[79]

Behavior-based interventions, such as cognitive behavioral therapy, have been shown to be effective not only for depression but also for the alleviation of other menopause-related concerns, such as sleep problems and VMS. Providing patients with choices to pursue medication, behavioral therapy, or both has been shown to improve outcomes.[80]

SUMMARY

Most women will not develop significant depressive symptoms or MDD during midlife years. It is imperative, however, that clinicians caring for women during midlife understand that there are windows of vulnerability for depression and to recognize the main contributing factors for the occurrence of midlife depression (new onset, recurrent). Furthermore, the impact of other concurrent conditions, such as anxiety, sleep problems, and cognitive complaints, should be considered for comprehensive diagnostic and therapeutic approaches.

Estrogen has neuromodulatory effects and may contribute to both the occurrence and the alleviation of depressive symptoms. Clinicians should be prepared to tailor therapeutic interventions for the management of symptomatic midlife women, using hormonal, pharmacologic, behavioral, and lifestyle change strategies.

CLINICAL CARE POINTS

- Management of depression during the midlife transition may required tailored treatment strategies, including hormonal and non-hormonal options.
- Transdermal estradiol has shown antidepressant properties among peri- and early postmenopausal women, but no in late postmenopause - suggesting a window for its efficacy.
- Therapeutic approaches should be multi-systemic and target core symptoms such as mood, anxiety, sleep, vasomotor symptoms.

DISCLOSURE

Dr C.N. Soares has received research and educational grants from the Ontario Brain Institute (OBI), the Ontario Research Funds–Research Excellence (ORF-RE), and the AHSC AFP Innovation Fund. He has served as a consultant for Sunovion, Merck, Otsuka and Lundbeck. Dr A.K. Shea has received honorarium from Pfizer. BioSyent and Sprout Pharmaceuticals. She has also received a research grant from Pfizer.

REFERENCES

1. Available at: https://www.who.int/news-room/fact-sheets/detail/depression. Accessed August 28, 2020.
2. Steiner M. Female-specific mood disorders. Clin Obstet Gynecol 1992;35(3): 599–611.
3. Soares CN, Zitek B. Reproductive hormone sensitivity and risk for depression across the female life cycle: a continuum of vulnerability? J Psychiatry Neurosci 2008;33(4):331–43.
4. Bloch M, Schmidt PJ, Danaceau M, et al. Effects of gonadal steroids in women with a history of postpartum depression. Am J Psychiatry 2000;157(6):924–30.
5. Soares CN. Mood disorders in midlife women: understanding the critical window and its clinical implications. Menopause 2014;21(2):198–206.
6. Kase NG, Gretz Friedman E, Brodman M, et al. The midlife transition and the risk of cardiovascular disease and cancer part I: magnitude and mechanisms [published online ahead of print, 2020 Jun 1]. Am J Obstet Gynecol 2020; S0002-9378(20):30607–14.
7. El Khoudary SR, Greendale G, Crawford SL, et al. The menopause transition and women's health at midlife: a progress report from the Study of Women's Health Across the Nation (SWAN). Menopause 2019;26(10):1213–27.
8. Pietrzak RH, Kinley J, Afifi TO, et al. Subsyndromal depression in the United States: prevalence, course, and risk for incident psychiatric outcomes. Psychol Med 2013;43(7):1401–14.
9. Bromberger JT, Matthews KA, Schott LL, et al. Depressive symptoms during the menopausal transition: the Study of Women's Health Across the Nation (SWAN). J Affect Disord 2007;103(1–3):267–72.
10. de Kruif M, Spijker AT, Molendijk ML. Depression during the perimenopause: a meta-analysis. J Affect Disord 2016;206:174–80.
11. Cohen LS, Soares CN, Vitonis AF, et al. Risk for new onset of depression during the menopausal transition: the Harvard study of moods and cycles. Arch Gen Psychiatry 2006;63(4):385–90.
12. Bromberger JT, Kravitz HM. Mood and menopause: findings from the study of Women's Health Across the Nation (SWAN) over 10 years. Obstet Gynecol Clin North Am 2011;38(3):609–25.
13. Shea AK, Sohel N, Gilsing A, et al. Depression, hormone therapy, and the menopausal transition among women aged 45 to 64 years using Canadian Longitudinal Study on aging baseline data. Menopause 2020;27(7):763–70.
14. Bromberger JT, Schott L, Kravitz HM, et al. Risk factors for major depression during midlife among a community sample of women with and without prior major depression: are they the same or different? Psychol Med 2015;45(8):1653–64.
15. Freeman EW, Sammel MD, Lin H, et al. Associations of hormones and menopausal status with depressed mood in women with no history of depression. Arch Gen Psychiatry 2006;63:375–82.
16. Epperson CN, Sammel MD, Bale TL, et al. Adverse childhood experiences and risk for first-episode major depression during the menopause transition. J Clin Psychiatry 2017;78(3):e298–307.
17. Gordon JL, Rubinow DR, Eisenlohr-Moul TA, et al. Estradiol variability, stressful life events, and the emergence of depressive symptomatology during the menopausal transition. Menopause 2016;23(3):257–66.

18. Bromberger JT, Kravitz HM, Youk A, et al. Patterns of depressive disorders across 13 years and their determinants among midlife women: SWAN mental health study. J Affect Disord 2016;206:31–40.

19. Clayton AH, Pinkerton JV. Vulnerability to depression and cardiometabolic risk associated with early ovarian disruption. Menopause 2013;20(6):598–9.

20. Hickey M, Schoenaker DA, Joffe H, et al. Depressive symptoms across the menopause transition: findings from a large population-based cohort study. Menopause 2016;23(12):1287–93.

21. Bromberger JT, Kravitz HM, Chang Y, et al. Does risk for anxiety increase during the menopausal transition? Study of Women's Health Across the Nation. Menopause 2013;20(5):488–95.

22. Freeman EW, Sammel MD. Anxiety as a risk factor for menopausal hot flashes: evidence from the Penn Ovarian Aging Cohort. Menopause 2016;23(90):942–9.

23. Mulhall S, Andel R, Anstey KJ. Variation in symptoms of depression and anxiety in midlife women by menopausal status. Maturitas 2018;108:7–12.

24. Maki PM, Henderson VW. Cognition and the menopause transition. Menopause 2016;23(7):803–5.

25. Henderson VW, Guthrie JR, Dudley EC, et al. Estrogen exposures and memory at midlife: a population-based study of women. Neurology 2003;60:1369–71.

26. Weber MT, Rubin LH, Maki PM. Cognition in perimenopause: the effect of transition stage. Menopause 2013;20(5):511–7.

27. Etgen T, Sander D, Bickel H, et al. Mild cognitive impairment and dementia: the importance of modifiable risk factors. Dtsch Arztebl Int 2011;108(44):743–50.

28. Karlamangla AS, Lachman ME, Han W, et al. Evidence for cognitive aging in midlife women: Study of Women's Health Across the Nation. PLoS One 2017; 12(1):e0169008.

29. Maki PM, Wu M, Rubin LH, et al. Hot flashes are associated with altered brain function during a memory task. Menopause 2020;27(3):269–77.

30. Alexander JL, Sommer BR, Dennerstein L, et al. Role of psychiatric comorbidity on cognitive function during and after the menopausal transition. Expert Rev Neurother 2007;7(11 Suppl):S157–80.

31. Freeman EW, Sammel MD, Gross SA, et al. Poor sleep in relation to natural menopause: a population-based 14-year follow-up of midlife women. Menopause 2015;22(7):719–26.

32. Kravitz HM, Zheng H, Bromberger JT, et al. An actigraphy study of sleep and pain in midlife women: the Study of Women's Health Across the Nation Sleep Study. Menopause 2015;22(7):710–8.

33. Naufel MF, Frange C, Andersen ML, et al. Association between obesity and sleep disorders in postmenopausal women. Menopause 2018;25(2):139–44.

34. Joffe H, Soares CN, Thurston RC, et al. Depression is associated with worse objectively and subjectively measured sleep, but not more frequent awakenings, in women with vasomotor symptoms. Menopause 2009;16(4):671–9.

35. Joffe H, Massler A, Sharkey KM. Evaluation and management of sleep disturbance during the menopause transition. Semin Reprod Med 2010;28(5):404–21.

36. Joffe H, Crawford SL, Freeman MP, et al. Independent contributions of nocturnal hot flashes and sleep disturbance to depression in estrogen-deprived women. J Clin Endocrinol Metab 2016;101(10):3847–55.

37. Lampio L, Polo-Kantola P, Himanen SL, et al. Sleep during menopausal transition: a 6-year follow-up. Sleep 2017;40(7). https://doi.org/10.1093/sleep/zsx090.

38. McEwen BS, Alves SE. Estrogen actions in the central nervous system. Endocr Rev 1999;20(3):279–307.

39. Lokuge S, Frey BN, Foster JA, et al. Depression in women: windows of vulnerability and new insights into the link between estrogen and serotonin. J Clin Psychiatry 2011;72(11):e1563–9.

40. Rubinow DR, Johnson SL, Schmidt PJ, et al. Efficacy of estradiol in perimenopausal depression: so much promise and so few answers. Depress Anxiety 2015;32(8):539–54.

41. Cyr M, Bosse R, Di Paolo T. Gonadal hormones modulate 5-hydroxytryptamine2A receptors: emphasis on the rat frontal cortex. Neuroscience 1998;83(3):829–36.

42. Hiroi R, McDevitt RA, Neumaier JF. Estrogen selectively increases tryptophan hydroxylase-2 mRNA expression in distinct subregions of rat midbrain raphe nucleus: association between gene expression and anxiety behavior in the open field. Biol Psychiatry 2006;60(3):288–95.

43. Pau KY, Hess DL, Kohama S, et al. Oestrogen upregulates noradrenaline release in the mediobasal hypothalamus and tyrosine hydroxylase gene expression in the brainstem of ovariectomized rhesus macaques. J Neuroendocrinol 2000;12(9): 899–909.

44. Srivastava DP, Woolfrey KM, Evans PD. Mechanisms underlying the interactions between rapid estrogenic and BDNF control of synaptic connectivity. Neuroscience 2013;239:17–33.

45. Schmidt PJ, Nieman L, Danaceau MA, et al. Estrogen replacement in perimenopause-related depression: a preliminary report. Am J Obstet Gynecol 2000;183(2):414–20.

46. Soares CN, Almeida OP, Joffe H, et al. Efficacy of estradiol for the treatment of depressive disorders in perimenopausal women: a double-blind, randomized, placebo-controlled trial. Arch Gen Psychiatry 2001;58(6):529–34.

47. MacQueen GM, Frey BN, Ismail Z, et al. Canadian Network for Mood and Anxiety Treatments (CANMAT) 2016 clinical guidelines for the management of adults with major depressive disorder: section 6. Special populations: youth, women, and the elderly. Can J Psychiatry 2016;61(9):588–603.

48. Morrison MF, Kallan MJ, Ten Have T, et al. Lack of efficacy of estradiol for depression in postmenopausal women: a randomized, controlled trial. Biol Psychiatry 2004;55(4):406–12.

49. Maki PM, Kornstein SG, Joffe H, et al. Guidelines for the evaluation and treatment of perimenopausal depression: summary and recommendations. Menopause 2018;25(10):1069–85.

50. Gordon JL, Rubinow DR, Eisenlohr-Moul TA, et al. Efficacy of transdermal estradiol and micronized progesterone in the prevention of depressive symptoms in the menopause transition: a randomized clinical trial. JAMA Psychiatry 2018; 75(2):149–57.

51. Kulkarni J, Gavrilidis E, Thomas N, et al. Tibolone improves depression in women through the menopause transition: a double-blind randomized controlled trial of adjunctive tibolone. J Affect Disord 2018;236:88–92.

52. Santoro N, Epperson CN, Mathews SB. Menopausal symptoms and their management. Endocrinol Metab Clin North Am 2015;44(3):497–515.

53. Zandi PP, Carlson MC, Plassman BL, et al. Hormone replacement therapy and incidence of Alzheimer disease in older women: the Cache County Study. JAMA 2002;288(17):2123–9.

54. Greendale GA, Huang MH, Wight RG, et al. Effects of the menopause transition and hormone use on cognitive performance in midlife women. Neurology 2009; 72(21):1850–7.

55. Almeida OP, Lautenschlager NT, Vasikaran S, et al. A 20-week randomized controlled trial of estradiol replacement therapy for women aged 70 years and older: effect on mood, cognition and quality of life. Neurobiol Aging 2006;27(1): 141–9.

56. The 2017 Hormone Therapy Position Statement of The North American Menopause Society. Menopause 2018;25(11):1362–87.

57. Gleason CE, Dowling NM, Wharton W, et al. Effects of hormone therapy on cognition and mood in recently postmenopausal women: findings from the randomized, controlled KEEPS-cognitive and affective study. PLoS Med 2015;12(6): e1001833 [discussion e].

58. Espeland MA, Shumaker SA, Leng I, et al. Long-term effects on cognitive function of postmenopausal hormone therapy prescribed to women aged 50 to 55 years. JAMA Intern Med 2013;173(15):1429–36.

59. Aichberger MC, Busch MA, Reischies FM, et al. Effect of physical inactivity on cognitive performance after 2.5 years of follow-up: longitudinal results from the Survey of Health, Ageing, and Retirement (SHARE). GeroPsych (Bern) 2010; 23(1):7–15.

60. Wu S, Ding Y, Wu F, et al. Omega-3 fatty acids intake and risks of dementia and Alzheimer's disease: a meta-analysis. Neurosci Biobehav Rev 2015;48:1–9.

61. Xu H, Wang Y, Yuan Y, et al. Gender differences in the protective effects of green tea against amnestic mild cognitive impairment in the elderly Han population. Neuropsychiatr Dis Treat 2018;14:1795–801.

62. Kang JH, Cook N, Manson J, et al. A randomized trial of vitamin E supplementation and cognitive function in women. Arch Intern Med 2006;166(22):2462–8.

63. Devore EE, Kang JH, Stampfer MJ, et al. The association of antioxidants and cognition in the Nurses' Health Study. Am J Epidemiol 2013;177(1):33–41.

64. Jiang X, Huang J, Song D, et al. Increased consumption of fruit and vegetables is related to a reduced risk of cognitive impairment and dementia: meta-analysis. Front Aging Neurosci 2017;9:18.

65. Weng PH, Chen JH, Chiou JM, et al. The effect of lifestyle on late-life cognitive change under different socioeconomic status. PLoS One 2018;13(6):e0197676.

66. Cintron D, Lahr BD, Bailey KR, et al. Effects of oral versus transdermal menopausal hormone treatments on self-reported sleep domains and their association with vasomotor symptoms in recently menopausal women enrolled in the Kronos Early Estrogen Prevention Study (KEEPS). Menopause 2018;25(2):145–53.

67. Geiger PJ, Eisenlohr-Moul T, Gordon JL, et al. Effects of perimenopausal transdermal estradiol on self-reported sleep, independent of its effect on vasomotor symptom bother and depressive symptoms. Menopause 2019;26(11):1318–23.

68. Ensrud KE, Guthrie KA, Hohensee C, et al. Effects of estradiol and venlafaxine on insomnia symptoms and sleep quality in women with hot flashes. Sleep 2015; 38(1):97–108.

69. Caufriez A, Leproult R, L'Hermite-Baleriaux M, et al. Progesterone prevents sleep disturbances and modulates GH, TSH, and melatonin secretion in postmenopausal women. J Clin Endocrinol Metab 2011;96(4):E614–23.

70. Freeman MP, Cheng LJ, Moustafa D, et al. Vortioxetine for major depressive disorder, vasomotor, and cognitive symptoms associated with the menopausal transition. Ann Clin Psychiatry 2017;29(4):249–57.

71. Frey BN, Haber E, Mendes GC, et al. Effects of quetiapine extended release on sleep and quality of life in midlife women with major depressive disorder. Arch Womens Ment Health 2013;16(1):83–5.

72. Gambacciani M, Ciaponi M, Cappagli B, et al. Effects of low-dose, continuous combined estradiol and noretisterone acetate on menopausal quality of life in early postmenopausal women. Maturitas 2003;44(2):157–63.

73. Joffe H, Groninger H, Soares CN, et al. An open trial of mirtazapine in menopausal women with depression unresponsive to estrogen replacement therapy. J Womens Health Gend Based Med 2001;10(10):999–1004.

74. Joffe H, Soares CN, Petrillo LF, et al. Treatment of depression and menopause-related symptoms with the serotonin-norepinephrine reuptake inhibitor duloxetine. J Clin Psychiatry 2007;68(6):943–50.

75. Kornstein SG, Jiang Q, Reddy S, et al. Short-term efficacy and safety of desvenlafaxine in a randomized, placebo-controlled study of perimenopausal and postmenopausal women with major depressive disorder. J Clin Psychiatry 2010;71(8): 1088–96.

76. Soares CN, Kornstein SG, Thase ME, et al. Assessing the efficacy of desvenlafaxine for improving functioning and well-being outcome measures in patients with major depressive disorder: a pooled analysis of 9 double-blind, placebo-controlled, 8-week clinical trials. J Clin Psychiatry 2009;70(10):1365–71.

77. Soares CN, Thase ME, Clayton A, et al. Desvenlafaxine and escitalopram for the treatment of postmenopausal women with major depressive disorder. Menopause 2010;17(4):700–11.

78. Soares CN, Frey BN, Haber E, et al. A pilot, 8-week, placebo lead-in trial of quetiapine extended release for depression in midlife women: impact on mood and menopause-related symptoms. J Clin Psychopharmacol 2010;30(5):612–5.

79. Kelly CM, Juurlink DN, Gomes T, et al. Selective serotonin reuptake inhibitors and breast cancer mortality in women receiving tamoxifen: a population based cohort study. BMJ 2010;340:c693.

80. McCurry SM, Guthrie KA, Morin CM, et al. Telephone-based cognitive behavioral therapy for insomnia in perimenopausal and postmenopausal women with vasomotor symptoms: a MsFLASH randomized clinical trial. JAMA Intern Med 2016; 176(7):913–20.

Burnout in Obstetricians-Gynecologists

Its Prevalence, Identification, Prevention, and Reversal

Roger P. Smith, MD[a],*, William F. Rayburn, MD, MBA[b]

KEYWORDS

- Burnout • Exhaustion • Stress • Prevention • Physicians
- Obstetrician-gynecologists

KEY POINTS

- Burnout is pervasive among physicians.
- Estimates are that 40% to 75% of obstetrician-gynecologists currently suffer from some form of professional burnout, making the lifetime risk a virtual certainty.
- The spectrum of professional burnout varies from physical or emotional fatigue to complete collapse, substance use, and suicidal ideation.
- A number of simple strategies for prevention and early reversal can decrease, if not eliminate, the risks of professional burnout.

INTRODUCTION

Whether it is dealing with global pandemics,[1–3] or just the unending bombardment of information, life may have seemed to have spiraled out of control. This focus can easily result in the exhaustion of physical or emotional strength or motivation, otherwise known as "burnout." Burnout is a physical or mental collapse caused by overwork or stress. All professionals are at risk of suffering from it—loss of control (real or imagined), conflicting demands on time from every direction, and a diminishing sense of worth erodes physician's lives.[4]

Estimates are that 40% to 75% of physicians currently suffer from professional burnout, making the lifetime risk a virtually certainty.[5–7] In an on-line study of more than 15,000 physicians who responded to a survey that included the prevalence of burnout, defined as a loss of enthusiasm for work, feelings of cynicism, and a low

[a] Parkland, FL, USA; [b] University of New Mexico School of Medicine, University of New Mexico, Building No. 2, MSC09 53701, Albuquerque, NM 87131, USA
* Corresponding author.
E-mail address: bgumalley@earthlink.net

Obstet Gynecol Clin N Am 48 (2021) 231–245
https://doi.org/10.1016/j.ogc.2020.11.008
0889-8545/21/© 2020 Elsevier Inc. All rights reserved.

sense of personal accomplishment, almost one-half of those surveyed demonstrated burnout[8] (**Fig. 1**). Although these surveys make for a dismal view of the profession, it does not mean that, with some simple steps, the causes and symptoms can be identified and simple steps implemented to reverse the threat.

The Problem Is Pervasive

Professional burnout is not new—what is new is the recognition of the pervasiveness of professional burnout.[9,10] Physicians, in general, have burnout rates that are twice the rate of working adults in general. No specialty within medicine is immune to burnout[5,11,12] (see **Fig. 1**). The results of burnout surveys have included many individual specialties, including plastic surgeons, headache medicine specialists, pediatric emergency physicians, pediatric intensivists, general pediatricians, multiple surgical specialists, and anesthesiologists.[13–22] The degree of pervasiveness is can be difficult to capture, however, because how it is defined varies widely.

Prevalence in Obstetricians-Gynecologists

Burnout has become more recognized as a variable that has not been taken into account in estimating a shortage of obstetrician-gynecologists. Vetter and colleagues[23] estimated obstetricians-gynecologist physician shortages of 17%, 24%, and 31% by

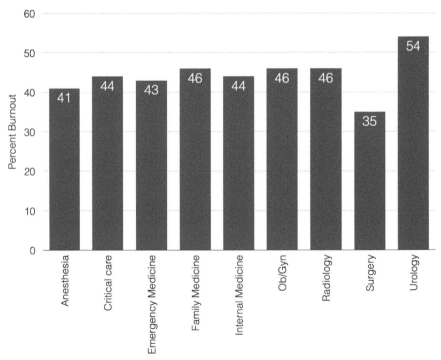

Fig. 1. Prevalence of physician burnout in select medical specialties. Selected results of an online survey of more than 15,000 physicians that included the prevalence of burnout (defined as a loss of enthusiasm for work, feelings of cynicism, and a low sense of personal accomplishment). (*Data from* Medscape National Physician Burnout & Suicide Report 2020. Available at: https://www.medscape.com/slideshow/2020-lifestyle-burnout-6012460#1. Accessed July 14, 2020.)

2030, 2040, and 2050, respectively. Burnout is associated with a decrease in clinical productivity and early retirement.[24] Implications may be more substantial with the increasing number of female obstetricians-gynecologists, now two-thirds of the workforce.[25]

A survey of gynecologic oncologists[26] found that 30% of study participants scored high for emotional exhaustion, 10% high for depersonalization, and 11% low for personal accomplishment—all markers for burnout. Overall, almost one-third (32%) of the physicians studied had scores indicating burnout. More concerning was that 33% screened positive for depression, 13% had a history of suicidal ideation, 15% screened positive for alcohol abuse, and 34% reported impaired quality of life. Almost 40% would not encourage their children to enter medicine and more than 10% said that they would not choose medicine as a career again if they had to do it over.

Although burnout among subspecialists in obstetrics and gynecology has been well-documented,[26,27] less well-understood is the difference, if any, between those who practice the full scope of obstetrics and gynecology and those who subspecialize. Weinstein[28] has speculated that practice patterns such as a "laborist" may result in fewer of the stresses of a private practice, with a more predictable and controllable schedule, although a decrease in burnout rates is unreported.

Residents and Young Physicians Are at Increased Risk

Professional burnout can occur at any point in a physician's career, with residents and those at mid career particularly vulnerable.[29] Resident burnout rates have been reported to be as high as 75%.[30,31] In 1 study, of the surveyed residents, 13% satisfied all 3 subscale scores for high burnout and more than 50% had high levels of depersonalization and emotional exhaustion.[32] Those practitioners with high levels of emotional exhaustion were less satisfied with their careers, regretted choosing their specialty, and had higher rates of depression—all consistent with both older[33,34] and more recent studies.[35]

A study of Australian trainees found a total incidence of burnout of 55.9%, with the highest rates in the first year of training[36] and, among orthopedic trainees, 53% were considered burned out.[37] In another study of 204 doctors in residency training in multiple specialties in a tertiary hospital, 45.6% of respondents reported burnout in the dimension of emotional exhaustion, 57.8% in the dimension of depersonalization, and 61.8% in the dimension of decreased personal accomplishment.[38]

Because of the documented impact of burnout on all graduate medical trainees, the Accreditation Council for Graduate Medical Education, the organization charged with the certification of all graduate medical education in the United States, has mandated that graduate medical education programs include a focus on resident and fellow wellness and fatigue mitigation. In the Accreditation Council for Graduate Medical Education Common Program Requirements, the Accreditation Council for Graduate Medical Education has committed to addressing physician well-being for individuals and as it relates to the learning and working environment with its program requirements VI.C (well-being) and VI.D (fatigue mitigation).[39] The requirements must be met by all graduate education programs in all specialties.

The impact of burnout for early to mid career practitioners is less well-studied. Based on the small differences found in studies across students, residents and early career physicians by Dyrbye and colleagues,[11,40] it is reasonable to assume that burnout continues to be at least as prevalent in these years. Furthermore, there is every reason to believe that burnout is common among senior obstetrician-gynecologists who tend to retire earlier, especially among women.[24]

IDENTIFYING THE CAUSE

In medicine and other professions, the likelihood of burnout happening depends on personal, developmental–psychodynamic, professional, and environmental factors, but the exact role of each in the development of burnout is incompletely understood.[41,42] The very same attributes that make successful physicians (type A behavior, obsessive–compulsive commitment to our profession, etc) increase the risk for professional burnout.[43] In general, autonomy, the power to make decisions, the workload, and working hours seem to be the greatest drivers of emotional exhaustion, the strongest predictor of burnout.[44]

Positive depression screening, pathologic sleepiness, and sleeping fewer than 7 hours a night were independent predictors of burnout in a study of medical students published in 2016.[45] In other studies, a high level of depersonalization (to make impersonal) has been inversely correlated with job satisfaction and personal accomplishment and strongly correlated with depression; both are risk factors for burnout.[32] A high level of personal accomplishment has been strongly correlated with job satisfaction and satisfaction in obstetrics and gynecology as a specialty, but was inversely correlated with a sense of depersonalization. No correlation between burnout and self-care activities was found. Similarly, younger age and greater job dissatisfaction have been found to predict higher depersonalization. Lower co-worker support and greater job dissatisfaction predict lower personal accomplishment.[46]

The issue of gender would seem to be of particular interest to obstetricians-gynecologists, where now nearly two-thirds of practitioners and more than 80% of residents are women. Unlike early reports, recent studies have found that women are at greater risk of professional burnout than their male counterparts.[25,47,48] This gender difference may be driven by unrealistic expectations, family pressure, work–life imbalance, or sleep disorders.

Sleep disorders are prevalent among physicians, especially among females, where rates have been found to be between 35% and 40%.[49,50] The importance of sleep disorders has been emphasized in many studies, which have shown that changing work schedules, night shifts, and the resultant fragmented sleep could have a severe cognitive and emotional impact on the performance of physicians on the day after a shift.

Work–life balance has been the subject of great debate and study showing the difficulties of balancing between work and family as important determinants of burnout.[51,52] Workload, a sense of control over one's work environment, and a shared core mission or vision (alignment of core values) were the greatest drivers of burnout in a study of practicing primary care physicians.[53] Experience from the novel coronavirus disease-2019 environment has certainly adversely affected workload and control over the environment.

In general, having some control over schedule and hours worked is associated with decreases in burnout and improved job satisfaction.[54] Professional autonomy, decision-making support and supervision for trainees, and social support have been found to decrease burnout in training programs,[55] physicians in academic settings tend to have higher rates of burnout in some studies,[56] but not in others.[57] This finding may not be surprising, because the academic environment is highly variable, often more bureaucratic (giving the individual less control), and frequently less efficient.

Despite this finding, having more control and a decreased workload are not always protective. Well-intentioned efforts to reduce workload, such as the electronic medical records or physician order entry systems, have actually made the problem worse,[58] although other forms of technology can be used to combat the effects of burnout.[59]

Even the seeming level of control that comes with being the chair of a department of obstetrics and gynecology does not decrease burnout rates.[60,61] Furthermore, the resilience of mental health professionals, who one might expect to be able to thwart their own threat, still report burnout rates that approach 25%.[62]

Stress versus Burnout

Stress is often seen as the primary cause of burnout, but there is no single cause of burnout.[13,29] Rather, a number of factors combine to cause the physical or mental collapse that is burnout. Stress can be a positive or negative factor in our performance. Too little stress leads to feeling underused, whereas with too much, collapse from the strain results. There is a middle ground where stress and expectations maintain focus and peak productivity—deadlines create focus and expectations provide standards to strive for. The key is the balance between control and demand: When there is a greater level of control, high demands can be handled. When there is a lack of that control, high demands result in what has been called "toxic stress," and collapse is likely to occur.

Physically, stress induces a dry mouth, dilated pupils, and the release of adrenalin and noradrenalin associated with the fight-or-flight reaction. Psychosocial stress influences cognitive abilities, such as long-term memory, and has impairing effects on cognitive flexibility in men more than women.[63] In 1 study, former patients with prolonged work-related stress improved with professional care, but they continued to perform worse than controls after 1 year.[64] In the acute phase, the greatest impairments were related to executive function and mental speed, but at follow-up, memory impairments also became apparent.

Burnout, as opposed to stress, is characterized by exhaustion, lack of enthusiasm and motivation, and feelings of ineffectiveness, with the added dimensions of frustration or cynicism. This situation results in disengagement, demotivation, and decreased workplace efficacy in a progressively intrusive manner (**Table 1**). Although chronic stress is identified as one of the key factors, as noted elsewhere in this article, no single element is sufficient to exceed the adaptive abilities of the individual. Burnout is generally more gradual, progressive, and insidious than is stress, making it more likely to go undetected until further along its continuum.

The Perils of Burnout

Physician burnout is associated with decreased productivity[65] and threatens the work–life balance among physicians, especially those in dual career relationships.[5,51] Among emergency physicians, burnout was significantly associated with higher frequencies of self-reported suboptimal care and strongly associated with actual decreases in professional work effort over the following 24 months.[66] Conditions where there are weak retention rates, high turnover, heavy workloads, low staffing levels, and/or staffing shortages increase the risk of burnout and, when burnout is present, are associated with a degraded quality of the care we provide.[67] Burnout is also associated with an increased risk for physical illness.[68]

Economically, the impact of physician's and other health professional's burnout can be very costly through early retirement, reduced work hours, job relocation, and additional costs of recruitment and retention.[69,70] Among residency program directors in radiation oncology surveyed, 11% of respondents met the criteria for low burnout, 83% for moderate burnout, and 6% for high burnout. Although 78% of the respondents reported feeling "satisfied" or "highly satisfied" with their current role, 85% planned to remain as program director for less than 5 years.[71]

Table 1
Symptoms associated with stages of professional burnout

	Early	Mid Stage	Advanced
Behavioral	Displacement of goals Emotional exhaustion: Feeling drained and depleted Starting workdays fatigued No longer look forward to work No longer "bounce back" from time off Working harder	Depersonalization: Lack of compassion for patients and colleagues More callous toward others Irritable at work Denial of emerging problems Needless competitive behaviors Passive–aggressive behaviors Slow response to pages Skipped meetings Tasks left uncompleted Temper outbursts	A sense of inner emptiness or exhaustion Cynicism Depersonalization Procrastination
Personal	A compulsion to prove yourself Anxiety Fatigue not relieved by rest Forgetfulness Impaired cognitive functions: Short attention span Memory for details is slipping Cognitive rigidity Irritability Neglecting your own needs Poor concentration	Dread going to work Difficulty relaxing or enjoying time off Diminished sense of accomplishment: Questioning the value of one's efforts Feeling that nothing has been accomplished Lost the "passion" for work Withdrawal Worry or anger that contaminates home life	Apathy Depression (including suicidal ideation) Withdrawal from friends and family
Physical	Bruxism (tooth grinding) Gastrointestinal problems Headaches Hypertension Insomnia Palpitations	Chronic sleep disturbances Increasing alcohol or other substance use More and more intrusive symptoms	Loss of libido

Stages of Professional Burnout.

When advanced, burnout is associated with depression and an increased risk of suicidal ideation. Suicidal ideation has been found to be more prevalent among physicians than in the general population.[72,73] In a meta-analysis, suicide was almost one and one-half times more frequent among male physicians compared with the general population, and twice as likely for female doctors.[74]

The impact of burnout goes beyond the emotional. Obstetricians must be sensitive to the fact that burnout in women is a predictor of infertility, miscarriage, and high-risk pregnancy. In a study of female Hungarian physicians with burnout, there were more complications of pregnancy, although a clear causal relationship could not be established,[75] despite older studies that have found a link between job stress, preterm delivery, and low birthweight for gestational age.[76] Clearly, the difficulties achieving, carrying, or delivering a healthy pregnancy themselves are sources of significant stress that could precipitate emotional collapse and burnout for the families involved.

Am I Burned Out?

Fatigue and stress are omnipresent, but that is not the same as burnout. The degree to which the physical, emotional, and professional symptoms are manifest depends on the depth or stage of burnout (see **Table 1**) making diagnosis problematic. The effective gold standard for diagnosing burnout is the Maslach Burnout Inventory.[77] This inventory operationalizes burnout as a 3-dimensional syndrome made up of exhaustion, cynicism, and inefficacy. The Maslach Burnout Inventory includes 3 scales: (1) emotional exhaustion (9 items), a state of chronic emotional and physical depletion; (2) depersonalization (5 items), a sense of disconnection from coworkers and clients; and (3) diminished personal accomplishment (8 items), a negative sense of self-value and ability.

Other diagnostic tools have been introduced,[78] but have not gained the wide acceptance of the Maslach Inventory. For example, West and colleagues[79] have validated single items from the Maslach Burnout Inventory emotional exhaustion and Maslach Burnout Inventory depersonalization subscales as stand-alone measures, and this approach has been confirmed by other investigators.[80] Some authors have argued that burnout and depression represent different, closely spaced, points along a spectrum and that any effort to separate them may be artificial.[81,82]

Unfortunately, the Maslach Burnout Inventory requires a fee, consists of 22 items, and requires interpretation by a qualified individual. A simpler screening test consists of 10 screening questions (**Box 1**)—if the individual can answer yes to 5 or more, they probably have burnout. For most individuals, a simple review of the symptoms and findings found in **Table 1** and **Box 1** will give a reasonable appraisal of the likelihood of burnout. This approach would seem reasonable for simple self-assessment or for broad screening of patients, coworkers, friends, or family.

Psychologists Herbert Freudenberger and Gail North studying burnout in women, have theorized that the burnout process can be divided into 12 phases.[83] This division has limited usefulness because the phases are not necessarily followed sequentially, some may be absent, and others present simultaneously and broadly mimic the symptoms and progression seen in the more general descriptions of characteristics, such as those shown in **Table 1**. It is easy to see how a progression of symptoms can represent a potentially spiraling series of behaviors and changes that result in complete dysfunction. It is also easy to understand that the characteristics that are associated with success in medical school, training, and practice, such as high expectations, placing the needs of others above our own, and a desire to prove oneself, virtually define the first 3 of these stages.

Box 1
Burnout screening questions (note: a "yes" to 5 or more questions is indicative of burnout.)

Do you have…
- A lack of pleasure in other activities (anhedonia)?
- Annoyance by simple things?
- Boredom?
- Cynicism?
- Depression before the work week?
- Dread before a return to work?
- Envy for those who are happy?
- Fatigue or low energy?
- No longer care about performance?
- Work affecting family?

PREVENTION

Because the early symptoms and signs of professional burnout are both common, awareness and prevention or early intervention are possible. Some simple steps can be taken to prevent or decrease the risk of burnout or to reverse its effects. A growing number of organizations, including The American College of Obstetricians and Gynecologists through its Council on Resident Education in Obstetrics and Gynecology, offer tool kits for established practitioners and our most vulnerable physicians in training.[84]

Because stress and fatigue are 2 of the greatest risk factors for burnout, decreasing these factors is a good place to start. When it comes to fatigue, the solution is easy—sleep. Physicians tend to sleep fewer hours than the general population and what is achieved is often not the type that is restful and restorative.[85] Just decreasing the number of hours worked is not enough, as a number of studies have found.[86] The rest must result in relaxation and renewal.

The impact of fewer duty hours in residency training might be anticipated to decrease both the fatigue and stress and, thus, the risk of burnout. In at least 1 study, this outcome has not been the case. In a study of internal medicine residents, the prevalence and incidence of year-end burnout did not differ significantly between those before and after the imposition of new work hour restrictions.[87] Interestingly, there was no difference in year-end prevalence of excessive sleepiness (as measured with the Epworth scale) among these same learners. Another study has found that organizations may be able to improve burnout, dissatisfaction, and retention rates by addressing communication and workflow, as well as initiating quality improvement projects targeting clinician concerns.[88]

Stress reduction may be a more difficult goal than is getting more sleep. Although studies indicate that experience or habituation to stressful situations can blunt the impact of stress,[89] this practice should not be seen as an adaptive way of dealing with stressful situations. In reality, there are several simple "A" approaches to reduce stress: Alter it (direct communication, problem solving, time management), Avoid it (delegate, know limits, walk away), or Accept it (build resistance, change perceptions).

Even though clinicians have busy clinical schedules, taking short breaks to rest, sing, laugh, or exercise can go a long way to decreasing stress. Shanafelt and colleagues[90] (who have contributed frequently to the burnout literature) found that even breaks as short as 10 minutes can be effective. Separating work from private life by taking a short break to resolve issues before heading home—avoiding baggage or homework—will go a long way to giving perspective from time off. This practice may also mean that tasks have to be delegated or shared or get carry-out for dinner. Set meaningful and realistic goals professionally and personally; do not expect or demand more than is possible. This approach will mean setting priorities—some tasks may have to wait. Finally, do not forget hobbies and activities that are enjoyable.

Physical activity has been shown to decrease feelings of fatigue and provide an improved sense of well-being,[91] although this effect seems to be blunted in the face of chronic stress,[92] limiting its value in ameliorating the impact of burnout when symptoms are advanced. Rewarding ourselves with enjoyable activities and hobbies has been shown to promote resiliency.[93]

REVERSING BURNOUT

Although a paucity of solutions have been proven to be effective for reversing burnout, one can reduce the effects, deal with the sources, and improve attitudes (**Box 2**). Rest and relaxation will go a long way to helping, but so will physical well-being, a healthy

---

Box 2
Burnout prevention and mitigation strategies

Reduce effects
- Health and fitness
- Personal coping strategies
- Rest and relaxation
- Social support

Deal with sources
- Assertiveness
- Be realistic, establish priorities
- Lobby for change
- Time management

Improve attitude
- Highlight the positive
- Let things go
- Look for good
- Reflect and take control

---

diet, exercise, and health checkups. Dealing with the sources of burnout by identifying the stressors, setting realistic priorities, and time management can also be helpful. Preferably with support from their colleagues, individuals should also advocate for changes that will increase their control and decrease unnecessary obstacles to completing goals. Look for the good and try to identify at least 1 instance during the day where your presence or acts made a difference.

Take advantage of mentors, friends, and loved ones to provide perspective, balance, and assistance.[94] Depression is a mood disorder that causes persistent feeling of sadness and loss of interest, leading to a variety of emotional and physical problems. Because depression and burnout may be virtually indistinguishable,[83,85] seek professional help and counseling early, sometimes through cognitive–behavioral therapy. This help can be in the forms of trained counselors, mentors, clergy, or others. They must be able to respect the individual's privacy and trust, but also bring either training or perspective. They can help to improve self-awareness and assist in developing coping strategies that are protective.

Do not attempt to "go it alone" or self-medicate with antidepressants, alcohol, or other substances—they will only compound the problem.[95] Multiple studies have shown that seeing burnout as a systemic problem worthy of enhanced communication and a systemic solution is important.[96,97] Modeling resilient behavior improves well-being for those around you.[98]

In the end, obstetricians and gynecologists really do have the tools to reduce, mitigate, or avoid the threat of professional burnout. Just as with the push to include patient satisfaction with any measure of the quality of medical care we provide, the quality of our own lives must matter. Burnout can be combated with self-awareness of internal and external stress factors, the use of coping strategies and well-being mechanisms, and a reliance on strong social, communication, and professional support networks to advocate for improved work conditions.

DISCLOSURE

Both authors have no disclosure of any commercial or financial conflicts of interest. There was no funding source for preparing this article.

REFERENCES

1. Bradley M, Chahar P. Burnout OF healthcare providers during COVID-19. Cleve Clin J Med 2020. https://doi.org/10.3949/ccjm.87a.ccc051.
2. Restauri N, Sheridan AD, Restauri N, et al. Burnout and posttraumatic stress disorder in the coronavirus disease 2019 (COVID-19) pandemic: intersection, impact, and interventions. J Am Coll Radiol 2020;17(7):921–6.
3. The American College of Obstetricians and Gynecologists. Emotional well-being during a pandemic: a guided discussion and best practice sharing of well-being interventions in the obstetrics and gynecology community. Available at: https://www.acog.org/education-and-events/webinars/emotional-well-being-during-a-pandemic-a-guided-discussion-and-best-practice-sharing-of-well-being-interventions-in-the-obstetrics-and-gynecology-community. Accessed July 18, 2020.
4. O'Connell VA, Youcha S, Pellegrini V. Physician burnout: the effect of time allotted for a patient visit on physician burnout among OB/GYN physicians. J Med Pract Manage 2009;24(5):300–13.
5. Shanafelt TD, Boone S, Tan L, et al. Burnout and satisfaction with work-life balance among US physicians relative to the general US population. Arch Intern Med 2012;172(18):1377–85.
6. Agency for Healthcare Research and Quality. Physician Burnout. Available at: https://www.ahrq.gov/sites/default/files/wysiwyg/professionals/clinicians-providers/ahrq-works/impact-burnout.pdf. Accessed July 15, 2020.
7. Rothenberger DA. Physician burnout and well-being: a systematic review and framework for action. Dis Colon Rectum 2017;60(6):567–76.
8. Medscape National Physician Burnout & Suicide Report 2020. Available at: https://www.medscape.com/slideshow/2020-lifestyle-burnout-6012460#1. Accessed July 14, 2020.
9. Lee YY, Medford AR, Halim AS. Burnout in physicians. J R Coll Physicians Edinb 2015;45(2):104–7.
10. Shanafelt TD, Hasan O, Dyrbye LN, et al. Changes in burnout and satisfaction with work-life balance in physicians and the general US working population between 2011 and 2014. Mayo Clin Proc 2015;90(12):1600–13.
11. Dyrbye LN, Burke SE, Hardeman RR, et al. Association of clinical specialty with symptoms of burnout and career choice regret among US resident physicians. JAMA 2018;320(11):1114–30.
12. Qureshi HA, Rawlani R, Mioton LM, et al. Burnout phenomenon in U.S. plastic surgeons: risk factors and impact on quality of life. Plast Reconstr Surg 2015;135(2):619–26.
13. Streu R, Hansen J, Abrahamse P, et al. Professional burnout among US plastic surgeons: results of a national survey. Ann Plast Surg 2014;72(3):346–50.
14. Evans RW, Ghosh K. A survey of headache medicine specialists on career satisfaction and burnout. Headache 2015;55(10):1448–57.
15. Bragard I, Dupuis G, Fleet R. Quality of work life, burnout, and stress in emergency department physicians: a qualitative review. Eur J Emerg Med 2015;22(4):227–34.
16. Arora M, Asha S, Chinnappa J, et al. Review article: burnout in emergency medicine physicians. Emerg Med Australas 2013;25(6):491–5.
17. Gorelick MH, Schremmer R, Ruch-Ross H, et al. Current workforce characteristics and burnout in pediatric emergency medicine. Acad Emerg Med 2016;23(1):48–54.

18. Garcia TT, Garcia PC, Molon ME, et al. Prevalence of burnout in pediatric intensivists: an observational comparison with general pediatricians. Pediatr Crit Care Med 2014;15(8):e347–53.

19. Shanafelt TD, Balch CM, Bechamps GJ, et al. Burnout and career satisfaction among American surgeons. Ann Surg 2009;250(3):463–71.

20. Rama-Maceiras P, Jokinen J, Kranke P. Stress and burnout in anaesthesia: a real world problem? Curr Opin Anaesthesiol 2015;28(2):151–8.

21. Pulcrano M, Evans SR, Sosin M. Quality of life and burnout rates across surgical specialties: a systematic review. JAMA Surg 2016;151(10):970–8.

22. McAbee JH, Ragel BT, McCartney S, et al. Factors associated with career satisfaction and burnout among US neurosurgeons: results of a nationwide survey. J Neurosurg 2015;123(1):161–73.

23. Vetter M, Salani R, Williams T, et al. The impact of burnout on the obstetrics and gynecology workforce. Clin Obstet Gynecol 2019;62:444–54.

24. Rayburn W, Petterson S, Strunk A. Considerations about retirement from clinical practice by obstetrician-gynecologists. Am J Obstet Gynecol 2015;213(3):335.e1–4.

25. Fronek H, Brubaker L. Burnout woman-style: the female face of burnout in obstetrics and gynecology. Clin Obstet Gynecol 2019;62(3):466–79.

26. Rath KS, Huffman LB, Phillips GS, et al. Burnout and associated factors among members of the Society of Gynecologic Oncology. Am J Obstet Gynecol 2015;213(6):824.e1–9.

27. Kawada T. Risk factors of burnout in gynecologic oncologist. Am J Obstet Gynecol 2016;214(4):550–1.

28. Weinstein L. Laborist to obstetrician/gynecologist-hospitalist: an evolution or a revolution? Obstet Gynecol Clin North Am 2015;42(3):415–7.

29. Dyrbye LN, Varkey P, Boone SL, et al. Physician satisfaction and burnout at different career stages. Mayo Clin Proc 2013;88(12):1358–67.

30. IsHak WW, Lederer S, Mandili C, et al. Burnout during residency training: a literature review. J Grad Med Educ 2009;1(2):236–42.

31. Morgan HK, Winkel AF, Nguyen AT, et al. Obstetrics and gynecology residents' perspectives on wellness: findings from a national survey. Obstet Gynecol 2019;133(3):552–7.

32. Govardhan LM, Pinelli V, Schnatz PF. Burnout, depression and job satisfaction in obstetrics and gynecology residents. Conn Med 2012;76(7):389–95.

33. Becker JL, Milad MP, Klock SC. Burnout, depression, and career satisfaction: cross-sectional study of obstetrics and gynecology residents. Am J Obstet Gynecol 2006;195(5):1444–9.

34. Castelo-Branco C, Figueras F, Eixarch E, et al. Stress symptoms and burnout in obstetric and gynaecology residents. BJOG 2007;114(1):94–8.

35. Iorga M, Socolov V, Muraru D, et al. Factors influencing burnout syndrome in obstetrics and gynecology physicians. Biomed Res Int 2017;2017:9318534.

36. Parr JM, Pinto N, Hanson M, et al. Medical graduates, tertiary hospitals, and burnout: a longitudinal cohort study. Ochsner J 2016;16(1):22–6.

37. Arora M, Diwan AD, Harris IA. Prevalence and factors of burnout among Australian orthopaedic trainees: a cross-sectional study. J Orthop Surg (Hong Kong) 2014;22(3):374–7.

38. Ogundipe OA, Olagunju AT, Lasebikan VO, et al. Burnout among doctors in residency training in a tertiary hospital. Asian J Psychiatr 2014;10:27–32.

39. Accreditation Council for Graduate Medical Education (ACGME). Common Program Requirements. Available at: https://www.acgme.org/What-We-Do/Accreditation/Common-Program-Requirements. Accessed July 15, 2020.
40. Dyrbye LN, West CP, Satele D, et al. Burnout among U.S. medical students, residents, and early career physicians relative to the general U.S. population. Acad Med 2014;89(3):443–51.
41. Thirioux B, Birault F, Jaafari N. Empathy Is a protective factor of burnout in physicians: new neuro-phenomenological hypotheses regarding empathy and sympathy in care relationship. Front Psychol 2016;7:763.
42. West CP, Dyrbye LN, Shanafelt TD. Physician burnout: contributors, consequences and solutions. J Intern Med 2018;283(6):516–29.
43. Nakagawa K, Yellowlees P. Inter-generational effects of technology: why millennial physicians may be less at risk for burnout than baby boomers. Curr Psychiatry Rep 2020;22(9):45.
44. Lee RT, Seo B, Hladkyj S, et al. Correlates of physician burnout across regions and specialties: a meta-analysis. Hum Resour Health 2013;11:48.
45. Wolf MR, Rosenstock JB. Inadequate sleep and exercise associated with burnout and depression among medical students. Acad Psychiatry 2016;41(2):174–9.
46. Kroll HR, Macaulay T, Jesse M. A preliminary survey examining predictors of burnout in pain medicine physicians in the United States. Pain Physician 2016;19(5):E689–96.
47. Győrffy Z, Dweik D, Girasek E. Workload, mental health and burnout indicators among female physicians. Hum Resour Health 2016;14:12.
48. Chesak SS, Cutshall S, Anderson A, et al. Burnout among women physicians: a call to action. Curr Cardiol Rep 2020;22(7):45.
49. Rodrigez-Muñoz A, Moreno-Jimenez B, Fernandez-Mendoza JJ, et al. Insomnia and quality of sleep among primary care physicians: a gender perspective. Rev Neurol 2008;47(3):119–23.
50. Vela-Bueno A, Moreno-Jiménez B, Rodríguez-Muñoz A, et al. Insomnia and sleep quality among primary care physicians with low and high burnout levels. J Psychosom Res 2008;64(4):435–42.
51. Dyrbye LN, Sotile W, Boone S, et al. A survey of U.S. physicians and their partners regarding the impact of work-home conflict. J Gen Intern Med 2014;29(1):155–61.
52. Roberts DL, Shanafelt TD, Dyrbye LN, et al. National comparison of burnout and work-life balance among internal medicine hospitalists and outpatient general internists. J Hosp Med 2014;9(3):176–81.
53. Gregory ST, Menser T. Burnout among primary care physicians: a test of the areas of worklife model. J Healthc Manag 2015;60(2):133–48.
54. Keeton K, Fenner DE, Johnson TR, et al. Predictors of physician career satisfaction, work-life balance, and burnout. Obstet Gynecol 2007;109(4):949–55.
55. Kimo Takayesu J, Ramoska EA, Clark TR, et al. Factors associated with burnout during emergency medicine residency. Acad Emerg Med 2014;21(9):1031–5.
56. Shanafelt TD, Gradishar WJ, Kosty M, et al. Burnout and career satisfaction among US oncologists. J Clin Oncol 2014;32(7):678–86.
57. Marshall AL, Dyrbye LN, Shanafelt TD, et al. Disparities in Burnout and Satisfaction with Work-Life Integration in U.S. Physicians by Gender and Practice Setting. Acad Med 2020. https://doi.org/10.1097/ACM.0000000000003521.
58. Shanafelt TD, Dyrbye LN, Sinsky C, et al. Between clerical burden and characteristics of the electronic environment with physician burnout and professional satisfaction. Mayo Clin Proc 2016;91(7):836–48.

59. Davis MJ. Using technology to combat clinician burnout. J Healthc Manag 2020; 65(4):265–72.
60. Gabbe SG, Melville J, Mandel L, et al. Burnout in chairs of obstetrics and gynecology: diagnosis, treatment, and prevention. Am J Obstet Gynecol 2002;186(4): 601–12.
61. Shanafelt TD, Makowski MS, Wang H, et al. Association of burnout, professional fulfillment, and self-care practices of physician leaders with their independently rated leadership effectiveness. JAMA Netw Open 2020;3(6):e207961.
62. Kok BC, Herrell RK, Grossman SH, et al. Prevalence of professional burnout among military mental health service providers. Psychiatr Serv 2016;67(1): 137–40.
63. Shields GS, Trainor BC, Lam JC, et al. Acute stress impairs cognitive flexibility in men, not women. Stress 2016;19(5):542–6.
64. Eskildsen A, Andersen LP, Pedersen AD, et al. Cognitive impairments in former patients with work-related stress complaints - one year later. Stress 2016;19(6): 559–66.
65. Dewa CS, Loong D, Bonato S, et al. How does burnout affect physician productivity? A systematic literature review. BMC Health Serv Res 2014;14:325.
66. Lu DW, Dresden S, McCloskey C, et al. Impact of burnout on self-reported patient care among emergency physicians. West J Emerg Med 2015;16(7):996–1001.
67. Humphries N, Morgan K, Conry MC, et al. Quality of care and health professional burnout: narrative literature review. Int J Health Care Qual Assur 2014;27(4): 293–307.
68. Honkonen T, Ahola K, Pertovaara M, et al. The association between burnout and physical illness in the general population–results from the Finnish Health 2000 Study. J Psychosom Res 2006;61(1):59–66.
69. Dewa CS, Jacobs P, Thanh NX, et al. An estimate of the cost of burnout on early retirement and reduction in clinical hours of practicing physicians in Canada. BMC Health Serv Res 2014;14:254.
70. Johnstone B, Kaiser A, Injeyan MC, et al. The relationship between burnout and occupational stress in genetic counselors. J Genet Couns 2016;25(4):731–41.
71. Aggarwal S, Kusano AS, Carter JN, et al. Stress and burnout among residency program directors in United States radiation oncology programs. Int J Radiat Oncol Biol Phys 2015;93(4):746–53.
72. Tyssen R, Vaglum P, Gronvold NT, et al. Suicidal ideation among medical students and young physicians: a nationwide and prospective study of prevalence and predictors. J Affect Disord 2001;64:69–79.
73. Bernal M, Haro JM, Bernet S, et al. Risk factors for suicidality in Europe: results from the ESEMED study. J Affect Disord 2007;101:27–34.
74. Schernhammer ES, Colditz GA. Suicidal rates among physicians: a quantitative and gender assessment (meta-analysis). Am J Psychiatry 2004;161(12): 2295–302.
75. Győrffy Z, Dweik D, Girasek E. Reproductive health and burn-out among female physicians: nationwide, representative study from Hungary. BMC Womens Health 2014;14:121.
76. Defoe DM, Power ML, Holzman GB, et al. The relation between psychosocial job strain, and preterm delivery and low birthweight for gestational age. Obstet Gynecol 2001;97(6):1015–8.
77. Maslach C, Jackson SE, Leiter MP. MBI: the Maslach Burnout Inventory: manual. Palo Alto: Consulting Psychologists Press; 1996.

78. Kristensen TS, Borritz M, Villadsen E, et al. The Copenhagen Burnout Inventory: a new tool for the assessment of burnout. Work Stress 2005;19:192–207.

79. West C, Dyrbye L, Sloan J, et al. Single item measures of emotional exhaustion and depersonalization are useful for assessing burnout in medical professionals. J Gen Intern Med 2009;24(12):1318–21.

80. Dolan ED, Mohr D, Lempa M, et al. Using a single item to measure burnout in primary care staff: a psychometric evaluation. J Gen Intern Med 2015;30(5):582–7.

81. Bianchi R, Boffy C, Hingray C, et al. Comparative symptomatology of burnout and depression. J Health Psychol 2013;18(6):782–7.

82. Bianchi R, Schonfeld IS, Laurent E. Is burnout a depressive disorder? A re-examination with special focus on atypical depression. Intl J Stress Mgmt 2014;21(4):307–24.

83. Freudenberger HJ, North G. Women's burnout: how to spot it, how to reverse it, and how to prevent it. New York: Doubleday; 1985.

84. Council on Resident Education in Obstetrics and Gynecology (CREOG). Physician Wellness Toolkit. Available at: https://www.acog.org/education-and-events/creog/curriculum-resources/physician-satisfaction-and-wellness-initiative/physician-wellness-toolkit. Accessed July 18, 2020.

85. Abrams RM. Sleep deprivation. Obstet Gynecol Clin North Am 2015;42(3): 493–506.

86. Williams D, Tricomi G, Gupta J, et al. Efficacy of burnout interventions in the medical education pipeline. Acad Psychiatry 2015;39(1):47–54.

87. Ripp JA, Bellini L, Fallar R, et al. The impact of duty hours restrictions on job burnout in internal medicine residents: a three-institution comparison study. Acad Med 2015;90(4):494–9.

88. Linzer M, Poplau S, Grossman E, et al. A cluster randomized trial of interventions to improve work conditions and clinician burnout in primary care: results from the Healthy Work Place (HWP) study. J Gen Intern Med 2015;30(8):1105–11.

89. Jezova D, Hlavacova N, Dicko I, et al. Psychosocial stress based on public speech in humans: is there a real life/laboratory setting cross-adaptation? Stress 2016;19(4):429–33.

90. Shanafelt TD, Oreskovich MR, Dyrbye LN, et al. Avoiding burnout: the personal health habits and wellness practices of US surgeons. Ann Surg 2012;255(4): 625–33.

91. Babbar S, Renner K, Williams K. Addressing obstetrics and gynecology trainee burnout using a yoga-based wellness initiative during dedicated education time. Obstet Gynecol 2019;133(5):994–1001.

92. Shields GS, Trainor BC, Lam JC, et al. Physical activity buffers fatigue only under low chronic stress. Stress 2016;19(5):535–41.

93. Perez GK, Haime V, Jackson V, et al. Promoting resiliency among palliative care clinicians: stressors, coping strategies, and training needs. J Palliat Med 2015; 18(4):332–7.

94. Dyrbye LN, Shanafelt TD, Gill PR, et al. Effect of a professional coaching intervention on the well-being and distress of physicians: a pilot randomized clinical trial. JAMA Intern Med 2019;179(10):1406–14.

95. Cecil J, McHale C, Hart J, et al. Behaviour and burnout in medical students. Med Educ Online 2014;19:25209.

96. Smith RP. Throw out the lifeline: it takes a village to combat burnout. Obstet Gynecol 2017;130(4):862–4.

97. Panagioti M, Panagopoulou E, Bower P, et al. Controlled interventions to reduce burnout in physicians a systematic review and meta-analysis. JAMA Intern Med 2017;177(2):195–205.
98. Dyrbye LN, Leep Hunderfund AN, Winters RC, et al. The relationship between residents' perceptions of residency program leadership team behaviors and resident burnout and satisfaction. Acad Med 2020. https://doi.org/10.1097/ACM.0000000000003538.

Moving?

Make sure your subscription moves with you!

To notify us of your new address, find your **Clinics Account Number** (located on your mailing label above your name), and contact customer service at:

Email: journalscustomerservice-usa@elsevier.com

800-654-2452 (subscribers in the U.S. & Canada)
314-447-8871 (subscribers outside of the U.S. & Canada)

Fax number: 314-447-8029

Elsevier Health Sciences Division
Subscription Customer Service
3251 Riverport Lane
Maryland Heights, MO 63043

*To ensure uninterrupted delivery of your subscription, please notify us at least 4 weeks in advance of move.

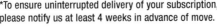